Progress in Endoscopic Ultrasonography

Editor

FRANK G. GRESS

GASTROINTESTINAL ENDOSCOPY CLINICS OF NORTH AMERICA

www.giendo.theclinics.com

Consulting Editor
CHARLES J. LIGHTDALE

October 2017 • Volume 27 • Number 4

ELSEVIER

1600 John F. Kennedy Boulevard • Suite 1800 • Philadelphia, Pennsylvania, 19103-2899

http://www.theclinics.com

GASTROINTESTINAL ENDOSCOPY CLINICS OF NORTH AMERICA Volume 27, Number 4
October 2017 ISSN 1052-5157, ISBN-13: 978-0-323-54664-5

Editor: Kerry Holland
Developmental Editor: Donald Mumford

Gastrointestinal Endoscopy Clinics of North America (ISSN 1052-5157) is published quarterly by Elsevier Inc., 360 Park Avenue South, New York, NY 10010-1710. Months of issue are January, April, July, and October. Business and Editorial Offices: 1600 John F. Kennedy Blvd., Suite 1800, Philadelphia, PA, 19103-2899. Periodicals postage paid at New York, NY and additional mailing offices. Subscription prices are $342.00 per year for US individuals, $560.00 per year for US institutions, $100.00 per year for US students and residents, $377.00 per year for Canadian individuals, $662.00 per year for Canadian institutions, $474.00 per year for international individuals, $662.00 per year for international institutions, and $245.00 per year for Canadian and foreign students/residents. To receive student/resident rate, orders must be accompanied by name of affiliated institution, date of term, and the *signature* of program/residency coordinator on institution letterhead. Orders will be billed at individual rate until proof of status is received. Foreign air speed delivery is included in all *Clinics* subscription prices. All prices are subject to change without notice. **POSTMASTER:** Send address change to *Gastrointestinal Endoscopy Clinics of North America*, Elsevier Health Sciences Division, Subscription Customer Service, 3251 Riverport Lane, Maryland Heights, MO 63043. **Customer Service: 1-800-654-2452 (US). From outside the United States, call 1-314-447-8871. Fax: 1-314-447-8029. E-mail: JournalsCustomerService-usa@elsevier.com (for print support) or JournalsOnlineSupport-usa@elsevier.com (for online support).**

Reprints. For copies of 100 or more, of articles in this publication, please contact the Commercial Reprints Department, Elsevier Inc., 360 Park Avenue South, New York, NY 10010-1710. Tel. 212-633-3874; Fax: 212-633-3820; E-mail: reprints@elsevier.com.

Gastrointestinal Endoscopy Clinics of North America is covered in *Excerpta Medica, MEDLINE/PubMed (Index Medicus), and MEDLINE/MEDLARS.*

Contributors

CONSULTING EDITOR

CHARLES J. LIGHTDALE, MD
Professor of Medicine, Division of Digestive and Liver Diseases, Columbia University Medical Center, New York, New York, USA

EDITOR

FRANK G. GRESS, MD
Professor, Department of Medicine, Clinical Chief and Chief, Interventional Endoscopy, Division of Digestive and Liver Diseases, Columbia University Medical Center, New York, New York, USA

AUTHORS

MOHAMMAD A. AL-HADDAD, MD, MSc, FACG, AGAF, FASGE
Associate Professor of Medicine, Division of Gastroenterology and Hepatology, Indiana University School of Medicine, Indianapolis, Indiana, USA

SUNIL AMIN, MD, MPH
Instructor, Division of Digestive and Liver Diseases, Department of Medicine, Columbia University Medical Center, New York, New York, USA

EVERSON LUIZ DE ALMEIDA ARTIFON, MD, PhD, FASGE
Department of Surgery, University of São Paulo, São Paulo, Brazil

HARRY R. ASLANIAN, MD, FASGE
Section of Digestive Diseases, Yale School of Medicine, New Haven, Connecticut, USA

TODD H. BARON, MD, FASGE
Professor of Medicine, Division of Gastroenterology and Hepatology, The University of North Carolina at Chapel Hill, Chapel Hill, North Carolina, USA

OMER BASAR, MD
Research Fellow, Pancreas Biliary Center, Gastrointestinal Unit, Massachusetts General Hospital, Boston, Massachusetts, USA

WILLIAM R. BRUGGE, MD
Director, Pancreas Biliary Center, Gastrointestinal Unit, Massachusetts General Hospital, Boston, Massachusetts, USA

SAHIN COBAN, MD
Research Scholar, Department of Medicine, University of Massachusetts Medical School, Worcester, Massachusetts, USA

JUAN ENRIQUE DOMÍNGUEZ-MUÑOZ, MD, PhD
Head, Department of Gastroenterology and Hepatology, Health Research Institute (IDIS), University Hospital of Santiago de Compostela, Santiago de Compostela, Spain

LARISSA L. FUJII-LAU, MD
The Queen's Medical Center, Honolulu, Hawaii, USA

TAMAS A. GONDA, MD
Assistant Professor, Division of Digestive and Liver Diseases, Department of Medicine, Columbia University, New York, New York, USA

FRANK G. GRESS, MD
Professor, Department of Medicine, Clinical Chief and Chief, Interventional Endoscopy, Division of Digestive and Liver Diseases, Columbia University Medical Center, New York, New York, USA

MEHRVASH HAGHIGHI, MD
Assistant Professor, Department of Pathology, Columbia University Medical Center, New York, New York, USA

JULIO IGLESIAS-GARCÍA, MD, PhD
Head, Endoscopy, Department of Gastroenterology and Hepatology, Health Research Institute (IDIS), University Hospital of Santiago de Compostela, Santiago de Compostela, Spain

MICHEL KAHALEH, MD, AGAF, FACG, FASGE
Department of Gastroenterology and Hepatology, Weill Cornell Medicine, New York Presbyterian Hospital, New York, New York, USA

MUHAMMAD ALI KHAN, MD
Department of Gastroenterology and Hepatology, The University of Tennessee Health Science Center, Memphis, Tennessee, USA

MASAYUKI KITANO, MD, PhD
Professor, Second Department of Internal Medicine, Wakayama Medical University, Wakayama, Japan

ALBERTO LARGHI, MD, PhD
Digestive Endoscopy Unit, Catholic University, Rome, Italy

JOSE LARIÑO-NOIA, MD
Department of Gastroenterology and Hepatology, Health Research Institute (IDIS), University Hospital of Santiago de Compostela, Santiago de Compostela, Spain

RYAN LAW, DO
Clinical Lecturer, Division of Gastroenterology, University of Michigan, Ann Arbor, Michigan, USA

DAVID S. LEE, MD
Division of Digestive and Liver Diseases, Department of Medicine, Columbia University Medical Center, New York, New York, USA

MICHAEL J. LEVY, MD
Division of Gastroenterology and Hepatology, Mayo Clinic, Rochester, Minnesota, USA

SRIHARI MAHADEV, MD, MS
Division of Digestive and Liver Diseases, Department of Medicine, Columbia University Medical Center, New York, New York, USA

FERNANDO PAVINATO MARSON, MD, PhD
Department of Surgery, University of São Paulo, São Paulo, Brazil, USA

SAURABH MUKEWAR, MD
Clinical Instructor, The Vatche and Tamar Manoukian Division of Digestive Diseases, David Geffen School of Medicine at UCLA, Los Angeles, California, USA

THIRUVENGADAM MUNIRAJ, MD, PhD, MRCP(UK)
Section of Digestive Diseases, Yale School of Medicine, New Haven, Connecticut, USA

VENKATARAMAN RAMAN MUTHUSAMY, MD, MAS
Director, Department of Endoscopy, Professor, Department of Clinical Medicine, The Vatche and Tamar Manoukian Division of Digestive Diseases, David Geffen School of Medicine at UCLA, Los Angeles, California, USA

CHRISTOPHER PACKEY, MD, PhD
Fellow in Gastroenterology, Department of Medicine, Columbia University Medical Center, New York, New York, USA

WIRIYAPORN RIDTITID, MD
Assistant Professor of Medicine, Division of Gastroenterology and Hepatology, Chulalongkorn University, King Chulalongkorn Memorial Hospital, Thai Red Cross Society, Bangkok, Thailand

MIHAI RIMBAŞ, MD, PhD
Department of Gastroenterology, Colentina Clinical Hospital, Internal Medicine Department, Carol Davila University of Medicine, Bucharest, Romania; Digestive Endoscopy Unit, Catholic University, Rome, Italy

MONICA SAUMOY, MD, MS
Department of Gastroenterology and Hepatology, Weill Cornell Medicine, New York Presbyterian Hospital, New York, New York, USA

AMRITA SETHI, MD
Associate Professor, Division of Digestive and Liver Diseases, Department of Medicine, Columbia University Medical Center, New York, New York, USA

YASUNOBU YAMASHITA, MD, PhD
Second Department of Internal Medicine, Wakayama Medical University, Wakayama, Japan

Contents

have an increasing role in the diagnosis through its characteristic imaging, image-enhancing techniques, and its ability to acquire tissue through either fine-needle aspiration or biopsy. This article reviews the diagnostic challenges of AIP and the current role of EUS.

Saurabh Mukewar and Venkataraman Raman Muthusamy

Therapeutic endosonography (EUS) may play an important role in the management of cancers. EUS-guided fiducial placement has a high success rate and can aid in stereotactic radiotherapy. EUS-guided tumor ablation therapies can help in palliation of locally advanced tumors. EUS-guided antitumor injection seems to be feasible and safe in animals; initial human studies suffer from small sample size and lack of controls. Randomized controlled trials have not shown benefit over conventional therapy. EUS celiac plexus neurolysis has gained popularity and is performed by interventional endosonographers. Large trials are needed to determine the most appropriate indications and overall usefulness of these therapies.

Mihai Rimbaş and Alberto Larghi

When endoscopic retrograde cholangiopancreatography (ERCP) fails to decompress the biliary system or the pancreatic duct, endoscopic ultrasonography (EUS)-guided biliary or pancreatic access and drainage can be used. Data show a high success rate and acceptable adverse event rate for EUS-guided biliary drainage. The outcomes of EUS-guided biliary drainage seem equivalent to percutaneous drainage and ERCP, whereas only retrospective studies are available for pancreatic duct drainage. In this article, revision of the technical and clinical status and the current evidence of interventional EUS-guided biliary and pancreatic duct access and drainage are presented.

Sunil Amin and Amrita Sethi

 Video content accompanies this article at http://www.giendo. theclinics.com.

Gastric outlet obstruction is a common complication of advanced upper gastrointestinal and pancreatic malignancies. Endoscopic ultrasound (EUS)-guided gastrojejunostomy is a new option that may provide a more durable solution than enteral stenting with shorter recovery time and lower cost than surgical gastrojejunostomy. Techniques to perform this procedure include direct EUS-guided puncture and balloon-assisted and free-hand methods. Use of cautery-tipped lumen-apposing metal stent results in higher rates of technical success and shorter procedure times. Prospective studies are needed to compare EUS-gastrojejunostomy with enteral stenting and surgical gastrojejusntomy, and to clarify indications, optimal patient selection, and most appropriate method of technically performing this procedure.

technique and increase familiarity with the rapidly changing devices. Trainees also must be given a graduated level of independence to perform each step and, eventually, be able to practice on a variety of endoscopic targets. With structured competency markers, trainees can learn methods to maximize success and minimize the risk of complications.

Sahin Coban, Omer Basar, and William R. Brugge

Endoscopic ultrasound (EUS) plays an important role as a diagnostic and therapeutic modality in gastroenterology. New developments have emerged, especially in the past decade, and are being introduced to endoscopists. The ability to readily visualize and access organs in the gastrointestinal tract has allowed endoscopists to perform new interventional procedures. EUS procedures have taken the place of conventional approaches for the treatment of various gastrointestinal diseases, including pancreatic cystic lesions. This article focuses on the advances and future of diagnostic and therapeutic EUS.

GASTROINTESTINAL ENDOSCOPY CLINICS OF NORTH AMERICA

RELATED INTEREST

Gastroenterology Clinics of North America, June 2015, (Vol. 44, No. 2)
Barrett's Esophagus
Prasad G. Iyer and Navtej S. Buttar, *Editors*

THE CLINICS ARE AVAILABLE ONLINE!
Access your subscription at:
www.theclinics.com

Foreword

Endoscopic Ultrasound Becomes a Major Interventional Tool

 CrossMark

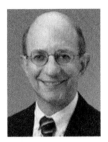

Charles J. Lightdale, MD
Consulting Editor

Over three decades, endoscopic ultrasound (EUS) has evolved from its origins as an imaging procedure for diagnosis and staging to its current role where it is used mostly for tissue acquisition and as a guide for endoscopic therapy. The forces leading to this change include the development of enhanced computed tomography (CT) and MRI for less invasive diagnosis and remarkable improvements in electronic linear array echo endoscopes that allow clear ultrasound visualization of needles directed through the biopsy port of the instruments. These developments also coincided with the recognition that imaging alone was not sufficient for diagnosis, and that pathologic diagnosis was essential. With tissue the issue, linear array EUS has become the method of choice for biopsy of lesions in proximity to the gastrointestinal tract, most notably in the pancreas, liver, and lymph nodes.

Dr Gress, the editor for this issue of *Gastrointestinal Endoscopy Clinics of North America* on progress in EUS, has been a long-time leader in the field and was an up-front proponent of linear array EUS for needle biopsy. He has contributed his own article for this issue on the early history of interventional EUS. Another remarkable development has been the recognition by instrument makers that interventional EUS could be an important new market. Hence the creation of improved EUS needles to obtain better samples for cytology and histology, and a growing toolbox of novel EUS-guided instruments for drainage and therapy.

Dr Gress has selected a comprehensive list of topics and an international group of expert authors for this issue. Important articles in this issue cover new instruments and techniques in EUS tissue acquisition and in handling and interpreting the obtained specimens. There seems little doubt that there will be even more need for EUS-guided fine-needle aspiration in this blossoming era of precision medicine with therapies, particularly in oncology, increasingly based on genetic analysis and biomarkers in tissue specimens. Not to ignore improvements in EUS imaging, there are also articles on

Gastrointest Endoscopy Clin N Am 27 (2017) xiii–xiv
http://dx.doi.org/10.1016/j.giec.2017.07.006
1052-5157/17/© 2017 Published by Elsevier Inc.

giendo.theclinics.com

EUS elastography and contrast-enhanced EUS. Articles also cover the role of EUS in diagnosis and therapy of pancreatic cysts, a common problem often discovered incidentally on CT and MRI scans, and the role of EUS in the diagnosis of autoimmune pancreatitis, which can often avoid major surgery. EUS-guided internal drainage procedures have proliferated and are presented in separate articles relating to the common bile duct and gallbladder, pancreatic fluid collections, and pelvic collections. Related to internal drainage, there is an article on the exciting use of EUS to help perform minimally invasive gastrojejunostomy. The nascent areas of EUS-guided cancer therapy and EUS-guided hemostasis are also presented.

The upshot of all this EUS interventional activity is that we need to have more and more trained endosonographers to fill the demand. The penultimate article in this issue is on training, and the good news is that almost all gastrointestinal advanced endoscopy fellowship programs teach EUS along with endoscopic retrograde cholangiopancreatography (ERCP), and in many programs, the number of EUS procedures performed is equal to or even greater than ERCP. In academic centers, EUS-trained interventionalists have already reached critical mass, but there is still plenty of room in the community for more. We have come a long way from the days when most gastroenterologists could not interpret EUS images at all. When I showed an EUS video in the 1990s, I remember one fellow who quipped: "Is that a storm over the Great Lakes?" No longer. The indications for EUS are well known. The images are discussed on rounds, and the questions are on the board exams. The final article discusses future directions for EUS, and we will see, but I suspect continuing growth. I am certain that the contents of this benchmark issue will be widely read and appreciated.

Charles J. Lightdale, MD
Department of Medicine
Columbia University Medical Center
161 Fort Washington Avenue
New York, NY 10032, USA

E-mail address:
CJL18@columbia.edu

Preface

Progress in Endoscopic Ultrasonography

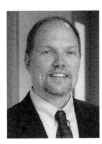

Frank G. Gress, MD
Editor

Endoscopic ultrasound (EUS) has come a long way since its initial reports in the gastro-enterology literature in 1980. Once a diagnostic and staging modality, EUS began a slow evolution from a purely diagnostic procedure to a therapeutic and interventional device. Over the last 20 years, EUS has seen a dramatic change in its role in the management of gastrointestinal disease, as innovative technology and accessories have emerged. These have included new and improved echoendoscopes with larger accessory channels allowing for the development of novel endoscopic tools and accessories that could be used for performing interventional procedures. Initially, early reports described the novel use of EUS to manage the intractable pain associated with chronic pancreatitis and pancreatic malignancy and to obtain cholangiogram and pancreatogram imaging in failed endoscopic retrograde cholangiopancreatography cases.

Now technical innovations allow us to perform minimally invasive EUS-guided procedures, such as EUS cystgastrostomy and EUS-guided drainage of the common bile duct, pancreatic duct, and even the gallbladder. EUS interventional techniques continue to evolve and include other new and emerging minimally invasive techniques, such as EUS-guided gastrojejunostomy and EUS necrosectomy.

The articles in this issue of *Gastrointestinal and Endoscopy Clinics of North America* represent the latest innovations in both diagnostic EUS imaging techniques and interventional EUS.

The aim of this issue was to bring together renowned experts from across the globe to discuss the latest techniques and innovations involving EUS. I am greatly indebted to the contributing authors for their articles, which allow us to disseminate this important knowledge and experience to a much wider audience. I hope the readers of this

Gastrointest Endoscopy Clin N Am 27 (2017) xv–xvi
http://dx.doi.org/10.1016/j.giec.2017.07.005
1052-5157/17/© 2017 Published by Elsevier Inc.

giendo.theclinics.com

issue enjoy and benefit, as much as I have, from this collection of superb articles from outstanding experts on the subject.

Frank G. Gress, MD
Division of Digestive and Liver Diseases
Columbia University Medical Center
161 Fort Washington Avenue
Herbert Irving Pavilion, HIP 13-1343
New York, NY 10032, USA

E-mail address:
fgg2109@columbia.edu

The Early History of Interventional Endoscopic Ultrasound

Frank G. Gress, MD

KEYWORDS

• Endoscopic ultrasound • Fine-needle aspiration • Gastrointestinal

KEY POINTS

- It has been a fascinating journey for endoscopic ultrasound (EUS) over the past approximately 30 years.
- Technological advances in the field of EUS have emerged, especially in the past decade, that have rapidly expanded the therapeutic potential of EUS, largely through the innovations of accessory technology that could not have happened without innovative changes to echoendoscopes.
- As interventional EUS continues to evolve, further expansion into previously uncharted areas will most certainly happen.

Endoscopic ultrasound (EUS) was developed by the Olympus Corporation in the late 1970s and 1980s in an attempt to improve ultrasound imaging of the pancreaticobiliary system. During this time period, prototypes were evaluated and studied primarily in Europe, in London, Munich, and Amsterdam. The initial EUS prototype was a 180° mechanical radial scanning instrument. There were just a few individuals performing EUS for most of the 1980s, including Lok Tio in Amsterdam at the Academic Medical Center, Thomas Rösch in Munich, and Charles Lightdale in New York. At that time, studies were performed largely to assess the potential role of EUS for evaluating gastrointestinal (GI) tract tumors and pancreaticobiliary disorders. These studies in the early days of EUS correlated EUS images with surgical resection specimens. It became clear toward the end of the 1980s that EUS was here to stay as it began to enter mainstream GI, with indications starting to appear for staging of GI tract tumors and pancreaticobiliary disorders.

By the early 1990s, there were 3 main centers in the United States performing EUS procedures: Charles Lightdale at Memorial Sloan Kettering Cancer Center, Michael Sivak at University Hospitals Case Medical Center, and Robert Hawes at the Indiana University (IU) Medical Center.

Division of Digestive and Liver Diseases, Columbia University Medical Center, 161 Fort Washington Avenue, New York, NY 10032, USA
E-mail address: fgg2109@cumc.columbia.edu

Gastrointest Endoscopy Clin N Am 27 (2017) 547–550
http://dx.doi.org/10.1016/j.giec.2017.06.015
1052-5157/17/© 2017 Elsevier Inc. All rights reserved.

giendo.theclinics.com

On a personal note, I arrived at the IU Medical Center to be their first EUS fellow with my mentor, Robert Hawes, in July 1993. Little did I know that my advanced year of therapeutic endoscopy training would bring me into the early period of therapeutic or interventional EUS. I will continue to share my own personal experience as I go forward in this article accounting the early years of therapeutic EUS.

In the early 1990s, Pentax Medical, in cooperation with Hitachi, developed the first linear-array EUS system. My first introduction with the Pentax linear echoendoscope came in 1993 during my EUS training in my advanced fellowship at IU. The Pentax representative, Bob Enerson, would bring the system (including scope and processor) to us in return for evaluating its clinical utility. These were exciting times for me because I was just beginning to master radial endosonography and the opportunity to look at EUS imaging in the linear perspective was fascinating to me. Linear endosonography brought a whole new landscape to EUS and the detailed imaging and the ability to track a needle in real time across the image plane into a target lesion was phenomenal.

It was at this time that Pentax started to partner with Wilson-Cook Endoscopy to develop an EUS fine-needle aspiration (FNA) needle that could be placed through the accessory channel of the linear EUS scope. The year was 1993 and IU was approached by Wilson-Cook to use their needle prototypes in return for evaluating its clinical utility. This needle began as an adaption of the Howell-type aspiration needle fashioned to the tip of a long plastic catheter, which was capable of going through the linear scope. This first EUS FNA needle, although it had limitations, was able to obtain cytology from the lymph node. Several renditions using various needle gauges were tested. Based on this early work with the EUS FNA needle, Robert Hawes and Maurits Wiersema published the first EUS-guided FNA report performed in the United States and it was only a short time behind the first EUS FNA performed in the world, which was done by Peter Vilmann in Denmark in 1992.[1–3]

The advent of EUS-guided FNA forever changed the landscape of EUS, shaping this emerging new technology from a purely diagnostic procedure to one that could do much more. With the development of EUS FNA, many reports on its clinical utility for sampling suspicious GI lesions and adjacent organs, including the liver, bile ducts, and pancreas, flooded the GI literature for more than a decade. During the 1990s many studies were published on the clinical utility of EUS-guided FNA for diagnosing many different types of GI malignancies. Further studies in the new millennium solidified the role of EUS FNA as the first-line modality for diagnosing pancreatic cancer.

EUS-guided FNA has further evolved into EUS-guided tissue acquisition and is now the procedure of choice for sampling GI tract lesions, such as subepithelial lesions and other structures adjacent to the GI tract, including lymph nodes, the pancreas, and liver, to name a few.

It was in 1995, as a junior faculty member at the IU Medical Center, that I had the chance to look beyond EUS FNA and attempt some of the earliest interventional/therapeutic techniques. Several studies demonstrated for the first time in 1995 and 1996 the feasibility of performing a pancreatogram or cholangiogram under EUS guidance.[4,5] This intrigued me, and during my time at IU, I worked with my colleagues there toward developing EUS-guided access techniques. This began initially as an attempt to access the pancreatic duct in a patient status post-Whipple having a failed endoscopic retrograde cholangiopancreatography (ERCP).[6] Although our first attempt at a "rendezvous procedure" failed due to the lack of the necessary tools to be successful at this, it demonstrated that we were now able to access the pancreatic duct and obtain pancreatograms in failed ERCP cases. Around the same time, EUS-guided cholangiography demonstrated that we could do the same with the common bile duct.

Not too long after these reports, investigators demonstrated the role of these techniques in cases where other standard approaches failed, such as ERCP.[6,7] Probably one of the most significant turning points was the development of EUS-guided pseudocyst drainage, which has revolutionized the way pancreatic fluid collections are managed.[8–10] The initial reports of this technique were described using early prototype accessories and it was not until the development of the therapeutic echoendoscope that major advances occurred in this area. This approach changed the way we manage these patients, from a surgical approach to a minimally invasive outpatient procedure.

Since then, EUS-guided biliary and pancreatic duct access and drainage techniques have emerged as attractive, less-invasive therapeutic alternatives after unsuccessful ERCP procedures. These techniques have evolved over time and are now reported as safe and technically and clinically successful in experienced hands for most patients.[11]

Another early therapeutic development was EUS-guided celiac plexus block, a technique for treating chronic pancreatitis pain.[12] This technique offered a new approach to managing the debilitating pain associated with chronic pancreatitis. Initially performed by fluoroscopy and CT-guided methods with mixed results and complications, EUS-guided celiac block has become a minimally invasive option for these patients as well as those suffering from intra-abdominal malignancies, such as pancreatic cancer.

Advances in therapeutic EUS were limited early on by a lack of large accessory channels in the linear EUS scopes, which prevented the development of effective EUS-guided accessories. It was not for a few years more until the first therapeutic linear EUS scope allowed for the development of better accessories to access the bile ducts and pancreatic ducts, sample cysts, and eventually place stents to drain pancreatic fluid collections and ultimately treat walled off pancreatic necrosis.[13]

It has been a fascinating journey for EUS over the past approximately 30 years. To see a technology advance from a purely diagnostic test to a therapeutic modality that can change the management of a patient, prevent surgery, and improve outcomes was, for me, personally, a very satisfying feeling. Technological advances in the field of EUS have emerged, especially in the past decade, that have rapidly expanded the therapeutic potential of EUS, largely through the innovations of accessory technology, that could not have happened without innovative changes to echoendoscopes, all of which have led to a broader range of indications for therapeutic endosonography. As interventional EUS continues to evolve, further expansion into previously uncharted areas will most certainly happen. Such advances are already being made in EUS-guided therapy for gallbladder disease, GI cancers, and management of obesity. I look forward to the next 30 years of EUS development!

REFERENCES

1. Vilmann P, Jacobsen GK, Henriksen FW, et al. Endoscopic ultrasonography with guided fine needle aspiration biopsy in pancreatic disease. Gastrointest Endosc 1992;38:172–3.

2. Giovannini M, Seitz JF, Monges G, et al. Guided puncture-cytology under electronic sectorial ultrasound endoscopy. Results in 26 patients. Gastroenterol Clin Biol 1993;17:465–70 [in French].

3. Wiersema MJ, Kochman ML, Chak A, et al. Mediastinal LN FNA Real-time endoscopic ultrasound-guided fine-needle aspiration of a mediastinal lymph node. Gastrointest Endosc 1993;39(3):429–31.

4. Harada N, Kouzu T, Arima M, et al. Endoscopic ultrasound-guided pancreatography: a case report. Endoscopy 1995;27:612–5.
5. Wiersema MJ, Sandusky D, Carr R, et al. Endosonography-guided cholangiopancreatography. Gastrointest Endosc 1996;43:102–6.
6. Gress F, Ikenberry S, Sherman S, et al. Endoscopic ultrasound-directed pancreatography. Gastrointest Endosc 1996;44(6):736–9.
7. Giovannini M, Moutardier V, Pesenti C, et al. Endoscopic ultrasound-guided bilio-duodenal anastomosis: a new technique for biliary drainage. Endoscopy 2001; 33(10):898–900.
8. Grimm H, Binmoeller KF, Soehendra N. Endosonography-guided drainage of a pancreatic pseudo-cyst. Gastrointest Endosc 1992;38:170–1.
9. Wiersema MJ. Endosonography-guided cystoduodenostomy with a therapeutic ultrasound endoscope. Gastrointest Endosc 1996;44:614–7.
10. Vilmann P, Hancke S, Pless T. One-step endosonography-guided drainage of a pancreatic pseudocyst: a new technique of stent delivery through the echo endoscope. Endoscopy 1998;30:730–3.
11. Shami V, Kahaleh M. Endoscopic ultrasonography (EUS)-guided access and therapy of pancreatico-biliary disorders: EUS-guided cholangio and pancreatic drainage. Gastrointest Endosc Clin N Am 2007;17(3):581–93.
12. Gress F, Schmitt C, Sherman S, et al. A prospective randomized comparison of endoscopic ultrasound- and computed tomography-guided celiac plexus block for managing chronic pancreatitis pain. Am J Gastroenterol 1999;94:900–5.
13. Baron TH. Treatment of pancreatic pseudocysts, pancreatic necrosis and pancreatic duct leaks. Gastrointest Endosc Clin N Am 2007;17(3):559–79.

New Imaging Techniques
Endoscopic Ultrasound-Guided Elastography

 CrossMark

Julio Iglesias-García, MD, PhD*, Jose Lariño-Noia, MD,
Juan Enrique Domínguez-Muñoz, MD, PhD

KEYWORDS

- Endoscopic ultrasound • Elastography • Stiffness • Diagnosis

KEY POINTS

- Endoscopic ultrasound (EUS) is considered a major imaging method in the management of several diseases of the gastrointestinal tract and surrounding structures.
- Elastography is a real-time method, based on ultrasound techniques, allowing the evaluation of tissue stiffness.
- EUS-guided elastography is considered an excellent tool in the differential diagnosis of solid pancreatic tumors and lymph nodes.
- There are emerging indications for EUS-guided elastography, such as the evaluation of liver lesions, subepithelial lesions, and left adrenal gland masses.

INTRODUCTION

The introduction of endoscopic ultrasound (EUS) in clinical practice is an important advancement in the management of a wide variety of diseases. EUS has been demonstrated to have significantly changed the diagnosis and/or management of up to 25% to 50% of cases.[1–4] Nevertheless, an accurate diagnosis cannot always be determined using only conventional B-mode EUS imaging. In many cases, EUS-guided tissue acquisition can provide a definitive diagnosis. Overall diagnostic accuracy of EUS-guided tissue acquisition can be considered to be very high, with sensitivities between 80% and 85%, and specificities approaching 100%.[5–7] However, EUS-guided tissue sampling is technically demanding and multiple punctures may be necessary to obtain a sufficient amount of tissue.[8,9] Furthermore, despite repeated sampling, cyto-histologic assessment can be falsely negative and EUS-guided tissue acquisition is

Disclosure Statement: J. Iglesias-García: International Advisor for Pentax-Medical, Boston-Scientific. J. Lariño-Noia: No disclosures. J.E. Domínguez-Muñoz: No disclosures.
Department of Gastroenterology and Hepatology, Health Research Institute (IDIS), University Hospital of Santiago de Compostela, c/Choupana s/n, Santiago de Compostela 15706, Spain
* Corresponding author.
E-mail address: julioiglesiasgarcia@gmail.com

associated with small but not insignificant morbidity rates.[10] Hence, new methods have been warranted, allowing for a more accurate but still noninvasive characterization of lesions, limiting the need for EUS-guided tissue sampling and guided biopsies of areas with the highest suspicion of malignancy in cases in which tissue sampling is still necessary. Among them, EUS-guided elastography has arisen as a very promising technique.

Elastography is a real-time method for evaluation of tissue stiffness. Initial investigations occurred in the 1990s. Currently, the strain technique is available to be used under EUS guidance.[11] Strain elastography is a qualitative method to evaluate tissue stiffness based on eternal or internal generated force, which in EUS is based on the internal force concept.[12] The method is based on stiff tissues presenting lower strain so that they deform less under compression when compared with soft tissues. With strain elastography, the compression-induced tissue deformations within a region of interest (ROI) are assessed in a comparative fashion. Several different diseases, including cancer, can induce alterations in tissue stiffness.[13–15] Elastography was initially developed for evaluation of lesions accessible from the body surface and was performed with external probes. Today, elastographic evaluation can be performed from inside the gastrointestinal tract combined with conventional EUS.[15] Promising results have been reported for EUS elastography in several studies, indicating its high accuracy in differentiating benign from malignant lesions in the pancreas and lymph nodes. The aim of this article is to review the technical aspects and clinical applications of EUS elastography and to identify related areas for further study.

TECHNIQUE
Preparation

No specific preparation is needed from the patient point of view for performing the EUS-guided elastography. Patient positioning does not differ from the position needed for the performance of a standard EUS exploration.

Approach and Theory

Elastography has emerged from the development of the fremitus technique in breast ultrasonography, which demonstrates that healthy breast tissue vibrates more than solid malignant lesions, despite their isoechoic appearance under B-mode ultrasound.[13] Elastography is based on the knowledge that many different pathologic processes, such as fibrosis, inflammation, and cancer, induce alterations in tissue stiffness.[13–15] Elastography evaluates this stiffness through the application of slight compression using an ultrasound transducer to the targeted tissue and recording the resulting tissue displacement from the region evaluated. Physiologic vascular pulsations and respiratory movements provide the vibrations and compressions necessary for the study. Measurement of displacement is made using an algorithm based on the extended combined autocorrelation method.[16] Elastography can be performed in real time using a conventional EUS probe attached to a processor with the specific software installed.[15] First-generation EUS elastography allowed only qualitative evaluation. Today, second-generation EUS elastography also allows for the quantitative evaluation of tissue stiffness with 2 different approaches: strain ratio and strain histogram.

Technique or Procedure

Two different systems of elastography are available. The first is based on the qualitative evaluation of the pattern obtained from the elastographic study, whereas the second is based on an evolution of the software, allowing a quantification of the stiffness.

Qualitative elastography

Qualitative elastography relies on the quantification of the compression-induced deformation of the structures in the B-mode image using the degree of deformation as an indicator of tissue stiffness. The technology is based on the detection of small structure deformations within the B-mode image caused by compression, so that the strain is smaller in hard tissues than in soft tissues.[13,17] To optimize and rely on the evaluation, large blood vessels should be avoided because movement of blood gives an artificial effect of large displacement or softness. A ROI is used to define the area of interest in a similar way to Doppler evaluation. Very little compression is necessary because the regular pressure variation from the pulsation of adjacent vessels will be enough. The size of the ROI is crucial because it needs to be sufficiently large to include both the pathologic tissue and surrounding normal tissue as reference. The best image quality has been documented to be when the area under study covers between 25% and 50% of the ROI.[18] Elasticity (on a scale of 1–255) is depicted using a color map (red, green, and blue), wherein hard tissue is shown in dark blue, tissue with intermediate hardness in green, medium soft tissue in yellow, and soft tissue in red. Elastography pattern is demonstrated by superimposing the color pattern on a conventional B-mode picture. Usually, a 2-panel image is used for presentation, including the conventional grey-scale B-mode image and the elastographic image, which represents different elasticity values marked with different colors, resulting in different elastographic patterns (**Fig. 1**). Specific settings for the EUS elastography software are commonly used (1/−/−/2/3/4 T-Elasto-H): reject function 1, e-smoothing 2, persistence 3, and e-dynamic range 4.[19] Different patterns and the diagnostic approach for malignancy are shown in **Table 1**.

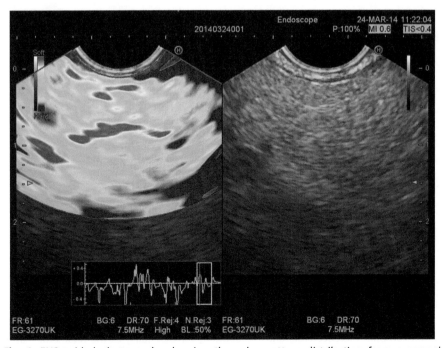

Fig. 1. EUS-guided elastography showing the color pattern distribution from a normal pancreas (*left*). Grey-scale B-mode image (*right*).

Table 1
Elastographic patterns classification for endoscopic ultrasound

Color and Pattern	Stiffness	Malignancy
Homogeneous green predominant	Soft	No
Heterogeneous green predominant	Intermediate	No
Heterogeneous blue predominant	Hard	Yes
Homogeneous blue predominant	Hard	Yes
Heterogeneous green and blue without predominant color	Intermediate hard	Undetermined

Quantitative elastography

Currently, there are 2 different methods allowing a quantitative elastographic evaluation: the strain ratio and the strain histogram.

Strain ratio calculation is based on standard qualitative EUS elastography data. Two different areas (A and B) are selected for quantitative elastographic analysis. Area A is selected so that it includes as much of the target lesion as possible without including the surrounding tissues. Area B is selected within a soft (red) reference area outside the target lesion, preferably the gut wall. The strain ratio is calculated as the quotient of B/A. However, the color map is just a guide because ratio is calculated using raw strain data and does not depend on color map display. A presumption of this method is that the investigated disease does not significantly alter the hardness of the reference connective or fat tissues (**Fig. 2**).[20]

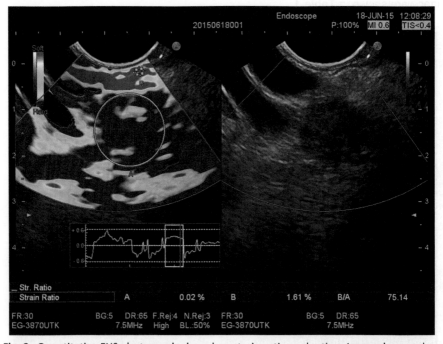

Fig. 2. Quantitative EUS elastography based on strain ratio evaluation. Image shows values from lesion and reference area, and the quotient corresponding to the final strain ratio evaluation (*left*). Grey-scale B-mode image (*right*). Picture corresponds to a pancreatic cancer.

Strain histogram is based on the qualitative EUS elastography data for a manually selected ROI within the standard elastography image. For the measurement, the largest measurement box that touches the inside boundary of lesion within the ROI must be selected.[21] The X-axis in the strain histogram represents the elasticity from 0 (hardest) to 255 (softest) of the tissue. This method analyses the range and distribution of strains within a large ROI. It shows several key parameters such as mean strain, standard deviation, percent of area (blue), and complexity (relation of circumference to area of blue patches) (**Fig. 3**).[22]

Table 2 shows the cut-off points for determine malignancy with strain ratio and strain histogram.

INDICATIONS OR CONTRAINDICATIONS

Because there are no formal contraindications for performing EUS-guided elastographic evaluation, the focus is on the accepted indications.

Over the past years, the role of EUS-guided elastography has been focused in the evaluation of solid pancreatic lesions and enlarged lymph. However, more indications are arising, highlighting the real importance of this technology and its progressive inclusion in clinical routine, such as left adrenal gland, subepithelial lesions, and focal left liver lesions.

Pancreatic Diseases

Today, EUS is considered a reference method for the diagnosis and staging of inflammatory, cystic, and neoplastic lesions of the pancreas.[4,23,24] In this setting, EUS elastography has arisen as great technique for the evaluation of pancreatic diseases.

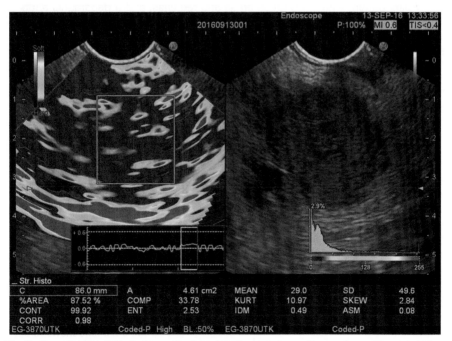

Fig. 3. Quantitative EUS elastography based strain histogram. Image shows the quantification of the color map at the area selected to be evaluated. Picture corresponds to a pancreatic cancer (*left*). Grey-scale B-mode image (*right*).

Table 2 Quantitative elastography classification for malignancy		
Quantification	Values	Malignancy
Strain Ratio	>10	Yes
Strain Histogram	<50	Yes

Differential diagnosis of solid pancreatic lesions

Malignant pancreatic tumors are generally harder than surrounding tissue (see previous discussion), which usually correspond to a blue pattern. The first ever study on EUS-guided elastography in pancreatic solid lesions was published by Giovannini and colleagues,[25] using the qualitative evaluation. Considering blue (hard) lesions as malignant, sensitivity and specificity for malignancy was 100% and 67%, respectively. Based on this study, a scoring system was defined. Score 1 and 2 (mainly green) were considered as benign, and scores 3 to 5 (mainly blue) were considered as malignant. In a subsequent multicenter trial, Giovannini and colleagues[26] reported EUS elastography findings in 121 cases with pancreatic masses. The sensitivity, specificity, positive predictive value, and negative predictive value of the differentiation between benign and malignant pancreatic masses were 92.3%, 80.0%, 93.3%, and 77.4%, respectively, with an overall accuracy of 89.2%. The interobserver agreement of the evaluation of 30 cases yielded a kappa score of 0.785 for the detection of malignancy. Iglesias-García and colleagues,[19] in 130 subjects with solid pancreatic masses and 20 controls, defined 4 patterns: a homogeneous green pattern present only in normal pancreas; a heterogeneous, predominantly green pattern with slight yellow and red lines present only in inflammatory pancreatic masses; a heterogeneous, predominantly blue pattern with small green areas and red lines, and a geographic appearance, present mainly in pancreatic malignant tumors (including pancreatic adenocarcinoma); and a homogeneous blue pattern, present only in pancreatic neuroendocrine malignant lesions. Using this classification, the sensitivity, specificity, positive and negative predictive values, and overall accuracy of EUS elastography for detecting malignancy were 100%, 85.5%, 90.7%, 100%, and 94.0%, respectively. All of the subjects were evaluated by 2 endosonographers who made the same interpretation in 121 out of 130 cases and 20 out of 20 controls, yielding a kappa value of 0.772. A study focused on the evaluation of the interobserver agreement concluded that EUS-guided elastography is reproducible in the evaluation of solid pancreatic lesions, even between endoscopists with no or limited experience.[27]

However, not all studies presented the same level of accuracy. Janssen and colleagues[28] reported a similar sensitivity (93.8%) but a significant lower specificity (65.4%). Their overall accuracy for malignancy detection was 73.5%. The investigators highlighted the problem on the evaluation of advanced chronic pancreatitis, which is difficult to differentiate from hard malignant lesions. Hirche and colleagues[29] could only perform an adequate elastographic evaluation in 56% of the subjects. In certain clinical situations, adequate elastography evaluation included difficulties such as including the entire lesion and enough surrounding tissues in the analyzed ROI in large (>35 mm) lesions, lesions distant from the transducer, and presence of fluid (eg, vessels, cysts) in the ROI. Overall, EUS elastography predicted the nature of pancreatic lesions with poor diagnostic sensitivity (41%), specificity (53%), and accuracy (45%).

More recent studies have analyzed the usefulness of quantitative EUS-elastography. Iglesias-García and colleagues[20] first published the results on the accuracy of the strain ratio evaluation for the differential diagnosis of solid pancreatic masses on 86 subjects. Quantitative EUS elastography with strain ratio presented a higher accuracy (97.7%) and specificity (92.9%) compared with the qualitative analysis. A strain ratio greater than 6.04 or a mass elasticity less than 0.05% defined a sensitivity of 100% for classifying tumors as malignant. The specificity could be improved to 100% with a strain ratio greater than 15.41 or a mass elasticity value less than 0.03%. In addition, EUS-guided elastography could differentiate pancreatic cancers from inflammatory masses (100% sensitivity and 96% specificity) and pancreatic cancers from neuroendocrine tumors (100% sensitivity and 88% specificity). With the same methodology, another prospective study evaluated 109 subjects. With the qualitative technique, all pancreatic cancers presented intense blue coloration; however, the inflammatory masses showed mixed colorations (green, yellow, and low-intensity blue). With the quantitative technique, the mean strain was 39.08 plus or minus 20.54 for pancreatic cancer and 23.66 plus or minus 12.65 for inflammatory masses ($P<.05$).[30] In the past years, several studies have been conducted with the aim to determine the accuracy of strain ratio for detecting malignancies. Different cut-off values have been defined, from 3.7 to 24. Diagnostic accuracy ranges from sensitivities of 67% to 98%, with lower levels of specificity, ranging from 45% to 71%.[31–37]

Săftoiu and colleagues[21] investigated quantitative EUS-guided elastography based on hue histograms. The sensitivity, specificity, positive predictive values, negative predictive values, and accuracy of the procedure in differentiating between benign and malignant pancreatic masses were 91.4%, 87.9%, 88.9%, 90.6%, and 89.7%, respectively, using 175 as the cut-off for the mean of the hue histogram. Recently, a multicenter study involving 258 subjects (211 with pancreatic adenocarcinoma and 47 with chronic pancreatitis) and using the same methodology showed a sensitivity, specificity, positive predictive values, negative predictive values, and accuracy were 93.4%, 66.0%, 92.5%, 68.9%, and 85.4%, respectively, using the same cut-off value (175) for the mean of the hue histogram.[38,39] Schrader and colleagues[38] investigated quantitative elastography based on the mean of the hue histogram in 86 subjects with malignant pancreatic masses and 28 controls without pancreatic disease. A 100% sensitivity and specificity for malignancy detection was obtained through the quantitative measurement of the blue color. However, this study did not include controls with benign pancreatic masses or chronic pancreatitis. No differences in terms of diagnostic accuracy have been documented between strain ratio and strain histogram. Iglesias-García and colleagues[22] reported that a strain ratio greater than 10 and a mean strain histogram value less than 50 were the optimal cutoff values for classification of lesions as malignant, with an overall accuracy of 98%.

Finally, several meta-analyses have been performed aiming to determine the role of EUS-guided elastography in the differential diagnosis of solid pancreatic masses. Two of these evaluated the role of the differentiation of malignant pancreatic tumors from inflammatory pancreatic masses, each including 13 studies with 1042 and 1044 subjects, showed a sensitivity of 95% and a specificity of 67% to 69%, with an area under the curve (AUC) of 0.86 to 0.90.[39,40] A third included 7 studies and 752 subjects, with a global sensitivity of 97%, a specificity of 76%, and an AUC of 0.95. This meta-analysis highlights the difficulties in differentiating adenocarcinoma and neuroendocrine tumor, which are both hard lesions.[41] A fourth meta-analysis found that the use of a color pattern for elastographic interpretation was associated with a sensitivity of 99% and a specificity of 69% to 76%.[42] By the use of hue histogram, the sensitivity was 92% and the specificity was slighter lower at 86%. **Fig. 4** shows the different images based on EUS-guided elastography in benign and malignant solid pancreatic lesions.

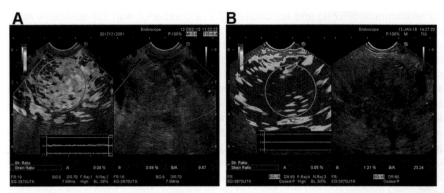

Fig. 4. Benign (*A*) and malignant (*B*) pancreatic solid lesions as evaluated by EUS-guided elastography (*left*). Grey-scale B-mode image (*right*).

Chronic pancreatitis

EUS can be considered the most sensitive method for the diagnosis of chronic pancreatitis. However, there are several challenges with this technique, mainly for the diagnosis of early stages of the disease. EUS elastography can provide additional relevant information of tissue stiffness and thus may benefit the diagnosis of this disease. In a study using the qualitative evaluation, subjects with chronic pancreatitis presented green areas with heterogenic, predominantly blue strands. These changes were clearly different from those observed in the control group (subjects without pancreatic diseases), with predominantly green and yellow homogeneous patterns. Iglesias-García and colleagues[43] published a prospective study in 191 subjects, with quantitative EUS elastography based on strain ratio evaluation. Strain ratio was measured in the head, body, and tail of the pancreas and the mean value was used for analysis. The investigators found a significant correlation between strain ratio and the number of EUS criteria for chronic pancreatitis ($r = 0.813$). By using a cutoff point for the strain ratio of 2.25, overall diagnostic accuracy was 91.1%. **Fig. 5** shows an EUS-guided elastographic evaluation from a patient with mild changes for chronic pancreatitis at B-mode. Measurement of pancreatic fibrosis can also be achieved by EUS-guided elastography. Itoh and colleagues[44] evaluated 58 consecutive subjects before pancreatectomy for both pancreatic tumors and upstream pancreas. Histologic fibrosis was graded into 4 categories (normal, mild fibrosis, marked fibrosis, and severe fibrosis). The results showed that fibrosis grade correlated significantly with strain histogram. Area under the ROC curves for the diagnosis of mild or higher-grade fibrosis, marked or higher-grade fibrosis, and severe fibrosis were 0.90, 0.90, and 0.90, respectively. This technique has also been used to evaluate the severity of chronic pancreatitis. Dominguez-Muñoz and colleagues[45] evaluated 115 subjects with chronic pancreatitis, 35 of them with exocrine pancreatic insufficiency (EPI), an advanced stage of the disease. Strain ratio levels were higher in subjects with EPI (4.89 vs 2.82–3.16; $P<.001$). There was a direct relationship between the strain ratio and the probability of EPI, which increases from 4.2% in subjects with a strain ratio less than 2.5% to 92.8% in those with a strain ratio greater than 5.5.

Lymph Node Evaluation

Differential diagnosis of lymph nodes is crucial, mainly to differentiate benign from malignant ones in the setting of the staging of several tumors. However, this differentiation based only in B-mode characteristic is truly challenging.[46] EUS-guided

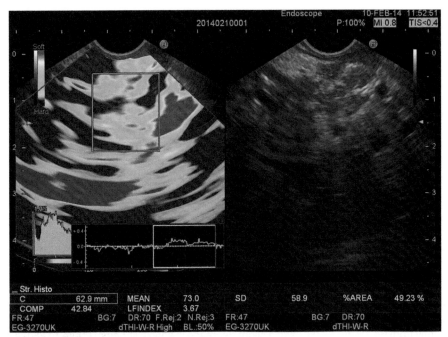

Fig. 5. EUS-guided elastography from a patient with mild changes in B-mode suggestive of chronic pancreatitis (*left*). Grey-scale B-mode image (*right*).

elastography can be also a helpful tool in this context. A study from Giovannini and colleagues[25] analyzed 31 lymph nodes from 25 subjects. By using the same score as described for pancreatic solid lesions, the results of the qualitative EUS elastography were consistent with malignancy in 22 cases, with benign masses in 7 cases, and indeterminate in 2 cases. No false-negative findings were found but 5 false-positives were documented. The sensitivity and specificity for determining malignancy were 100% and 50%, respectively. A subsequent multicenter study, also by Giovannini and colleagues,[26] investigated 101 lymph nodes (57 malignant and 44 benign). The elastographic images were interpreted as benign in 38 cases, indeterminate in 10 cases, and malignant in 53 cases. Considering benign lesions test as negative and indeterminate and malignant lesions as positive, the sensitivity, specificity, positive predictive value, and negative predictive value for the detection of malignancy were 91.8%, 82.5%, 88.8%, and 86.8%, respectively, whereas the overall accuracy was 88.1%. The interobserver agreement of the evaluation of 30 cases yielded a kappa score of 0.657 for the detection of malignant lymph nodes. Janssen and colleagues[47] evaluated the feasibility of qualitative EUS elastography of the dorsal mediastinum, comparing the elastographic patterns of lymph nodes to the gold standard (EUS-guided tissue acquisition). A total of 66 lymph nodes were examined (37 benign and 29 malignant under histologic evaluation). In 31 of 37 benign lymph nodes, elastography showed a homogeneous pattern (intermediate elasticity). Predominantly hard tissues were found in 23 of the 29 malignant lymph nodes. Overall accuracy ranged from 84.6% to 86.4% for malignancy. Interestingly, interobserver agreement was perfect (kappa = 0.84). Lariño-Noia and colleagues[48] presented as an abstract their results in 63. Three different elastographic patterns were identified: a predominantly blue pattern, a predominantly green pattern, and a mixed pattern (blue and green without predominance). The probability of a benign histology in lymph nodes with a green pattern was 100%, and the probability of malignant histology with a predominantly blue pattern was 92.3%. A mixed pattern yielded a probability of malignancy of 50%. Săftoiu and colleagues[49] analyzed whether EUS-elastography may differentiate between benign and malignant lymph nodes by using qualitative pattern and quantitative histogram analyses. The qualitative pattern analysis showed a high sensitivity (91.7%), specificity (94.4%), and accuracy (92.86%). By defining an elasticity ratio based on separate red-green-blue channel histogram values, diagnostic accuracy even increased to a sensitivity, specificity, and accuracy of 95.8, 94.4, and 95.2%, respectively.[49] In a second study, using a dynamic hue histogram, sensitivity, specificity, and overall accuracy was 85.4, 91.9, and 88.5%, respectively.[50] **Fig. 6** demonstrate the elastographic pattern of a benign lymph node.

Recent studies have tried to evaluate the specific role of EUS-guided elastography for assessing lymph nodes malignancy in cancer staging. Knabe and colleagues,[51] aimed to assess whether EUS-guided elastography was able to improve lymph node staging in patients with esophageal cancer. The investigators evaluated the proportions of color pixels in 40 lymph nodes evaluated, assessed using computer analysis of the elastography images. Sensitivity, specificity, and positive predictive values of EUS-guided elastography alone were 100%, 64.1%, and 75%, respectively, compared with the values of 91.3%, 64.7%, and 74%, respectively, obtained for B-mode criteria. When computer analysis of the elastographic images was added, with a cut-off value randomly set to 50% blue pixels, the specificity improved significantly from 64.1% to 86.7%, with a slight decrease in sensitivity, from 100% to 88.9%. Positive predictive value improved from 75% to 86%. Larsen and colleagues,[52]

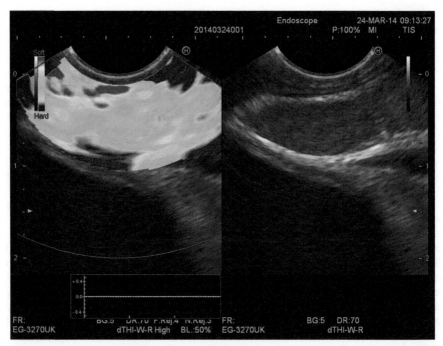

Fig. 6. EUS-guided elastography of a benign, reactive, lymph node (*left*). Grey-scale B-mode image (*right*).

analyzed 56 lymph nodes in subjects with upper gastrointestinal cancer, using surgical histologic evaluation as gold-standard. Values of sensitivity, specificity, accuracy, positive predictive value, and negative predictive value of 86%, 71%, 77%, 66%, and 89%, respectively, were obtained for EUS; 59%, 82%, 73%, 68%, and 76%, respectively, for EUS-guided elastography using a 5-pattern scoring system; and 55%, 82%, 71%, 67%, and 74%, respectively, for strain ratio calculation (cut-off value 4.5). In a study from Paterson and colleagues[53] evaluating esophageal cancer subjects, strain ratio (cut-off value of $\geq$7.5 for malignancy) yielded a sensitivity, specificity, positive predictive value, negative predictive value, and accuracy of 83%, 96%, 95%, 86%, and 90%, respectively, significantly higher than that obtained with standard B-mode–defined criteria.

Finally, Xu and colleagues,[54] conducted a meta-analysis to evaluate the accuracy of EUS-guided elastography by pooling data of existing trials. Seven studies involving 368 subjects with 431 lymph nodes were included. Pooled sensitivity of EUS-guided elastography for the differential diagnosis of benign and malignant lymph nodes was 88% and the specificity was 85%.

Transrectal Endoscopic Ultrasound–Guided Elastography

The value of transrectal EUS-guided elastography has been investigated for the diagnosis and evaluation of prostate cancer, rectal cancer, inflammatory bowel disease, and fecal incontinence. In prostate cancer, elastography has been demonstrated to be superior to transrectal EUS alone, and it improves the specificity of prostate biopsies by highlighting areas highly suspected of malignancy. The sensitivity of transrectal elastography in the diagnosis of prostate cancer ranges from 68% to 92%, and its specificity ranges from 62% to 87% in subjects clinically suspected of prostate cancer.[55,56]

Transrectal elastography for differentiating between benign and malignant rectal tumors has been evaluated in a study that involved 69 subjects with rectal tumors. By using strain ratio, differentiation between adenomas and adenocarcinomas yielded a sensitivity of 93%, a specificity of 96%, and an accuracy of 94%.[57] This method has even proven to be highly reproducible.[58] In a recent pilot study, EUS evaluation of rectal wall thickness and the strain ratio have been investigated for diagnosing inflammatory bowel disease and differentiating Crohn disease from ulcerative colitis. Subjects with Crohn disease had significantly higher strain ratios than both the controls and subjects with ulcerative colitis but there was no difference between the strain ratios of subjects with ulcerative colitis and the controls.[59] Finally, Allgayer and colleagues[60] evaluated the elastography of anal sphincters in 50 subjects with fecal incontinence, finding no correlation between the elastographic appearance of sphincters and the functional and clinical parameters.

Subepithelial Masses

Imaging the layers of the gastrointestinal (GI) tract is among the major indications for EUS examination. In the case of subepithelial masses, EUS-guided elastography can provide information on stiffness, which may help increase the diagnostic confidence and accuracy of the staging. So far, there have been only few reports concerning the use of EUS elastography in characterizing subepithelial masses. Based on EUS-guided elastography, benign subepithelial masses usually show an intermediate stiffness with homogenous strain pattern. In the other hand, malignant subepithelial masses show a heterogeneously stiff pattern. Gastrointestinal stromal tumors are difficult cases.[61]

Liver

No proper data are yet available on the role of EUS-guided elastography for the evaluation of liver stiffness. However, some reports have shown a potential role of this methodology for the evaluation of solid liver lesions, such as liver metastasis. At least 1 case report has been published showing that malignant solid liver lesions can be characterized as presenting a typical stiff pattern, similar to those described in pancreatic solid masses.[62] An example of a malignant lesion as shown by EUS-guided elastography is shown in **Fig. 7**.

Adrenal Glands

The left adrenal gland presents a good access for EUS. In fact, EUS is the preferred way to biopsy enlargements of the gland. The main indication is in the staging of lung cancer. Initially, only case reports have been published with this indication, showing that malignant infiltrations tend to be stiffer than benign tumors, inflammatory processes, and fatty deposits. Iglesias-García and colleagues[63] presented the first study in which the probability of malignancy of a left adrenal mass showing a blue-predominant (stiff) pattern is 91.3%, whereas it is as low as 10% in the presence of a green-predominant (soft) pattern.

COMPLICATIONS AND MANAGEMENT

Because this method is based on a specific software associated with ultrasound devices, no specific complications have been documented related to EUS-guided elastography. The only probable complications could be those related to the performance of the EUS.

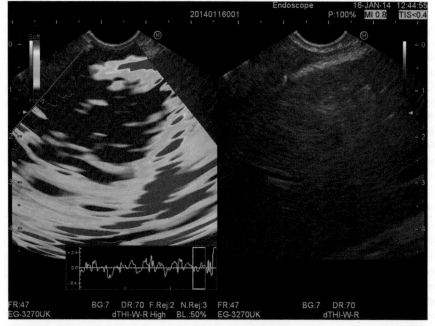

Fig. 7. EUS-guided elastography obtained from a metastatic left liver lobe lesion (primary pancreatic cancer) (*left*). Grey-scale B-mode image (*right*).

CURRENT CONTROVERSIES

Main controversies on EUS-guided elastography area related to the limitations of this technology. First, both qualitative and quantitative EUS-guided elastography are considered to be exploratory-dependent, the main issues being the bias on the selection of the ROI for the analysis and also the inside areas to be analyzed. These 2 points could cause intraobserver and interobserver variability. Another point is the difficulty of controlling the tissue compression because an excessive pressure applied to the tissues by the probe may alter the strain measured. It is crucial for optimizing the elastographic analysis to control the motion artifacts, which can be considered to be very complex under EUS guidance. Strain can be very easily altered by the vessels, cysts, and bones in the selected areas, thus these structures should be avoided in the ROI. Finally, for quantitative assessments, there is a need for standardization of the methodology of selection of the areas to be analyzed because strain value may be affected if there is insufficient surrounding normal tissue as reference in the ROI. Another similar problem for the calculation of the strain ratio is that the reference area has not been properly defined and different studies use different areas for the analysis, which may affect the overall result. In this context, the use of the strain histogram may improve this limitation. Overall, there is a need to standardize the technique, to make it more reproducible, and thus, increase the use and indications.

Of course, EUS-guided elastography requires a specific period of training to perform a high-quality study. The length of training has not been yet established. However, once the endosonographer has been properly trained, the technique does not significantly increase the time of the complete procedure.

FUTURE CONSIDERATIONS

The use of EUS elastography for determining the infiltration of adjacent organs in the staging of gastric and esophageal cancers is currently being evaluated in ongoing studies. Further studies will evaluate the usefulness of EUS elastography in diagnosing the aforementioned diseases and other indications. The authors believe that EUS elastography will be integral part of the EUS evaluation of any pathologic condition that may alter tissue stiffness, including inflammation, fibrosis, and cancer.

Furthermore, EUS-guided elastography may be useful to identify the hard (most likely to be malignant) areas within the pancreatic masses and lymph nodes for targeted EUS-guided tissue acquisition. New studies are needed to further define the role of EUS-guided elastography for this indication. Although new indications have arisen, such as lesions located in the liver, biliary tract, adrenal glands, and GI tract, additional evidence is required to define the role of EUS elastography in these clinical applications. Future perspectives include monitoring treatment response in antiangiogenic therapy with elastography technique and applications of EUS elastography.

SUMMARY

As a minimally invasive method, EUS plays an important role in the evaluation of several GI tract diseases, mainly for assessing malignancies of the GI tract and nearby organs. Elastography adds valuable information to EUS by providing a qualitative and quantitative evaluation of tissue stiffness, thus reflecting the potential malignant or benign nature of the disease. Pancreas and lymph nodes are the 2 most investigated organs with EUS-guided elastography. In fact, both qualitative and quantitative techniques have been proven useful in the differentiation between benign and malignant solid pancreatic masses and lymph nodes, and differentiation between normal pancreatic tissues and chronic pancreatitis, all with a high accuracy. This method can be also combined with other imaging techniques, such as contrast-enhanced EUS, which may be helpful to further improve the accuracy of EUS assessment.

EUS-guided elastography is not yet ready to replace EUS-guided tissue acquisition in any of its indications; however, EUS-guided elastography may play an important role for making clinical decisions, such as whether biopsies are necessary for a patient and which lymph nodes are most likely to be malignant and thus selected for biopsy. In addition, a suspicious finding based on elastography can be helpful for guiding further clinical management when EUS-guided tissue acquisition is inconclusive or negative.

Emergent indications include the use of EUS elastography for the characterization of lesions located in the liver, biliary tract, adrenal glands, and gastrointestinal tract.

REFERENCES

1. Dye CE, Waxman I. Endoscopic ultrasound. Gastroenterol Clin North Am 2002; 31(3):863–79.
2. Tamerisa R, Irisawa A, Bhutani MS. Endoscopic ultrasound in the diagnosis, staging, and management of gastrointestinal and adjacent malignancies. Med Clin North Am 2005;89(1):139–58.
3. Luthra AK, Evans JA. Review of current and evolving clinical indications for endoscopic ultrasound. World J Gastrointest Endosc 2016;8(3):157–64.
4. Iglesias-García J, Lindkvist B, Lariño-Noia J, et al. The role of EUS in relation to other imaging modalities in the differential diagnosis between mass forming chronic pancreatitis, autoimmune pancreatitis and ductal pancreatic adenocarcinoma. Rev Esp Enferm Dig 2012;104(6):315–21.
5. Bhatia V, Varadarajulu S. Endoscopic ultrasonography-guided tissue acquisition: how to achieve excellence? Dig Endosc 2017;29(4):417–30.
6. Huang JY-L, Chang KJ. Improvements and innovations in endoscopic ultrasound guided fine needle aspiration. J Hepatobiliary Pancreat Sci 2015;22(7):E37–46.
7. Dumonceau J-M, Koessler T, van Hooft JE, et al. Endoscopic ultrasonography-guided fine needle aspiration: relatively low sensitivity in the endosonographer population. World J Gastroenterol 2012;18(19):2357–63.
8. Jhala NC, Jhala D, Eltoum I, et al. Endoscopic ultrasound-guided fine-needle aspiration biopsy: a powerful tool to obtain samples from small lesions. Cancer 2004;102(4):239–46.
9. Dumonceau J-M, Polkowski M, Larghi A, et al. Indications, results, and clinical impact of endoscopic ultrasound (EUS)-guided sampling in gastroenterology: European Society of Gastrointestinal Endoscopy (ESGE) Clinical Guideline. Endoscopy 2011;43(10):897–912.
10. Polkowski M, Larghi A, Weynand B, et al. Learning, techniques, and complications of endoscopic ultrasound (EUS)-guided sampling in gastroenterology: European Society of Gastrointestinal Endoscopy (ESGE) Technical Guideline. Endoscopy 2012;44(2):190–206.
11. Cui X-W, Chang J-M, Kan Q-C, et al. Endoscopic ultrasound elastography: current status and future perspectives. World J Gastroenterol 2015;21(47): 13212–24.
12. Dietrich CF. Elastography, the new dimension in ultrasonography. Praxis (Bern 1994) 2011;100(25):1533–42 [in German].
13. Itoh A, Ueno E, Tohno E, et al. Breast disease: clinical application of US elastography for diagnosis. Radiology 2006;239(2):341–50.

14. Thomas A, Kümmel S, Gemeinhardt O, et al. Real-time sonoelastography of the cervix: tissue elasticity of the normal and abnormal cervix. Acad Radiol 2007; 14(2):193–200.
15. Iglesias-García J, Domínguez-Muñoz JE. Endoscopic ultrasound image enhancement elastography. Gastrointest Endosc Clin N Am 2012;22(2):333–48.
16. Shiina T, Nightingale KR, Palmeri ML, et al. WFUMB guidelines and recommendations for clinical use of ultrasound elastography: part 1: basic principles and terminology. Ultrasound Med Biol 2015;41(5):1126–47.
17. Frey H. Realtime elastography. A new ultrasound procedure for the reconstruction of tissue elasticity. Radiol 2003;43(10):850–5 [in German].
18. Havre RF, Elde E, Gilja OH, et al. Freehand real-time elastography: impact of scanning parameters on image quality and in vitro intra- and interobserver validations. Ultrasound Med Biol 2008;34(10):1638–50.
19. Iglesias-García J, Larino-Noia J, Abdulkader I, et al. EUS elastography for the characterization of solid pancreatic masses. Gastrointest Endosc 2009;70(6): 1101–8.
20. Iglesias-García J, Larino-Noia J, Abdulkader I, et al. Quantitative endoscopic ultrasound elastography: an accurate method for the differentiation of solid pancreatic masses. Gastroenterology 2010;139(4):1172–80.
21. Săftoiu A, Vilmann P, Gorunescu F, et al. Neural network analysis of dynamic sequences of EUS elastography used for the differential diagnosis of chronic pancreatitis and pancreatic cancer. Gastrointest Endosc 2008;68(6):1086–94.
22. Iglesias-García J, Lindkvist B, Lariño-Noia J, et al. Differential diagnosis of solid pancreatic masses: contrast-enhanced harmonic (CEH-EUS), quantitative-elastography (QE-EUS), or both? United European Gastroenterol J 2017;5(2): 236–46.
23. Iglesias-García J, Lariño-Noia J, Lindkvist B, et al. Endoscopic ultrasound in the diagnosis of chronic pancreatitis. Rev Esp Enferm Dig 2015;107(4):221–8.
24. Kawaguchi Y, Mine T. Endoscopic approach to the diagnosis of pancreatic cystic tumor. World J Gastrointest Oncol 2016;8(2):159–64.
25. Giovannini M, Hookey LC, Bories E, et al. Endoscopic ultrasound elastography: the first step towards virtual biopsy? Preliminary results in 49 patients. Endoscopy 2006;38(4):344–8.
26. Giovannini M, Thomas B, Erwan B, et al. Endoscopic ultrasound elastography for evaluation of lymph nodes and pancreatic masses: a multicenter study. World J Gastroenterol 2009;15(13):1587–93.
27. Soares J-B, Iglesias-García J, Goncalves B, et al. Interobserver agreement of EUS elastography in the evaluation of solid pancreatic lesions. Endosc Ultrasound 2015;4(3):244–9.
28. Janssen J, Schlörer E, Greiner L. EUS elastography of the pancreas: feasibility and pattern description of the normal pancreas, chronic pancreatitis, and focal pancreatic lesions. Gastrointest Endosc 2007;65(7):971–8.
29. Hirche TO, Ignee A, Barreiros AP, et al. Indications and limitations of endoscopic ultrasound elastography for evaluation of focal pancreatic lesions. Endoscopy 2008;40(11):910–7.
30. Itokawa F, Itoi T, Sofuni A, et al. EUS elastography combined with the strain ratio of tissue elasticity for diagnosis of solid pancreatic masses. J Gastroenterol 2011; 46(6):843–53.
31. Figueiredo FAF, da Silva PM, Monges G, et al. Yield of contrast-enhanced power doppler endoscopic ultrasonography and strain ratio obtained by

eus-elastography in the diagnosis of focal pancreatic solid lesions. Endosc Ultrasound 2012;1(3):143–9.

32. Dawwas MF, Taha H, Leeds JS, et al. Diagnostic accuracy of quantitative EUS elastography for discriminating malignant from benign solid pancreatic masses: a prospective, single-center study. Gastrointest Endosc 2012;76(5):953–61.

33. Lee TH, Cho YD, Cha S-W, et al. Endoscopic ultrasound elastography for the pancreas in Korea: a preliminary single center study. Clin Endosc 2013;46(2): 172–7.

34. Havre RF, Ødegaard S, Gilja OH, et al. Characterization of solid focal pancreatic lesions using endoscopic ultrasonography with real-time elastography. Scand J Gastroenterol 2014;49(6):742–51.

35. Rustemovic N, Opacic D, Ostojic Z, et al. Comparison of elastography methods in patients with pancreatic masses. Endosc Ultrasound 2014;3(Suppl 1):S4.

36. Kongkam P, Lakananurak N, Navicharern P, et al. Combination of EUS-FNA and elastography (strain ratio) to exclude malignant solid pancreatic lesions: a prospective single-blinded study. J Gastroenterol Hepatol 2015;30(11):1683–9.

37. Mayerle J, Beyer G, Simon P, et al. Prospective cohort study comparing transient EUS guided elastography to EUS-FNA for the diagnosis of solid pancreatic mass lesions. Pancreatol 2016;16(1):110–4.

38. Schrader H, Wiese M, Ellrichmann M, et al. Diagnostic value of quantitative EUS elastography for malignant pancreatic tumors: relationship with pancreatic fibrosis. Ultraschall Med 2012;33(7):E196–201.

39. Pei Q, Zou X, Zhang X, et al. Diagnostic value of EUS elastography in differentiation of benign and malignant solid pancreatic masses: a meta-analysis. Pancreatol 2012;12(5):402–8.

40. Mei M, Ni J, Liu D, et al. EUS elastography for diagnosis of solid pancreatic masses: a meta-analysis. Gastrointest Endosc 2013;77(4):578–89.

41. Xu W, Shi J, Li X, et al. Endoscopic ultrasound elastography for differentiation of benign and malignant pancreatic masses: a systemic review and meta-analysis. Eur J Gastroenterol Hepatol 2013;25(2):218–24.

42. Li X, Xu W, Shi J, et al. Endoscopic ultrasound elastography for differentiating between pancreatic adenocarcinoma and inflammatory masses: a meta-analysis. World J Gastroenterol 2013;19(37):6284–91.

43. Iglesias-García J, Domínguez-Muñoz JE, Castiñeira-Alvariño M, et al. Quantitative elastography associated with endoscopic ultrasound for the diagnosis of chronic pancreatitis. Endoscopy 2013;45(10):781–8.

44. Itoh Y, Itoh A, Kawashima H, et al. Quantitative analysis of diagnosing pancreatic fibrosis using EUS-elastography (comparison with surgical specimens). J Gastroenterol 2014;49(7):1183–92.

45. Dominguez-Muñoz JE, Iglesias-García J, Castiñeira Alvariño M, et al. EUS elastography to predict pancreatic exocrine insufficiency in patients with chronic pancreatitis. Gastrointest Endosc 2015;81(1):136–42.

46. Bhutani MS, Hawes RH, Hoffman BJ. A comparison of the accuracy of echo features during endoscopic ultrasound (EUS) and EUS-guided fine-needle aspiration for diagnosis of malignant lymph node invasion. Gastrointest Endosc 1997; 45(6):474–9.

47. Janssen J, Dietrich CF, Will U, et al. Endosonographic elastography in the diagnosis of mediastinal lymph nodes. Endoscopy 2007;39(11):952–7.

48. Lariño-Noia J, Iglesias-García J, Alvarez-Castro A, et al. Usefulness of endoscopic ultrasound (EUS) elastography for the detection of malignant infiltration

of mediastinal and abdominal lymph nodes [abstract]. Gastroenterology 2009; 136(5 Suppl 1):AB231.

49. Săftoiu A, Vilmann P, Hassan H, et al. Analysis of endoscopic ultrasound elastography used for characterisation and differentiation of benign and malignant lymph nodes. Ultraschall Med 2006;27(6):535–42.

50. Săftoiu A, Vilmann P, Ciurea T, et al. Dynamic analysis of EUS used for the differentiation of benign and malignant lymph nodes. Gastrointest Endosc 2007;66(2): 291–300.

51. Knabe M, Günter E, Ell C, et al. Can EUS elastography improve lymph node staging in esophageal cancer? Surg Endosc 2013;27(4):1196–202.

52. Larsen MH, Fristrup C, Hansen TP, et al. Endoscopic ultrasound, endoscopic sonoelastography, and strain ratio evaluation of lymph nodes with histology as gold standard. Endoscopy 2012;44(8):759–66.

53. Paterson S, Duthie F, Stanley AJ. Endoscopic ultrasound-guided elastography in the nodal staging of oesophageal cancer. World J Gastroenterol 2012;18(9): 889–95.

54. Xu W, Shi J, Zeng X, et al. EUS elastography for the differentiation of benign and malignant lymph nodes: a meta-analysis. Gastrointest Endosc 2011;74(5): 1001–9, 4.

55. Kamoi K, Okihara K, Ochiai A, et al. The utility of transrectal real-time elastography in the diagnosis of prostate cancer. Ultrasound Med Biol 2008;34(7): 1025–32.

56. Kapoor A, Kapoor A, Mahajan G, et al. Real-time elastography in the detection of prostate cancer in patients with raised PSA level. Ultrasound Med Biol 2011; 37(9):1374–81.

57. Waage JER, Havre RF, Odegaard S, et al. Endorectal elastography in the evaluation of rectal tumours. Colorectal Dis 2011;13(10):1130–7.

58. Waage JER, Rafaelsen SR, Borley NR, et al. Strain Elastography evaluation of rectal tumors: inter- and intraobserver reproducibility. Ultraschall Med 2015; 36(6):611–7.

59. Rustemovic N, Cukovic-Cavka S, Brinar M, et al. A pilot study of transrectal endoscopic ultrasound elastography in inflammatory bowel disease. BMC Gastroenterol 2011;11:113.

60. Allgayer H, Ignee A, Zipse S, et al. Endorectal ultrasound and real-time elastography in patients with fecal incontinence following anorectal surgery: a prospective comparison evaluating short- and long-term outcomes in irradiated and non-irradiated patients. Z Gastroenterol 2012;50(12):1281–6.

61. Ignee A, Jenssen C, Hocke M, et al. Contrast-enhanced (endoscopic) ultrasound and endoscopic ultrasound elastography in gastrointestinal stromal tumors. Endosc Ultrasound 2017;6(1):55–60.

62. Iglesias García J, Lariño-Noia J, Souto R, et al. Endoscopic ultrasound (EUS) elastography of the liver. Rev Esp Enferm Dig 2009;101(10):717–9.

63. Iglesias-García J, de la Iglesia-García D, Lariño-Noia J, et al. Accuracy of qualitative ultrasound-guided elastography for the diagnosis of malignancy of left adrenal gland masses [abstract]. United European Gastroenterol J 2016; 4(5 Suppl):A410.

New Imaging Techniques for Endoscopic Ultrasonography

Contrast-Enhanced Endoscopic Ultrasonography

Masayuki Kitano, MD, PhD*, Yasunobu Yamashita, MD, PhD

KEYWORDS

- Contrast • EUS • CH-EUS • Harmonic imaging • Enhancement • Sonazoid
- SonoVue • Definity • Pancreatic lesions

KEY POINTS

- Contrast-enhanced harmonic endoscopic ultrasonography (CH-EUS) visualizes macrovesicles and parenchymal perfusion in digestive diseases.
- CH-EUS is useful for diagnosis of pancreatic solid lesions by their characterization using enhancement patterns.
- CH-EUS is complementary to EUS-guided fine-needle aspiration for diagnosing pancreatic cancer.
- CH-EUS accurately discriminates mural nodules from mucous clots in intraductal mucinous neoplasms.
- CH-EUS is useful for estimation of malignant potential of gastrointestinal stromal tumors.

INTRODUCTION

Endoscopic ultrasonography (EUS) was developed in the 1980s to overcome the problems caused by intervening gas, bone, and fat, which affect transabdominal ultrasound (US) imaging. EUS is thought to be among most reliable and efficient diagnostic modalities for digestive diseases because its spatial resolution is superior to any other modality. However, conventional EUS suffers limitations in the diagnosis of digestive diseases because most solid lesions are depicted as a hypoechoic masses, making it difficult to differentiate benign and malignant lesions. Evaluation of vascularity is a way to improve the characterization of digestive lesions and this can be achieved using the recently developed technique of contrast-enhanced harmonic EUS (CH-EUS). This

Second Department of Internal Medicine, Wakayama Medical University, Wakayama, Japan
* Corresponding author. Second Department of Internal Medicine, Wakayama Medical University, 811-1 Kimiidera, Wakayama 641-0012, Japan.
E-mail address: kitano@wakayama-med.ac.jp

Gastrointest Endoscopy Clin N Am 27 (2017) 569–583
http://dx.doi.org/10.1016/j.giec.2017.06.002
1052-5157/17/© 2017 Elsevier Inc. All rights reserved.

technology has increased the use of CH-EUS in the diagnostic field, and its utility has been widely reported. Moreover, CH-EUS has advantages over contrast-enhanced (CE) MR imaging and computed tomography (CT) in patients with contraindications such as renal failure or contrast allergy. CH-EUS also allows for dynamic and repeat examinations. This article focuses on updates on current applications of this new imaging technique.

HISTORY OF CONTRAST-ENHANCED ENDOSCOPIC ULTRASONOGRAPHY

In 1986, Matsuda and Yabuuchi[1] were the first to report the concept of abdominal CE-US with an intra-arterial infusion of carbon dioxide (CO_2) being used as the contrast material. CE-EUS was first reported in 1995 by Kato and colleagues,[2] again using an intra-arterial CO_2 infusion. However, this method was limited in that CE-EUS was only performed during angiographic examinations. EUS with color and power Doppler functions then became possible, and the subsequent development of contrast agents that could be delivered through peripheral veins enabled the acquisition of images without angiography in the mid-1990s.[3] CE-Doppler EUS (CD-EUS) increases the sensitivity to signals from vessels by generating pseudo-Doppler signals from microbubbles.[4–7] However, CD-EUS suffers from artifacts that include blooming, overpainting, and motion artifacts.[5–7] Recently, the visualization of microvessels and parenchymal perfusion by decreasing artifacts was achieved by CE-harmonic imaging.[8,9] CH-EUS allows the detection of signals from microbubbles produced by intravenously administered contrast agents and allows filtering of signals originating from different tissues by selectively detecting harmonic components.

CONTRAST AGENTS

Contrast agents consist of gas-filled microbubbles of approximately 2 to 5 μm in diameter encapsulated by a phospholipid or lipid shell. After contrast agents are administered through a peripheral vein, they are not metabolized in the human body and are eliminated from the lungs. When the microbubbles in the contrast agent receive transmitted US waves, the microbubbles are disrupted or resonate, thereby producing the signal detected in the US image.

Three generations of contrast agents have been developed that vary in their transpulmonary passage and half-life in the human body. The first-generation agents, such as Levovist (mix of galactose and palmitic acid with air; Bayer Schering Pharma, Germany), are microbubbles filled with air. These generally require high acoustic power to produce oscillation or break the microbubbles. Second-generation agents, including SonoVue (sulfur hexafluoride microbubbles; Bracco, Italy), Definity (octafluoropropane microbubbles; Bristol-Myers Squibb Medical Imaging, USA) and Sonazoid (perfluorobutane microbubbles [GE Healthcare, USA; Daiichi Sankyo, Tokyo, Japan]), produce harmonic signals at lower acoustic power. They are, therefore, suitable for EUS imaging because EUS involves a small transducer and low acoustic power. A difference between these second-generation agents is that, after a preliminary vascular phase, Sonazoid has a late hepatosplenic phase due to trapping of microbubbles by Kupffer cells. Third-generation agents, such as EchoGen (dodecafluoropentane liquid; Sonus Pharmaceuticals, Bothell, WA), are capable of phase shifting from lipid to gas when they reach body temperature, although they have not yet been widely used in EUS. Adverse reactions to US contrast agents are rare in humans.[10]

CATEGORIES OF CONTRAST-ENHANCED ENDOSCOPIC ULTRASONOGRAPHY
Contrast-Enhanced Color and Power Doppler Endoscopic Ultrasonography

US contrast agents induce a phase shift (pseudo-Doppler signals) that enhances the Doppler signals from the vessels. Thus, infusion of a contrast agent increases the sensitivity with which color and power Doppler imaging depicts Doppler signals from vessels.[7,11] However, there are several limitations to CD-EUS, including blooming artifacts, poor spatial resolution, low sensitivity to slow flow, and vulnerability to motion artifacts. Recently, a novel directional power Doppler method called directional eFLOW has been developed.[12] This method permits the blood flow in minute vessels to be detected in more detail than can be achieved with conventional power or color Doppler. In the directional eFLOW mode (**Fig. 1**), fewer blooming artifacts are observed because the broadband transmission is optimized and the real repeating frequency is increased.

Contrast-Enhanced Harmonic Endoscopic Ultrasonography

The underlying principle of contrast harmonic imaging is as follows: when exposed to US beams, microbubbles in the contrast agent are disrupted or resonate, thereby releasing many harmonic signals.[7] When the tissue and microbubbles receive transmitted US waves, both produce harmonic components that are integer multiples of the fundamental frequency; the harmonic content from microbubbles is higher than that from tissue and selective depiction of the second harmonic component visualizes signals from microbubbles more strongly than those from tissue[13] (**Fig. 2**). This technology can, therefore, detect signals from microbubbles in vessels with very slow flow without Doppler-related artifacts and is used to characterize vascularity.[9,14] Moreover, CH-EUS can be subjected to quantitative analyses using inflow time mapping and time-intensity curve (TIC) patterns to characterize lesions.[15]

Critical points to perform CH-EUS

Mechanical index (MI) is set to 0.2–0.4. Before infusion of contrast agent, echo image of CH-EUS should be dark to the extent that little signals from the tissue can be observed. Focus point should be set at the bottom. Dual screen with fundamental B-mode and CH-EUS images should be displayed. Before performing CH-EUS, the target lesion should be imaged as close as possible, because penetration of ultrasound beam with CH-EUS is inferior to that with fundamental B-mode. A bolus

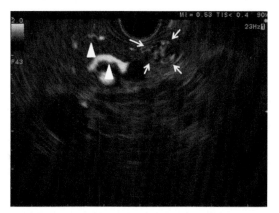

Fig. 1. Contrast-enhanced-directional eFLOW (pancreatic neuroendocrine tumor). eFLOW EUS detected the tumor (*arrows*) with color signals and fine vessel structure (*arrowheads*) in surrounding pancreatic tissue.

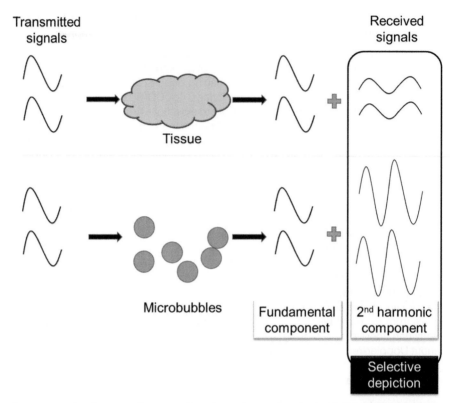

Fig. 2. Principle of contrast harmonic imaging. When exposed to US beams, microbubbles in the contrast agent are disrupted or resonate, and release many harmonic signals. When tissue and microbubbles receive the transmitted US waves, both produce harmonic components that are integer multiples of the fundamental frequency; the harmonic components from the microbubbles are higher than those from the tissue. Selective depiction of the second harmonic component visualizes signals from microbubbles more strongly than those from tissue.

injection of contrast agent (Sonazoid, 15 μL/kg body; Sonovue, 2.4–4.8 mL/body; Definity, 10 μL/kg body) is given through a peripheral vein. Signals from contrast agent appear from 10 to 15 seconds and peak to approximately 20 seconds.

SOLID PANCREATIC LESIONS

EUS is thought to be among most reliable and efficient diagnostic modalities for pancreatic diseases because it has superior spatial resolution to any other relevant modality.[16,17] Despite its ability to detect small pancreatic lesions with high sensitivity, EUS alone is limited in its ability to distinguish pancreatic cancer from non-neoplastic pancreatic masses because most pancreatic solid lesions are depicted as a hypoechoic mass, regardless of histology.[18] Therefore, CH-EUS is useful to diagnose those lesions with vascularity.

Characterization

CH-EUS images of pancreatic cancers were found to have a hypovascular pattern and lower intensity of enhancement relative to the surrounding pancreatic tissue (**Fig. 3A**). Kitano and colleagues[19] reported on the largest series of 277 subjects

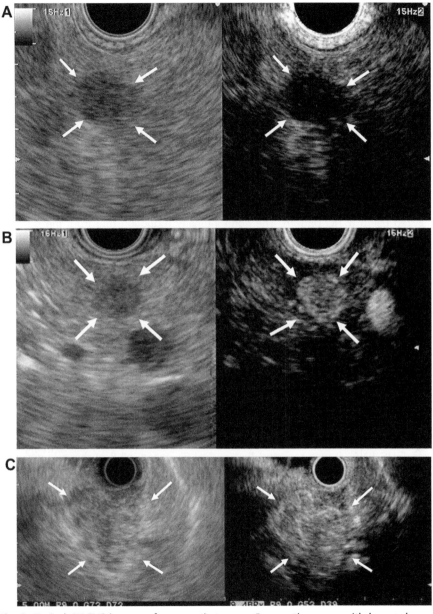

Fig. 3. Typical CH-EUS images of pancreatic tumors. Pancreatic cancer with hypoenhance-ment. The pancreatic lesion was detected as a low echoic lesion (*arrows*) with fundamental B-mode EUS (*A, left*). CH-EUS detected a pancreatic lesion with hypoenhancement (*arrows*) in comparison with that of the surrounding pancreatic tissue (*A, right*). Neuroendocrine tumor with hyperenhancement. The pancreatic lesion was detected as a low echoic lesion (*arrows*) with fundamental B-mode EUS (*B, left*). CH-EUS detected a pancreatic lesion with hyperenhancement (*arrows*) in comparison with that of the surrounding pancreatic tissue (*B, right*). Inflammatory mass with isoenhancement. The pancreatic lesion was detected as a low echoic lesion (*arrows*) with fundamental B-mode EUS (*C, left*). CH-EUS detected a pancreatic lesion with isoenhancement (*arrows*) in comparison with that of the surrounding pancreatic tissue (*C, right*).

with a solid pancreatic lesion who underwent CH-EUS. A depiction of hypoenhancement on CH-EUS with Sonazoid diagnosed pancreatic cancer with a sensitivity and specificity of 95% and 89%, respectively. When compared with CE-multidetector CT (MDCT), CH-EUS yielded a significantly higher accuracy in the diagnosis of pancreatic cancers less than 2 cm in size, with a sensitivity and specificity of 91% and 94%, respectively. In this report, 36 of 46 (78%) inflammatory masses (see **Fig. 3**C) had an isovascular pattern, whereas 15 of 19 (78%) neuroendocrine tumors (NETs) had a hypervascular pattern[19] (see **Fig. 3**B). Three other groups reported that CH-EUS with SonoVue could be used to diagnose pancreatic cancers with high sensitivity (93%, 89%, and 96%, respectively).[18,20,21] Matsubara and colleagues[22] defined autoimmune pancreatitis (AIP) and the presence of an inflammatory mass as inflammatory pancreatic pseudotumor (IPPT), and reported that 21 of 27 (78%) IPPTs (AIP, 14; inflammatory mass, 13) had an isovascular pattern (see **Fig. 3**C). In their study, vascularity on CH-EUS was analyzed using a TIC pattern. The echo intensity reduction rate from the peak at 1 minute was greater in pancreatic cancer than in mass-forming pancreatitis, AIP, and NET ($P<.05$). Another study achieved similar results, with 104 of 109 (94%) pancreatic cancers being hypovascular, 8 of 11 (72%) inflammatory masses, and 8 of 9 (89%) AIPs being isovascular, and 5 of 8 (63%) NETs being hypervascular.[23] In this study, CH-EUS images were analyzed at 2 time points to obtain early-phase and late-phase images. The additional analysis of early-phase, and the combination of early-phase and late-phase images, revealed novel aspects of the potential utility of CH-EUS for pancreatic tumor patients. Finally, a correlation between CH-EUS images and the histopathology of resected pancreatic cancer specimens was found. Analysis of early-phase images enabled a clinically relevant comparison between CH-EUS images and pancreatic cancer histology. A hypovascular pattern in the early phase corresponded with heterogeneous tumor cells with necrotic tissue, fibrous tissue, and few vessels, whereas an isovascular pattern in the early phase corresponded with homogeneous tumor cells with abundant vessels and no necrotic or fibrous tissues. In a study on EUS-guided fine-needle aspiration (EUS-FNA), it was reported that, out of 61 cases, all 8 of those in which a diagnosis was not possible from the obtained sample exhibited a hypovascular pattern. Therefore, the results may be helpful in current clinical settings involving EUS-FNA assessment. Moreover, fewer needle passes are required to obtain samples with CH-EUS. In fact, no matter how useful EUS-FNA is for obtaining a diagnostic yield of pancreatic cancers, the biopsy specimens from EUS-FNA are sometimes inadequate for appropriate pathologic diagnosis because of possible sampling errors. Hou and colleagues[24] reported that the percentage of adequate biopsy specimens in an EUS-FNA with CH-EUS (**Fig. 4**) group (96.6%) was greater than that in an EUS-FNA group (86.7%). In another study by Kitano and colleagues,[19] all those pancreatic cancers that were false-negative according to EUS-FNA were detected as hypoenhancing tumors on CH-EUS, and the combination of CH-EUS and EUS-FNA increased the sensitivity of EUS-FNA for pancreatic cancer from 92% to 100%.

Tumor Staging

Tumor staging (T staging) with regard to vascular invasion is important to determine the appropriate treatment strategy for pancreatic cancer. However, it is sometimes difficult to distinguish tumor from peritumoral inflammation with conventional EUS. Imazu and colleagues[25] reported that CH-EUS was significantly superior to EUS for T staging, with overall accuracies of 92% and 69%, respectively ($P<.05$). In particular,

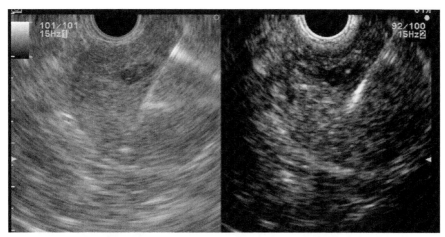

Fig. 4. EUS-guided fine-needle aspiration with CH-EUS. Compared with fundamental B-mode EUS (*left*), CH-EUS (*right*) detected the pancreatic lesion more clearly and helped differentiate the pathologic area with contrast-uptake.

CH-EUS more clearly detected the portal wall (**Fig. 5**) and was, therefore, more specific for portal invasion than EUS (100% vs 83%).

Node Staging

Node staging (N staging) is an important factor in evaluating the prognosis and determining the treatment approach. Miyata and colleagues[26] reported on the use of CH-EUS on pancreatobiliary carcinoma subjects with visible lymph nodes. Heterogeneous enhancement was observed in 39 of 47 malignant lesions, whereas homogeneous enhancement was observed in 79 of 87 benign lesions (**Fig. 6**). CH-EUS allowed determination of malignant from benign lymph nodes with a sensitivity, specificity, and accuracy of 83%, 91%, and 88%, respectively.

PREDICTING CHEMOTHERAPY RESPONSE

Antitumor agents have been introduced in an attempt to improve the survival of patients with advanced pancreatic cancer. Even identical chemotherapy regimens bring

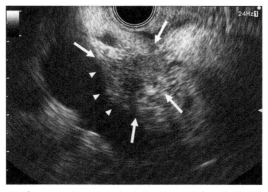

Fig. 5. CH-EUS image of pancreatic cancer invasion to portal wall. CH-EUS clearly shows the interface between portal vein and tumor (*arrows*) is disappeared (*arrowheads*).

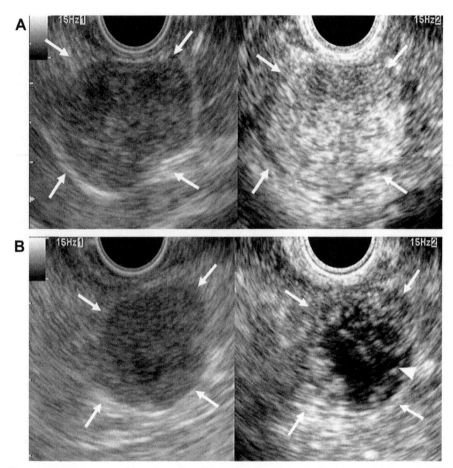

Fig. 6. CH-EUS images of lymph nodes. (*A*) Benign lymph node. Fundamental B mode EUS (*A, left*) shows low echoic lymph node (*arrows*). CH-EUS (*A, right*) reveals homogeneous enhancement in the lymph node (*arrows*). (*B*) Malignant lymph node. Fundamental B mode EUS (*B, left*) shows low echoic lymph node (*arrows*). CH-EUS (*B, right*) reveals heterogeneous enhancement with avasculare area (*arrowhead*) in the lymph node (*arrows*).

about different outcomes in different patients. Some patients experience improvements in survival and tumor response, whereas other patients only suffer from inconvenience and increased toxicity. Therefore, obtaining an understanding of the prognostic factors before treatment would be helpful for selecting the subgroups of patients predicted to have improved survival with chemotherapy and for determining efficient treatment strategies for expected survival. Yamashita and colleagues[27] reported on CH-EUS in subjects with advanced unresectable pancreatic cancer who were scheduled to undergo chemotherapy. Thirty-nine subjects were divided into 2 groups according to the intratumoral vessel flow observed with CH-EUS; these were vessel sign–positive and vessel sign–negative groups. Both progression-free survival and overall survival were significantly longer in the positive versus negative vessel sign group (*P* = .037 and *P* = .027, respectively). Multivariate analysis demonstrated that a positive vessel sign was an independent factor associated with longer overall survival (hazard ratio = 0.22, 95% CI 0.08–0.53).

CYSTIC PANCREATIC LESIONS

The decision to surgically treat intraductal papillary mucinous neoplasms (IPMNs) must be made carefully because IPMNs are slow-growing tumors having a range of histologic features from benign to malignant, they are likely to occur in elderly patients, and resection requires invasive procedures such as pancreaticoduodenectomy. The presence or absence of mural nodules is an important factor in the decision-making process for surveillance versus surgical intervention for IPMNs. However, it is sometimes difficult to precisely evaluate the presence of mural nodules. In particular, the discrimination of mural nodules from mucous clots is a major source of concern because neither MDCT nor EUS are satisfactory for this discrimination.[28] Therefore, IPMN patients with avascular mural lesions on CH-EUS may undergo observation without surgery, unless other criteria for resection are fulfilled (**Fig. 7**). Harima and colleagues[29] reported that diagnostic accuracies for mural nodules were 92% by CT, 72% by EUS, and 98% by CH-EUS, with CH-EUS detecting significantly more mural nodules than CT or EUS (CT vs CH-EUS, $P<.05$; EUS vs CH-EUS, $P<.01$). Another important question is whether CH-EUS can differentiate benign from malignant IPMNs. Ohno and colleagues[30] classified mural nodules into 4 types according to CH-EUS findings. Papillary nodules (type III) and invasive nodules (type IV) were more associated with invasive cancer, with rates of 88.9% and 91.7%, respectively. Kamata and colleagues[31] compared CH-EUS and fundamental B-mode EUS in the differential diagnosis of pancreatic cysts according to presence of mural nodules. If presence of mural nodule was considered to indicate malignancy, CH-EUS was significantly more accurate than fundamental B-mode EUS. In particular, specificity of CH-EUS (75%) is remarkably higher than that of fundamental B-mode EUS (40%).

BILIARY TRACT DISEASE

The differential diagnosis of benign and malignant lesions in the biliary tract is challenging on EUS because they have similar echogenicity and morphology. Therefore, CH-EUS is useful to diagnose those lesions with vascularity.

In biliary tract disease, the evaluation of vascularity by CH-EUS can be useful for distinguishing true mural lesions from sludge. Determination of the presence of vascularity in these lesions seems to be helpful for distinguishing these entities.[32] The efficacy of CH-EUS in the differential diagnosis of gallbladder lesions has been investigated by Imazu and colleagues.[33] They reported that depiction of inhomogeneous enhancement of the gallbladder with wall thickening on CH-EUS diagnosed malignancy with a sensitivity and specificity of 89.6% and 98%, respectively. In another study, Choi and colleagues[34] reported that an irregular pattern and the presence of perfusion defects aided in the differentiation of malignant from benign gallbladder polyps with sensitivities of 90.3% and 90.3%, and specificities of 96.6% and 94.9%, respectively (**Fig. 8**). Therefore, CH-EUS is useful for detecting malignant gallbladder lesion with inhomogeneous enhancement and/or irregular vasculature. Another study reported that CH-EUS is useful in the evaluation of T staging in gallbladder cancer, allowing detection of the depth of tumor invasion. The accuracy of CH-EUS for estimating the depth of tumor invasion was higher (92.9%) than that of EUS (78.6%).[35]

GASTROINTESTINAL TRACT

Gastrointestinal submucosal tumors include benign and malignant types. It can sometimes be difficult to distinguish gastrointestinal stromal tumor (GIST) from benign

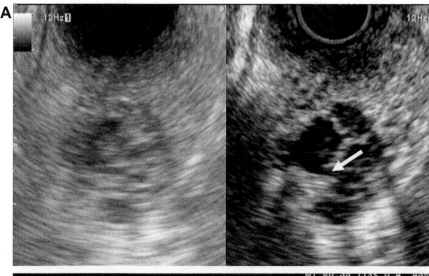

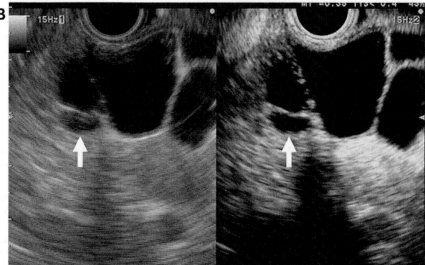

Fig. 7. CH-EUS for an intraductal papillary mucinous neoplasm with mural lesion. (*A*) A mural nodule case. Fundamental B-mode EUS (*A, left*) shows a hyperechoic lesion in a cyst. CH-EUS (*A, right*) clearly detects a mural nodule with vascularity (*arrow*) in the lesion. (*B*) A representative mucous clot case. Fundamental B-mode EUS (*B, left*) shows a hyperechoic lesion (*arrow*) in a cyst cavity. CH-EUS (*B, right*) detects no vascularity in the lesion (*arrow*).

tumor using EUS factors such as echo pattern, echogenicity, and internal features. One study found that CH-EUS images of most diagnosed GISTs had a hypervascular pattern, whereas leiomyomas and lipomas had a hypovascular pattern. Kannengiesser and colleagues[36] reported that CH-EUS can discriminate GISTs from benign lesions with high accuracy. In their study, they found that 8 hypervascular tumors were all GISTs, whereas the 9 hypovascular tumors included 4 lipomas and 5 leiomyomas.

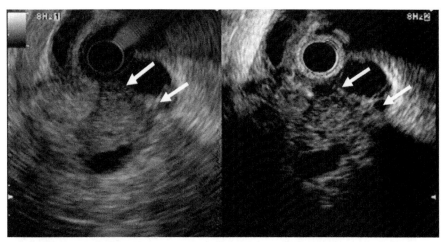

Fig. 8. CH-EUS for gallbladder cancer. Fundamental B-mode EUS (*left*) shows a sessile polyp (*arrows*) protruding into the lumen of the gallbladder. CH-EUS (*right*) reveals heterogeneous enhancement in the polyp.

Although 10% to 30% of GISTs are clinically malignant, all GISTs are known to have some degree of malignant potential and several risk classifications have been developed, with the modified-Fletcher classification having been frequently used.[37] This classification includes 4 factors: tumor size, tumor site, the mitotic count, and the presence of tumor rupture. Among several prognostic factors for GISTs, 1 of the most important is the mitotic count of a histologic sample. However, although EUS-FNA is the gold standard for the diagnosis of submucosal lesions, EUS-FNA samples are often insufficient for a mitotic count. Conventional EUS allows evaluation of the tumor size, lobular border, heterogeneity, cystic spaces, and hyperechoic foci of GISTs; and a previous report indicated the values predictive of a higher malignant potential. Palazzo and colleagues[38] reported that tumor size (>30 mm), a lobular border, heterogeneity, and a cystic space on EUS have sensitivities of 77%, 50%, 27%, and 41%, and specificities of 59%, 91%, 67%, and 94%, respectively. The evaluation of vascularity has been another approach used to estimate the malignant potential of GISTs. Sakamoto and colleagues[39] assessed the malignant risk of GISTs with CH-EUS. All 16 high-risk GISTs demonstrated irregular vessels and heterogeneous enhancement on CH-EUS, whereas only 5 of the 13 low-risk GISTs exhibited these features (**Fig. 9**). CH-EUS predicted malignant GISTs with a sensitivity, specificity, and accuracy of 100%, 63%, and 83%, respectively, which compared with a 63% sensitivity, 92% specificity, and 83% accuracy for the diagnosis of high-grade malignant GISTs on EUS-FNA. The relationship between the detection of vessels on CH-EUS and prediction of the malignant potential of GISTs was reported in another report.[40] Five of 6 cases with positive intratumoral vessels (83%) were intermediate or high-risk GISTs, whereas all 7 intratumoral vessel negative cases (100%) were categorized as very-low or low risk. The visualization of vessels was significantly correlated with the risk classification ($P = .005$). The investigators compared the visualization of intratumoral vessels on CH-EUS with the presence of microscopic vessels in histology and vascular endothelial growth factor (VEGF) expression by immunohistochemistry. The results revealed that intratumoral vessels observed on CH-EUS were consistent with large vessels on histology and

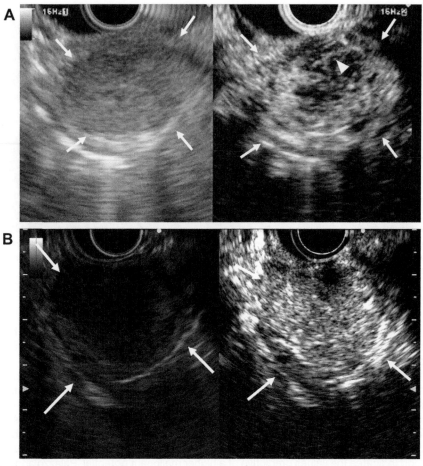

Fig. 9. CH-EUS for GIST. (*A*) A representative case of high-risk malignant GIST. GIST is detected as a low echoic lesion (*arrows*) with fundamental B-mode EUS (*A, left*). CH-EUS (*A, right*) detects irregular vessels flowing (*arrowhead*) from the periphery to center of a tumor (*arrows*) with heterogeneous enhancement. (*B*) A representative case for low-risk malignant GIST. GIST is detected as a low echoic lesion (*arrows*) with fundamental B-mode EUS (*B, left*). CH-EUS (*B, right*) detects a homogeneous enhanced tumor(*arrows*) without flowing vessels.

marked VEGF expression. The presence of large neovascular vessels and VEGF expression fully corresponded with the intermediate or high-risk degree of the GISTs. Moreover, the visualization of intratumoral vessels with CH-EUS was significantly correlated with the presence of neovascular vessels and VEGF expression ($P = .005$ and $P = .005$, respectively). CH-EUS was used to successfully visualize the neovascular vessels of GISTs, and the vessels were relevantly correlated with VEGF expression and the higher malignant potential of the GISTs. Thus, the vessel findings on CH-EUS can predict the malignant potential of GISTs based on the molecular importance of angiogenesis in the development of GISTs. This study showed that targeted CH-EUS may enable in vivo molecular imaging of neovascular vessels and VEGF expression in the tumor vascular endothelium, and that it may be used for noninvasive longitudinal evaluation of tumor angiogenesis in preclinical studies.

SUMMARY

With the recent progress in CH-EUS, it is likely to play a more important role in the differential diagnosis of upper gastrointestinal tract and pancreatobiliary lesions. Moreover, the developments will expand to a wide variety of biomedical indications, especially in oncology. In the future, CH-EUS may become a useful alternative tool for pathologic evaluations involving tumor angiogenesis, the prediction of therapeutic response, and therapeutic approaches using ultrasonography-triggered drug and gene delivery.

REFERENCES

1. Matsuda Y, Yabuuchi I. Hepatic tumors: US contrast enhancement with CO_2 microbubbles. Radiology 1986;161:701–5.
2. Kato T, Tsukamoto Y, Naitoh Y, et al. Ultrasonographic and endoscopic ultrasonographic angiography in pancreatic mass lesions. Acta Radiol 1995;36:381–7.
3. Hirooka Y, Naitoh Y, Goto H, et al. Usefulness of contrast-enhanced endoscopic ultrasonography with intravenous injection of sonicated serum albumin. Gastrointest Endosc 1997;46:166–9.
4. Hocke M, Schulze E, Gottschalk P, et al. Contrast-enhanced endoscopic ultrasound in discrimination between focal pancreatitis and pancreatic cancer. World J Gastroenterol 2006;12:246–50.
5. Sakamoto H, Kitano M, Suetomi Y, et al. Utility of contrast-enhanced endoscopic ultrasonography for diagnosis of small pancreatic carcinomas. Ultrasound Med Biol 2008;34:525–32.
6. Sanchez MV, Varadarajulu S, Napoleon B. EUS contrast agents: what is available, how do they work, and are they effective? Gastrointest Endosc 2009;69:571–7.
7. Kudo M. Various contrast-enhanced imaging modes after administration of Levovist. In: Kudo M, editor. Contrast harmonic imaging in the diagnosis and treatment of hepatic tumors. Tokyo (Japan): Springer; 2003. p. 22–30.
8. Kitano M, Kudo M, Sakamoto H, et al. Preliminary study of contrast-enhanced harmonic endosonography with second-generation contrast agents. J Med Ultrason (2001) 2008;35:11–8.
9. Kitano M, Sakamoto H, Matsui U, et al. A novel perfusion imaging technique of the pancreas: contrast-enhanced harmonic EUS (with video). Gastrointest Endosc 2008;67:141–50.
10. Reddy NK, Ioncică AM, Săftoiu A, et al. Contrast-enhanced endoscopic ultrasonography. World J Gastroenterol 2011;17:42–8.
11. Kitano M, Sakamoto H, Kudo M. Endoscopic ultrasound: contrast enhancement. Gastrointest Endosc Clin N Am 2012;22:349–58.
12. Das K, Kudo M, Kitano M, et al. Diagnostic value of endoscopic ultrasound-guided directional eFLOW in solid pancreatic lesions. J Med Ultrason (2001) 2013;40:211–8.
13. Kitano M, Sakamoto H, Komaki T, et al. New techniques and future perspective of EUS for the differential diagnosis of pancreatic malignancies: contrast harmonic imaging. Dig Endosc 2011;23(Suppl 1):46–50.
14. Sakamoto H, Kitano M, Kamata K, et al. Diagnosis of pancreatic tumors by endoscopic ultrasonography. World J Radiol 2010;28:122–34.
15. Hirooka Y, Itoh A, Kawashima H, et al. Contrast-enhanced endoscopic ultrasonography in digestive diseases. J Gastroenterol 2012;47:1063–72.

16. Ahmad NA, Kochman ML, Lewis JD, et al. Endosonography is superior to angiography in the preoperative assessment of vascular involvement among patients with pancreatic carcinoma. J Clin Gastroenterol 2001;32:54–8.
17. DeWitt J, Devereaux B, Chriswell M, et al. Comparison of endoscopic ultrasonography and multidetector computed tomography for detecting and staging pancreatic cancer. Ann Intern Med 2004;141:753–63.
18. Lee TY, Cheon YK, Shim CS. Clinical role of contrast-enhanced harmonic endoscopic ultrasound in differentiating solid lesions of the pancreas: a single-center experience in Korea. Gut Liver 2013;7:559–604.
19. Kitano M, Kudo M, Yamao K, et al. Characterization of small solid tumors in the pancreas: the value of contrast-enhanced harmonic endoscopic ultrasonography. Am J Gastroenterol 2012;107:303–10.
20. Fusaroli P, Spada A, Mancino MG, et al. Contrast harmonic echo-endoscopic ultrasound improves accuracy in diagnosis of solid pancreatic masses. Clin Gastroenterol Hepatol 2010;8(7):629–34.
21. Napoleon B, Alvarez-Sanchez MV, Gincoul R, et al. Contrast-enhanced harmonic endoscopic ultrasound in solid lesions of the pancreas: results of a pilot study. Endoscopy 2010;42(7):564–70.
22. Matsubara H, Itoh A, Kawashima H, et al. Dynamic quantitative evaluation of contrast-enhanced endoscopic ultrasonography in the diagnosis of pancreatic diseases. Pancreas 2011;40(7):1073–9.
23. Yamashita Y, Kato J, Ueda K, et al. Contrast-enhanced endoscopic ultrasonography for pancreatic tumors. Biomed Res Int 2015;2015:491782.
24. Hou X, Jin Z, Xu C, et al. Contrast-enhanced harmonic endoscopic ultrasound-guided fine-needle aspiration in the diagnosis of solid pancreatic lesions: a retrospective study. PLoS One 2015;10(3):e0121236.
25. Imazu H, Uchiyama Y, Matsunaga K, et al. Contrast-enhanced harmonic EUS with novel ultrasonographic contrast (Sonazoid) in the preoperative T-staging for pancreaticobiliary malignancies. Scand J Gastroenterol 2010;45:732–8.
26. Miyata T, Kitano M, Omoto S, et al. Contrast-enhanced harmonic endoscopic ultrasonography for assessment of lymph node metastases in pancreatobiliary carcinoma. World J Gastroenterol 2016;22(12):3381–91.
27. Yamashita Y, Ueda K, Itonaga M, et al. Tumor vessel depiction with contrast-enhanced endoscopic ultrasonography predicts efficacy of chemotherapy in pancreatic cancer. Pancreas 2013;42:990–5.
28. Zhong N, Zhang L, Takahashi N, et al. Histologic and imaging features of mural nodules in mucinous pancreatic cysts. Clin Gastroenterol Hepatol 2012;10(2):192–8.
29. Harima H, Kaino S, Shinoda S, et al. Differential diagnosis of benign and malignant branch duct intraductal papillary mucinous neoplasm using contrast-enhanced endoscopic ultrasonography. World J Gastroenterol 2015;21(20):6252–60.
30. Ohno E, Hirooka Y, Itoh A, et al. Intraductal papillary mucinous neoplasms of the pancreas: differentiation of malignant and benign tumors by endoscopic ultrasound findings of mural nodules. Ann Surg 2009;249:628–34.
31. Kamata K, Kitano M, Omoto S, et al. Contrast-enhanced harmonic endoscopic ultrasonography for differential diagnosis of pancreatic cysts. Endoscopy 2016;48:35–41.
32. Cui XW, Ignee A, Braden B, et al. Biliary papillomatosis and new ultrasound imaging modalities. Z Gastroenterol 2012;50:226–31.

33. Imazu H, Mori N, Kanazawa K, et al. Contrast-enhanced harmonic endoscopic ultrasonography in the differential diagnosis of gallbladder wall thickening. Dig Dis Sci 2014;59(8):1909–16.
34. Choi JH, Seo DW, Choi JH, et al. Utility of contrast-enhanced harmonic EUS in the diagnosis of malignant gallbladder polyps (with videos). Gastrointest Endosc 2013;78:484–93.
35. Hirooka Y, Naitoh Y, Goto H, et al. Contrast-enhanced endoscopic ultrasonography in gallbladder diseases. Gastrointest Endosc 1998;48:406–10.
36. Kannengiesser K, Mahlke R, Petersen F, et al. Contrast-enhanced harmonic endoscopic ultrasound is able to discriminate benign submucosal lesions from gastrointestinal stromal tumors. Scand J Gastroenterol 2012;47:1515–20.
37. Joensuu H. Risk stratification of patients diagnosed with gastrointestinal stromal tumor. Hum Pathol 2008;39(10):1411–9.
38. Palazzo L, Landi B, Cellier C, et al. Endosonographic features predictive of benign and malignant gastrointestinal stromal tumors. Gut 2000;46(1):88–92.
39. Sakamoto H, Kitano M, Matsui S, et al. Estimation of malignant potential of GI stromal tumors by contrast-enhanced harmonic EUS (with videos). Gastrointest Endosc 2011;73(2):227–37.
40. Yamashita Y, Kato J, Ueda K, et al. Contrast-enhanced endoscopic ultrasonography can predict a higher malignant potential of gastrointestinal stromal tumors by visualizing large newly formed vessels. J Clin Ultrasound 2015;43(2):89–97.

New Developments in Endoscopic Ultrasound Tissue Acquisition

Thiruvengadam Muniraj, MD, PhD, MRCP(UK)*,
Harry R. Aslanian, MD, FASGE

KEYWORDS

- Endoscopic ultrasound-guided fine-needle aspiration (EUS-FNA)
- Endoscopic ultrasound-guided Tru-Cut biopsy (EUS-TCB)
- Endoscopic ultrasound-guided tissue acquisition (EUS-TA)

KEY POINTS

- EUS FNA is the primary procedure of choice for tissue acquisition from pancreas, subepithelial lesions and solid tissues adjacent to GI tract.
- EUS guided tissue acquisition will play a major role in targeted 'personalized therapy' in cancer management in the future.
- Newer needles with novel needle tip design may be utilized to obtain better core samples for histological diagnosis.

Endoscopic ultrasound (EUS)-guided tissue acquisition (EUS-TA) has greatly evolved since the first EUS-guided fine-needle aspiration (FNA) was reported nearly 25 years ago.[1–3] EUS-TA has become the procedure of choice for sampling of the pancreas, subepithelial lesions, and other structures adjacent to the gastrointestinal (GI) tract.[4–8] This review focuses on recent developments in procedural techniques and needle technologies for EUS-TA.

The common indications for EUS-TA include diagnosis and staging of solid and cystic lesions within and adjacent to the GI tract, including pancreaticobiliary, esophageal, gastric and rectal malignancies, GI subepithelial lesions, abdominal and mediastinal lymphadenopathy and cystic lesions, lung cancer, and adrenal masses[9] (**Box 1**).

Multiple factors may contribute to the outcomes of EUS-TA. These factors include site selection for sampling, sampling technique (utilization of the stylet and suction), location and nature of the lesion, needle size and type (aspiration or biopsy needle), utilization of rapid on-site cytopathology evaluation,[31–33] experience level of the endosonographer,[34] and various methods of handling and processing the sample obtained.[31]

Disclosure Statement: No disclosures.
Section of Digestive Diseases, Yale School of Medicine, 333 Cedar Street-1080 LMP, PO Box 208019, New Haven, CT 06520-8019, USA
* Corresponding author.
E-mail address: Thiruvengadam.muniraj@yale.edu

Gastrointest Endoscopy Clin N Am 27 (2017) 585–599
http://dx.doi.org/10.1016/j.giec.2017.06.008
1052-5157/17/© 2017 Elsevier Inc. All rights reserved.

giendo.theclinics.com

Box 1
Common indications for endoscopic ultrasound–guided tissue acquisition

1. Pancreatic mass (solid and cystic)[10–12]

2. Bile duct strictures[13,14]

3. Focal solid liver lesions (metastasis, hepatocellular carcinoma)[15]

4. Diffuse esophageal or gastric wall thickening[16–18]

5. Nodal staging in the setting of esophageal, gastric,[19,20] rectal, or lung cancer[21]

6. Subepithelial tumors (gastrointestinal stromal tumor, schwannoma, leiomyoma, neuroendocrine tumor, others)[22,23]

7. Evaluation of lymphadenopathy (mediastinal, abdominal, pelvic)[24]

8. Adrenal gland lesions[25,26] (left adrenal more common)

9. Prostate mass[27]

10. Peritoneal carcinomatosis[21,28]

11. Splenic mass[29]

12. Perivascular tumor extension,[30] tumor thrombus, extramural tumor recurrence[22]

EUS-TA can be performed by fine-needle aspiration (EUS-FNA) or fine-needle biopsy (EUS-FNB). Differences in the needle tip design are currently the primary distinguishing feature between FNA and FNB, because the procedural techniques are similar.

An ideal EUS-TA technique optimizes safety and diagnostic accuracy. Diagnostic accuracy for malignancy has typically been defined by the cytologic diagnosis. Although tissue histology has been recognized as important for the diagnosis of autoimmune pancreatitis (AIP),[35] Hodgkin lymphoma,[36] and some mesenchymal tumors and well-differentiated adenocarcinomas,[37] the utility of histology for pancreas sampling has been less clear. The expectation that tumor genotyping will play an increasingly important role in cancer therapy in the next several years, particularly relative to pancreatic cancer treatment, suggests that the objectives of tissue histology and the ability to obtain a cell block for additional studies should be included among the goals of EUS-TA. The role of "personalized medicine" in cancer therapy remains a process in evolution, as does the amount of tissue needed for molecular profiling. Although repeatedly smaller amounts of DNA are required to achieve "Next Generation Sequencing," a current benchmark of adequate tissue is 1 mm of tissue, 8 to 10 slides, or 5×5-mm surface area, with at least 20% tumor tissue, which may potentially be facilitated with FNB needles.

CONSIDERATIONS FOR ENDOSCOPIC ULTRASOUND–GUIDED TISSUE ACQUISITION

When a target lesion is identified, the endosonographer must determine which portion of the lesion is optimal for sampling to achieve the highest diagnostic yield and what scope position to approach the lesion from (gastric, duodenal bulb, or second duodenum). Considerations in choosing a scope position and needle trajectory include avoiding vascular structures and the pancreas and bile ducts, the degree of scope torque and stability of the scope position, and maintaining a transduodenal approach for a potentially resectable pancreatic head mass. Although the risk of tumor seeding via the EUS needle tract is very low, rare instances of seeding of the stomach wall have been reported.[38] (The proximal duodenum is resected as part of a Whipple resection, whereas the stomach is not.) The endosonographer then chooses a needle size (25, 22, 20, or 19 gauge are currently available), needle type (FNA vs FNB), and the technique of needle utilization (stylet placement, needle manipulation in the lesion, and the degree of suction applied), and if rapid onsite cytologic evaluation (ROSE) will be used.

EUS-TA practices vary widely across institutions and among endosonographers. The degree of cytologic expertise at a particular institution may impact some of these choices because the endosonographer must provide a sample that can provide diagnostic information relative to the expectations of the interpreting pathologists. For example, if FNA samples of solid pancreatic masses are regularly interpreted as malignant on onsite evaluation with 25-G FNA needles and there is no clear need for histology or a cell block, this may favor the use of ROSE and smaller FNA needles. If, however, the endosonographer finds that ROSE rarely yields an onsite diagnosis and larger samples are requested by pathologists to achieve a malignant diagnosis, larger FNA needles or FNB needles, without ROSE, may be favored.

FINE-NEEDLE ASPIRATION NEEDLE SIZE: SMALL VERSUS LARGE

EUS FNA needles measuring 22 G and 25 G have been extensively investigated for outcomes such as cytologic adequacy and diagnostic yield of malignancy in solid lesions. For FNA of solid lesions, most endosonographers use 25-G or 22-G needles, and 22-G needles for cystic lesions. Although most randomized trials have shown no significant difference in diagnostic accuracy,[39] meta-analyses have identified a trend of higher sensitivity for malignant diagnosis of pancreatic masses with 25-G needles.[40–42] There are limited studies comparing 19-G needles and other needle sizes. One prospective, randomized study found that 19-G needles in comparison to 22-G needles provided better diagnostic accuracy and superior cellular material for solid pancreatic masses.[43] There was, however, a significantly higher technical failure rate (96% vs 79%, $P = .01$) with the 19-G needle for FNA of pancreatic head masses,[44] because of torque on the scope and limited needle maneuverability.[45] A prospective comparison of the 19-G Tru-Cut FNB needle (Cook Medical, Winston-Salem, NC, USA), and 22-G and 25-G FNA needles for aspiration of pancreatic mass lesions reported overall diagnostic accuracy of the 25-G, 22-G, and 19-G Tru-Cut needles to be 91.7%, 79.7%, and 54.1%, respectively. For uncinate masses, the diagnostic accuracy of the 25G was much better than 22G, and 19G Trucut needles. There was no significant difference between the 3 needle types for evaluation of pancreatic body and tail masses.[43] Newer generations of 19-G FNA needles have used nitinol to increase flexibility and maneuverability to overcome limitations accessing the pancreas head. Nineteen-gauge FNA needles have been shown to reliably obtain adequate histology when performing liver biopsy.[46–49] Additional studies have shown a high rate of diagnostic accuracy and tissue histology with 19-G needles, including subepithelial lesions, which typically have a lower diagnostic yield with 25- and 22-G FNA needles[50–53] (Table 1).

Table 1 Meta-analysis of 22-G versus 25-G needles for solid lesions				
Meta-Analysis	n	Needle	Pooled Sensitivity	P
Affolter et al,[41] 2013	1026	22 vs 25	0.78 (95% CI 0.74–0.81) vs 0.91 (95% CI 0.87–0.94)	.01
Madhoun et al,[42] 2013	1292	22 vs 25	0.85 (95% CI 0.82–0.88) vs 1 (95% CI 0.98–1)	.0003

FINE-NEEDLE ASPIRATION NEEDLES AND TISSUE HISTOLOGY

Most studies evaluating 25-G and 22-G FNA needles have focused on cytologic diagnosis rather than tissue histology. FNA needles measuring 25 G and 22 G have demonstrated low to moderate yields for tissue histology, ranging between 33% and 74%.[54–56] In several reports, the yield of 19-G FNA needles for histology has been high (94%–98%) for a variety of tissues, including lymph nodes, subepithelial lesions, and pancreatic masses.[53,57,58]

HISTOLOGIC DIAGNOSIS OF AUTOIMMUNE PANCREATITIS

A definitive diagnosis of AIP cannot be achieved with a cytology sample.[35] The ability to achieve a histologic diagnosis of AIP with 22-G FNA needles has varied across several studies,[59,60] without an increased yield with 19-G needles identified.[61] Some studies demonstrated safety and an increased diagnostic yield with 19-G (Tru-Cut) FNB in the diagnosis of AIP.[62–64]

FINE-NEEDLE BIOPSY NEEDLES

The first core biopsy EUS needle was the 19-G Tru-Cut needle (Quick-Core; Cook Medical, Limerick, Ireland). It utilized a spring-loaded firing mechanism. Although some endosonographers were able to achieve high diagnostic yields,[65] many struggled to achieve similar results because of limited flexibility of the needle. The Tru-Cut was replaced by the ProCore FNB (EchoTip Procore; Cook Medical, Bloomington, IN, USA) needles, which are available in a range (19, 20, 22, 25 G) of sizes and have a beveled side cut of the distal needle shaft to create an additional tissue acquisition site. A multicenter randomized trial identified the newer Procore 19-G needle to be superior to the Tru-Cut needle with higher diagnostic accuracy (88% vs 62%; $P = .02$) and frequency of diagnostic histology (85% vs 57%; $P = .006$).[66] Modifications to the 20-G Procore needle from the original Procore design include a flexible needle sheath and a reverse direction of the bevel cut.

Additional FNB needles use a novel needle tip design (Sharkcore; Medtronic, Minneapolis, MN, USA) and a Franseen needle tip design (Acquire; Boston Scientific, Natick, MA, USA) (**Fig. 1**). Considerations for the endosonographer in choosing between FNA and FNB needles and sizes include safety, the rate and ease (number of passes and ability to pass the needle to the target) of obtaining diagnostic material, and the necessity of and ability to obtain histology and a cell block. The optimal manner to process FNB samples is discussed elsewhere in this issue and is a subject of ongoing study[47,67] (**Table 2**).

ENDOSCOPIC ULTRASOUND FINE-NEEDLE BIOPSY
Diagnostic Yield and Ability to Obtain Tissue Histology

The 25-G Procore was shown to have high diagnostic accuracy (96%), while obtaining histology samples in 32% of cases.[55] A trial of the 22-G Procore needle in 61 pancreatic masses obtained adequate histologic samples in 88.5%.[68] Nineteen-gauge Procore FNB needles were shown to have a diagnostic accuracy of 85%, with adequate histologic samples in 89% among 114 lesions in a multicenter study. Transduodenal needle passage through the scope was noted to provide some challenges.[69] A multicenter, retrospective review of 250 lesions of different type, sampled with the 25- or 22-G Sharkcore (Medtronic, Dublin, Ireland) FNB needle, reported a cytologic diagnostic yield of 85% and a pathologic diagnostic yield of 88%.[70] Patients with small subepithelial tumors (mean size 16 mm) undergoing EUS-FNB had a diagnostic yield of 75%, although core samples were only obtained in 25% of cases.[71]

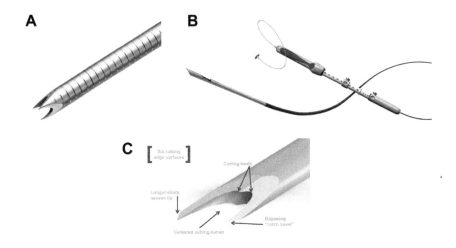

Fig. 1. (*A*) The 22-G Acquire EUS-FNB needle tip; (*B*) 20-G EchoTip Procore EUS-FNB needle tip; (*C*) 22-G Sharkcore EUS-FNB needle tip. (*Courtesy of* (*A*) Boston Scientific, Natick, MA, USA; (*B*) Cook Medical, Bloomington, IN, USA and (*C*) All rights reserved. Used with the Permission of Medtronic.)

Number of Needle Passes

Several studies have found that EUS-FNB decreases the number of needle passes to obtain adequate cellularity.[51,52,72,73]

Optimal Fine-Needle Aspiration and Fine-Needle Biopsy Technique

Studies of FNA needles have shown the passage of the needle with or without the stylet makes no difference in overall yield.[74–78] The optimal amount of suction for solid lesions differs between published reports. High diagnostic yields have been achieved with no suction for lymph node sampling[79] and with the stylet pull technique (pulling the stylet while moving the needle within the target lesion to achieve approximately 3 mL of suction[80]) for solid lesions. The stylet pull technique may be well suited to 25-G FNA needles to give less blood in the sample for onsite review, however, typically

Table 2
Endoscopic ultrasound fine-needle biopsy needles available in the United States

Manufacturer	Needle Name	Size (G)	Comments
Boston Scientific	Acquire	22, 25	Franseen needle design with a crown tip with 3 points to provide stability at the puncture site, and 3 symmetric surfaces that manifest as 3 cutting edges, heels designed for tissue capture
Cook Medical	Echo Tip Procore	19, 20, 22, 25	Has a reverse bevel to aid collection of core sample by shearing material from target during retrograde movement of needle in the lesion Needle has dimpling to improve visualization
Medtronic	SharkCore	19, 22, 25	Has multiple parallel cutting surfaces at the needle tip

without differences in the final diagnostic yield in comparison to the application of suction.[81–84] A novel "wet-suction" technique (where the EUS needle is flushed with 5 mL of saline solution to replace the column of air within the lumen of needle with saline solution before needle aspiration)[85] was shown to increase cellularity and cell block specimen adequacy (85.5% vs 75.2%; $P<.035$)[86] with 22-G FNA needles. A "fanning technique," which involves altering the trajectory of the needle while moving within the lesion, has been shown to increase diagnostic yield.[87]

The application of these findings to FNB has not been well studied; however, most endosonographers use their preferred FNA techniques in the performance of FNB. Suction has widely been applied during 19-G FNA liver biopsy, and suction appears to be more commonly used with FNB needles.[82] The benefits of stylet replacement with FNB needles are uncertain; however, it may be useful to clear any tissue persistently stuck at the tip or side bevel of FNB needles that persists after flushing with air or water. The fanning technique appears to also be useful when using FNB needles.[88] Given the likely increased shearing with FNB needles, increased bloodiness may be expected within an existing FNB needle track.

Rapid On-Site Evaluation and Fine-Needle Biopsy Needles

A "touch-prep" or smearing of a small portion of FNB samples appears to facilitate the performance of ROSE. ROSE adds additional time to EUS-TA, and its overall utility has been questioned, if there is no associated difference in final diagnostic yield. In a recent randomized controlled trial (RCT), there was no significant difference in the diagnostic yield of malignancy, proportion of inadequate specimens, and accuracy in patients with pancreatic masses undergoing EUS-FNA with or without ROSE.[89] Of note, 22-G FNA needles were used and 4 passes were required to achieve a malignant ROSE diagnosis, which is higher than some reports using 25-G FNA needles (which may provide a sample with less blood to facilitate on-site review).[55,90,91]

The utility of ROSE in FNB has not been extensively evaluated. In clinical practice, most endosonographers favor the use of FNB needles with samples sent directly for cytology or histology in the absence of an onsite cytopathologist.[92] Krishnan and colleagues[93] studied the utility of ROSE for EUS-FNB sampling and noted a specimen adequacy of 58% (95% confidence interval [CI], 45.1–71.2) and final diagnostic yield of 83% (95% CI, 71.9–91.5). Although the specificity of ROSE was 100%, the limited sensitivity of 65% suggested that ROSE may not be beneficial with EUS-FNB sampling. A retrospective study of 43 patients compared EUS-FNB without ROSE to matched control patients who underwent EUS-FNA with or without ROSE and found no difference in final diagnostic accuracy between groups (84% vs 85%).[94]

FNB performed without ROSE may provide a similar yield to FNA with ROSE, with less passes, while avoiding the extra time required for ROSE. In an RCT crossover study of FNA versus FNB needles, the diagnostic yield for solid pancreatic masses was the same; however, FNB had a higher yield (88.2% vs 54.5%, $P = .006$) and more specimen adequacy (82.8% vs 60.0%, $P = .006$) with a cost saving with FNB for solid lesions overall.[95] Potential benefits of achieving an ROSE diagnosis of malignancy that may be difficult to quantify include the ability to deliver a diagnosis to the patient at the conclusion of the EUS procedure in the endoscopy suite and the ability of the endosonographer to expedite patient referral.[32]

ENDOSCOPIC ULTRASOUND FINE-NEEDLE ASPIRATION VERSUS FINE-NEEDLE BIOPSY

Several studies have shown a similar diagnostic yield for malignancy with FNA and FNB needles.[91,96–98] A systematic review of 10 randomized studies comparing FNA with FNB identified a superior yield with FNB in 4 studies and no difference in diagnostic yield in 6 studies.[99] A recent randomized controlled crossover trial compared the diagnostic yield of EUS-FNB (Echotip Procore; Cook Medical, Winston-Salem, NC, USA) with EUS-FNA needles in patients presenting with pancreatic and nonpancreatic masses and demonstrated a significantly overall higher diagnostic yield with specimens obtained by EUS-FNB compared with EUS-FNA needles (90% vs 67.1%, P = .002). There was, however, no difference between the 2 groups for pancreatic masses. A retrospective, case control study of a total of 156 lesions (39 FNB and 117 FNA) found that FNB needles of similar size had a significantly higher yield for histologic core samples (95 vs 59%, P = .01) and required a fewer number of passes (median 2 vs 4 passes; P = .01).[73]

FNB may provide benefit for nonpancreatic solid masses and lesions where FNA has been nondiagnostic.[95,99] A prospective study compared 22-G FNA versus FNB needle for gastric subepithelial lesions and demonstrated a significantly higher yield with EUS-FNB (75% vs 20%; P<.010).[51]

A comparison of 6 different needles (a novel 19-G FNB needle, 19- and 22-G FNB needles, 19-G FNA needle, and two 18-G percutaneous needles) used to perform 288 samples of cadaveric human liver tissue found that the novel 19-G FNB needle had significantly increased mean portal tracts compared with existing 19-G FNA needles and core needles. The 22-G FNB needle also provided adequate tissue and significantly more portal tracts than the remaining needles (equivalent portal tracts to one of the 18-G percutaneous needles). Overall, the use of FNB needles with a fanning technique was associated with an increased number of portal tracts obtained.[88]

Endoscopic Ultrasound–Guided Fine Needle Vein Puncture

Circulating tumor cells (CTCs) and free circulating DNA/RNA from tumors may enter the bloodstream and can be isolated from blood samples.[100,101] The detection of CTCs in blood has been termed a "liquid biopsy."[102–104] The CellSearch EpCAM-positive–dependent system and isolation by size of epithelial tumor cells are 2 platforms currently used to isolate CTCs in Pancreatic Cancer.[103,104] EUS–fine needle vein (FNV) can be used to obtain a liquid biopsy, and molecular assays may aid in the early detection and monitoring of cancer therapy, including identification of mutations that confer resistance to therapy. EUS-FNV of portal venous blood has been shown to be feasible and safe with a 19-G FNA needle advanced transhepatically to analyze CTCs.[105] Higher levels of pancreatic adenocarcinoma cells were identified in portal venous samples versus peripheral blood samples[105] (**Fig. 2**).

Through-the-Needle Imaging and Forceps

Devices including cytology brushes,[106] fiberoptic fibers,[107–109] confocal microscopy probes,[109,110] and forceps have been passed through 19-G EUS FNA needles to evaluate cystic and solid lesions. Cytology brushes were shown to increase diagnostic yield in pancreatic cystic lesions; however, increased bleeding[111] and mild acute pancreatitis[106] were noted, and these are not commonly used. Small forceps (Moray Microforceps; US Endoscopy, Mentor, OH, USA) passed through 19-G needles have been safely used and found to provide diagnostic histology in case reports of pancreatic cystic lesions[112–115] (**Fig. 3**). Comparisons of forceps samples to other EUS-TA techniques have not been reported to date.

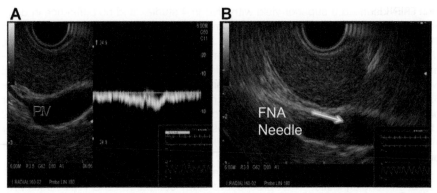

Fig. 2. EUS-guided access of the portal vein. (*A*) The portal vein is identified under EUS guidance with Doppler wave verification; (*B*) EUS-guided, transhepatic, FNA puncture of the portal vein with a 19-G EUS FNA needle for portal venous blood acquisition. PV, portal vein. (*From* Catenacci DV, Chapman CG, Xu P, et al. Acquisition of portal venous circulating tumor cells from patients with pancreaticobiliary cancers by endoscopic ultrasound. Gastroenterology 2015;149:1795.e4; with permission.)

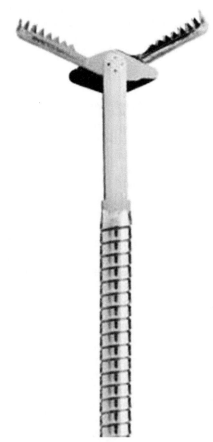

Fig. 3. Moray microforceps. (Moray® micro forceps – permission granted by US Endoscopy, Mentor, Ohio.)

REFERENCES

1. Vilmann P, Jacobsen GK, Henriksen FW, et al. Endoscopic ultrasonography with guided fine needle aspiration biopsy in pancreatic disease. Gastrointest Endosc 1992;38:172–3.
2. Giovannini M, Seitz JF, Monges G, et al. Guided puncture-cytology under electronic sectorial ultrasound endoscopy. Results in 26 patients. Gastroenterol Clin Biol 1993;17:465–70 [in French].
3. Giovannini M, Seitz JF, Monges G, et al. Fine-needle aspiration cytology guided by endoscopic ultrasonography: results in 141 patients. Endoscopy 1995;27: 171–7.
4. Vilmann P, Hancke S, Henriksen FW, et al. Endosonographically-guided fine needle aspiration biopsy of malignant lesions in the upper gastrointestinal tract. Endoscopy 1993;25:523–7.
5. Wegener M, Adamek RJ, Wedmann B, et al. Endosonographically guided fine-needle aspiration puncture of paraesophagogastric mass lesions: preliminary results. Endoscopy 1994;26:586–91.
6. Chang KJ, Katz KD, Durbin TE, et al. Endoscopic ultrasound-guided fine-needle aspiration. Gastrointest Endosc 1994;40:694–9.
7. Binmoeller KF, Thul R, Rathod V, et al. Endoscopic ultrasound-guided, 18-gauge, fine needle aspiration biopsy of the pancreas using a 2.8 mm channel convex array echoendoscope. Gastrointest Endosc 1998;47:121–7.
8. Binmoeller KF, Brand B, Thul R, et al. EUS-guided, fine-needle aspiration biopsy using a new mechanical scanning puncture echoendoscope. Gastrointest Endosc 1998;47:335–40.
9. Dumonceau JM, Polkowski M, Larghi A, et al. Indications, results, and clinical impact of endoscopic ultrasound (EUS)-guided sampling in gastroenterology: European Society of Gastrointestinal Endoscopy (ESGE) Clinical Guideline. Endoscopy 2011;43:897–912.
10. Khalid A, Nodit L, Zahid M, et al. Endoscopic ultrasound fine needle aspirate DNA analysis to differentiate malignant and benign pancreatic masses. Am J Gastroenterol 2006;101:2493–500.
11. Alomari AK, Ustun B, Aslanian HR, et al. Endoscopic ultrasound-guided fine-needle aspiration diagnosis of secondary tumors involving the pancreas: an institution's experience. Cytojournal 2016;13:1.
12. Eloubeidi MA, Chen VK, Eltoum IA, et al. Endoscopic ultrasound-guided fine needle aspiration biopsy of patients with suspected pancreatic cancer: diagnostic accuracy and acute and 30-day complications. Am J Gastroenterol 2003;98:2663–8.
13. Eloubeidi MA, Chen VK, Jhala NC, et al. Endoscopic ultrasound-guided fine needle aspiration biopsy of suspected cholangiocarcinoma. Clin Gastroenterol Hepatol 2004;2:209–13.
14. Lee JH, Salem R, Aslanian H, et al. Endoscopic ultrasound and fine-needle aspiration of unexplained bile duct strictures. Am J Gastroenterol 2004;99:1069–73.
15. Singh P, Mukhopadhyay P, Bhatt B, et al. Endoscopic ultrasound versus CT scan for detection of the metastases to the liver: results of a prospective comparative study. J Clin Gastroenterol 2009;43:367–73.
16. Gines A, Pellise M, Fernandez-Esparrach G, et al. Endoscopic ultrasonography in patients with large gastric folds at endoscopy and biopsies negative for malignancy: predictors of malignant disease and clinical impact. Am J Gastroenterol 2006;101:64–9.

17. Thomas T, Kaye PV, Ragunath K, et al. Endoscopic-ultrasound-guided mural trucut biopsy in the investigation of unexplained thickening of esophagogastric wall. Endoscopy 2009;41:335–9.

18. Aithal GP, Anagnostopoulos GK, Kaye P. EUS-guided Trucut mural biopsies in the investigation of unexplained thickening of the esophagogastric wall. Gastrointest Endosc 2005;62:624–9.

19. Marsman WA, Brink MA, Bergman JJ, et al. Potential impact of EUS-FNA staging of proximal lymph nodes in patients with distal esophageal carcinoma. Endoscopy 2006;38:825–9.

20. Pech O, May A, Gunter E, et al. The impact of endoscopic ultrasound and computed tomography on the TNM staging of early cancer in Barrett's esophagus. Am J Gastroenterol 2006;101:2223–9.

21. Gress FG, Savides TJ, Sandler A, et al. Endoscopic ultrasonography, fine-needle aspiration biopsy guided by endoscopic ultrasonography, and computed tomography in the preoperative staging of non-small-cell lung cancer: a comparison study. Ann Intern Med 1997;127:604–12.

22. Fu K, Eloubeidi MA, Jhala NC, et al. Diagnosis of gastrointestinal stromal tumor by endoscopic ultrasound-guided fine needle aspiration biopsy–a potential pitfall. Ann Diagn Pathol 2002;6:294–301.

23. Philipper M, Hollerbach S, Gabbert HE, et al. Prospective comparison of endoscopic ultrasound-guided fine-needle aspiration and surgical histology in upper gastrointestinal submucosal tumors. Endoscopy 2010;42:300–5.

24. Catalano MF, Rosenblatt ML, Chak A, et al. Endoscopic ultrasound-guided fine needle aspiration in the diagnosis of mediastinal masses of unknown origin. Am J Gastroenterol 2002;97:2559–65.

25. Patil R, Ona MA, Papafragkakis C, et al. Endoscopic ultrasound-guided fine-needle aspiration in the diagnosis of adrenal lesions. Ann Gastroenterol 2016; 29:307–11.

26. DeWitt J, Alsatie M, LeBlanc J, et al. Endoscopic ultrasound-guided fine-needle aspiration of left adrenal gland masses. Endoscopy 2007;39:65–71.

27. Gleeson FC, Clain JE, Karnes RJ, et al. Endoscopic-ultrasound-guided tissue sampling facilitates the detection of local recurrence and extra pelvic metastasis in pelvic urologic malignancy. Diagn Ther Endosc 2012;2012:219521.

28. Levy MJ, Abu Dayyeh BK, Fujii LL, et al. Detection of peritoneal carcinomatosis by EUS fine-needle aspiration: impact on staging and resectability (with videos). Gastrointest Endosc 2015;81:1215–24.

29. Eloubeidi MA, Varadarajulu S, Eltoum I, et al. Transgastric endoscopic ultrasound-guided fine-needle aspiration biopsy and flow cytometry of suspected lymphoma of the spleen. Endoscopy 2006;38:617–20.

30. Levy MJ, Gleeson FC, Zhang L. Endoscopic ultrasound fine-needle aspiration detection of extravascular migratory metastasis from a remotely located pancreatic cancer. Clin Gastroenterol Hepatol 2009;7:246–8.

31. Klapman JB, Logrono R, Dye CE, et al. Clinical impact of on-site cytopathology interpretation on endoscopic ultrasound-guided fine needle aspiration. Am J Gastroenterol 2003;98:1289–94.

32. Oza VM, Cai G, Aslanian HR. Clinical utility of rapid on-site cytopathology. Gastrointest Endosc 2017;85:261.

33. Iglesias-Garcia J, Dominguez-Munoz JE, Abdulkader I, et al. Influence of on-site cytopathology evaluation on the diagnostic accuracy of endoscopic ultrasound-guided fine needle aspiration (EUS-FNA) of solid pancreatic masses. Am J Gastroenterol 2011;106:1705–10.

34. Mertz H, Gautam S. The learning curve for EUS-guided FNA of pancreatic cancer. Gastrointest Endosc 2004;59:33–7.
35. Muniraj T, Sah RP, Chari ST. Autoimmune pancreatitis: an update, in Pancreatitis: Medical and surgical management. In: Adams DB, Cotton PB, Zyromski NJ, editors. Chichester, UK: John Wiley & Sons Ltd; 2017.
36. Eloubeidi MA, Mehra M, Bean SM. EUS-guided 19-gauge trucut needle biopsy for diagnosis of lymphoma missed by EUS-guided FNA. Gastrointest Endosc 2007;65:937–9.
37. Karadsheh Z, Al-Haddad M. Endoscopic ultrasound guided fine needle tissue acquisition: where we stand in 2013? World J Gastroenterol 2014;20:2176–85.
38. Paquin SC, Gariepy G, Lepanto L, et al. A first report of tumor seeding because of EUS-guided FNA of a pancreatic adenocarcinoma. Gastrointest Endosc 2005;61:610–1.
39. Lee JH, Stewart J, Ross WA, et al. Blinded prospective comparison of the performance of 22-gauge and 25-gauge needles in endoscopic ultrasound-guided fine needle aspiration of the pancreas and peri-pancreatic lesions. Dig Dis Sci 2009;54:2274–81.
40. Yusuf TE, Ho S, Pavey DA, et al. Retrospective analysis of the utility of endoscopic ultrasound-guided fine-needle aspiration (EUS-FNA) in pancreatic masses, using a 22-gauge or 25-gauge needle system: a multicenter experience. Endoscopy 2009;41:445–8.
41. Affolter KE, Schmidt RL, Matynia AP, et al. Needle size has only a limited effect on outcomes in EUS-guided fine needle aspiration: a systematic review and meta-analysis. Dig Dis Sci 2013;58:1026–34.
42. Madhoun MF, Wani SB, Rastogi A, et al. The diagnostic accuracy of 22-gauge and 25-gauge needles in endoscopic ultrasound-guided fine needle aspiration of solid pancreatic lesions: a meta-analysis. Endoscopy 2013;45:86–92.
43. Sakamoto H, Kitano M, Komaki T, et al. Prospective comparative study of the EUS guided 25-gauge FNA needle with the 19-gauge Trucut needle and 22-gauge FNA needle in patients with solid pancreatic masses. J Gastroenterol Hepatol 2009;24:384–90.
44. Song TJ, Kim JH, Lee SS, et al. The prospective randomized, controlled trial of endoscopic ultrasound-guided fine-needle aspiration using 22G and 19G aspiration needles for solid pancreatic or peripancreatic masses. Am J Gastroenterol 2010;105:1739–45.
45. Itoi T, Itokawa F, Kurihara T, et al. Experimental endoscopy: objective evaluation of EUS needles. Gastrointest Endosc 2009;69:509–16.
46. DeWitt J, LeBlanc J, McHenry L, et al. Endoscopic ultrasound-guided fine needle aspiration cytology of solid liver lesions: a large single-center experience. Am J Gastroenterol 2003;98:1976–81.
47. Stavropoulos SN, Im GY, Jlayer Z, et al. High yield of same-session EUS-guided liver biopsy by 19-gauge FNA needle in patients undergoing EUS to exclude biliary obstruction. Gastrointest Endosc 2012;75:310–8.
48. Diehl DL, Johal AS, Khara HS, et al. Endoscopic ultrasound-guided liver biopsy: a multicenter experience. Endosc Int open 2015;3:E210–5.
49. Pineda JJ, Diehl DL, Miao CL, et al. EUS-guided liver biopsy provides diagnostic samples comparable with those via the percutaneous or transjugular route. Gastrointest Endosc 2016;83:360–5.
50. El Chafic AH, Loren D, Siddiqui A, et al. Comparison of fine-needle aspiration and fine-needle biopsy for EUS-guided sampling of suspected GI stromal tumors. Gastrointest Endosc 2017. [Epub ahead of print].

51. Kim GH, Cho YK, Kim EY, et al. Comparison of 22-gauge aspiration needle with 22-gauge biopsy needle in endoscopic ultrasonography-guided subepithelial tumor sampling. Scand J Gastroenterol 2014;49:347–54.
52. Han JP, Lee TH, Hong SJ, et al. EUS-guided FNA and FNB after on-site cytological evaluation in gastric subepithelial tumors. J Dig Dis 2016;17:582–7.
53. Larghi A, Verna EC, Ricci R, et al. EUS-guided fine-needle tissue acquisition by using a 19-gauge needle in a selected patient population: a prospective study. Gastrointest Endosc 2011;74:504–10.
54. Lee JK, Lee KT, Choi ER, et al. A prospective, randomized trial comparing 25-gauge and 22-gauge needles for endoscopic ultrasound-guided fine needle aspiration of pancreatic masses. Scand J Gastroenterol 2013;48:752–7.
55. Iwashita T, Nakai Y, Samarasena JB, et al. High single-pass diagnostic yield of a new 25-gauge core biopsy needle for EUS-guided FNA biopsy in solid pancreatic lesions. Gastrointest Endosc 2013;77:909–15.
56. Rong L, Kida M, Yamauchi H, et al. Factors affecting the diagnostic accuracy of endoscopic ultrasonography-guided fine-needle aspiration (EUS-FNA) for upper gastrointestinal submucosal or extraluminal solid mass lesions. Dig Endosc 2012;24:358–63.
57. Yasuda I, Tsurumi H, Omar S, et al. Endoscopic ultrasound-guided fine-needle aspiration biopsy for lymphadenopathy of unknown origin. Endoscopy 2006;38:919–24.
58. Varadarajulu S, Bang JY, Hebert-Magee S. Assessment of the technical performance of the flexible 19-gauge EUS-FNA needle. Gastrointest Endosc 2012;76:336–43.
59. Imai K, Matsubayashi H, Fukutomi A, et al. Endoscopic ultrasonography-guided fine needle aspiration biopsy using 22-gauge needle in diagnosis of autoimmune pancreatitis. Dig Liver Dis 2011;43:869–74.
60. Kanno A, Masamune A, Fujishima F, et al. Diagnosis of autoimmune pancreatitis by EUS-guided FNA using a 22-gauge needle: a prospective multicenter study. Gastrointest Endosc 2016;84:797–804.e1.
61. Iwashita T, Yasuda I, Doi S, et al. Use of samples from endoscopic ultrasound-guided 19-gauge fine-needle aspiration in diagnosis of autoimmune pancreatitis. Clin Gastroenterol Hepatol 2012;10:316–22.
62. Mizuno N, Bhatia V, Hosoda W, et al. Histological diagnosis of autoimmune pancreatitis using EUS-guided trucut biopsy: a comparison study with EUS-FNA. J Gastroenterol 2009;44:742–50.
63. Morishima T, Kawashima H, Ohno E, et al. Prospective multicenter study on the usefulness of EUS-guided FNA biopsy for the diagnosis of autoimmune pancreatitis. Gastrointest Endosc 2016;84:241–8.
64. Levy MJ, Smyrk TC, Takahashi N, et al. Idiopathic duct-centric pancreatitis: disease description and endoscopic ultrasonography-guided trucut biopsy diagnosis. Pancreatology 2011;11:76–80.
65. Gleeson FC, Clayton AC, Zhang L, et al. Adequacy of endoscopic ultrasound core needle biopsy specimen of nonmalignant hepatic parenchymal disease. Clin Gastroenterol Hepatol 2008;6:1437–40.
66. DeWitt J, Cho CM, Lin J, et al. Comparison of EUS-guided tissue acquisition using two different 19-gauge core biopsy needles: a multicenter, prospective, randomized, and blinded study. Endosc Int open 2015;3:E471–8.
67. Witt BL, Adler DG, Hilden K, et al. A comparative needle study: EUS-FNA procedures using the HD ProCore(™) and EchoTip(®) 22-gauge needle types. Diagn Cytopathol 2013;41:1069–74.

68. Larghi A, Iglesias-Garcia J, Poley JW, et al. Feasibility and yield of a novel 22-gauge histology EUS needle in patients with pancreatic masses: a multicenter prospective cohort study. Surg Endosc 2013;27:3733–8.
69. Iglesias-Garcia J, Poley JW, Larghi A, et al. Feasibility and yield of a new EUS histology needle: results from a multicenter, pooled, cohort study. Gastrointest Endosc 2011;73:1189–96.
70. DiMaio CJ, Kolb JM, Benias PC, et al. Initial experience with a novel EUS-guided core biopsy needle (SharkCore): results of a large North American multicenter study. Endosc Int open 2016;4:E974–9.
71. Schlag C, Menzel C, Gotzberger M, et al. Endoscopic ultrasound-guided tissue sampling of small subepithelial tumors of the upper gastrointestinal tract with a 22-gauge core biopsy needle. Endosc Int open 2017;5:E165–71.
72. Lee YN, Moon JH, Kim HK, et al. Core biopsy needle versus standard aspiration needle for endoscopic ultrasound-guided sampling of solid pancreatic masses: a randomized parallel-group study. Endoscopy 2014;46:1056–62.
73. Kandel P, Tranesh G, Nassar A, et al. EUS-guided fine needle biopsy sampling using a novel fork-tip needle: a case-control study. Gastrointest Endosc 2016; 84:1034–9.
74. Sahai AV, Paquin SC, Gariepy G. A prospective comparison of endoscopic ultrasound-guided fine needle aspiration results obtained in the same lesion, with and without the needle stylet. Endoscopy 2010;42:900–3.
75. Rastogi A, Wani S, Gupta N, et al. A prospective, single-blind, randomized, controlled trial of EUS-guided FNA with and without a stylet. Gastrointest Endosc 2011;74:58–64.
76. Wani S, Early D, Kunkel J, et al. Diagnostic yield of malignancy during EUS-guided FNA of solid lesions with and without a stylet: a prospective, single blind, randomized, controlled trial. Gastrointest Endosc 2012;76:328–35.
77. Abe Y, Kawakami H, Oba K, et al. Effect of a stylet on a histological specimen in EUS-guided fine-needle tissue acquisition by using 22-gauge needles: a multicenter, prospective, randomized, controlled trial. Gastrointest Endosc 2015;82: 837–44.e1.
78. Gimeno-Garcia AZ, Paquin SC, Gariepy G, et al. Comparison of endoscopic ultrasonography-guided fine-needle aspiration cytology results with and without the stylet in 3364 cases. Dig Endosc 2013;25:303–7.
79. Wallace MB, Kennedy T, Durkalski V, et al. Randomized controlled trial of EUS-guided fine needle aspiration techniques for the detection of malignant lymphadenopathy. Gastrointest Endosc 2001;54:441–7.
80. Aslanian HR. EUS-needle aspirate yield of different media and needle type with stylet slow pull and syringe suction. Gastrointest Endosc 2013;77(5S):AB359.
81. Nakai Y, Isayama H, Chang KJ, et al. Slow pull versus suction in endoscopic ultrasound-guided fine-needle aspiration of pancreatic solid masses. Dig Dis Sci 2014;59:1578–85.
82. Chen JY, Ding QY, Lv Y, et al. Slow-pull and different conventional suction techniques in endoscopic ultrasound-guided fine-needle aspiration of pancreatic solid lesions using 22-gauge needles. World J Gastroenterol 2016;22:8790–7.
83. El Haddad R, Barret M, Beuvon F, et al. The slow-pull capillary technique increases the quality of endoscopic ultrasound fine needle biopsy samples in solid pancreatic lesions. Eur J Gastroenterol Hepatol 2016;28:911–6.
84. Kin T, Katanuma A, Yane K, et al. Diagnostic ability of EUS-FNA for pancreatic solid lesions with conventional 22-gauge needle using the slow pull technique: a prospective study. Scand J Gastroenterol 2015;50:900–7.

85. Antonini F, Fuccio L, Fabbri C, et al. Endoscopic ultrasound-guided tissue acquisition of pancreatic masses with core biopsy needles using wet suction technique. Endoscopic ultrasound 2017;6:73–4.

86. Attam R, Arain MA, Bloechl SJ, et al. "Wet suction technique (WEST)": a novel way to enhance the quality of EUS-FNA aspirate. Results of a prospective, single-blind, randomized, controlled trial using a 22-gauge needle for EUS-FNA of solid lesions. Gastrointest Endosc 2015;81:1401–7.

87. Bang JY, Magee SH, Ramesh J, et al. Randomized trial comparing fanning with standard technique for endoscopic ultrasound-guided fine-needle aspiration of solid pancreatic mass lesions. Endoscopy 2013;45:445–50.

88. Schulman AR, Thompson CC, Odze R, et al. Optimizing EUS-guided liver biopsy sampling: comprehensive assessment of needle types and tissue acquisition techniques. Gastrointest Endosc 2017;85:419–26.

89. Wani S, Mullady D, Early DS, et al. The clinical impact of immediate on-site cytopathology evaluation during endoscopic ultrasound-guided fine needle aspiration of pancreatic masses: a prospective multicenter randomized controlled trial. Am J Gastroenterol 2015;110:1429–39.

90. Siddiqui UD, Rossi F, Rosenthal LS, et al. EUS-guided FNA of solid pancreatic masses: a prospective, randomized trial comparing 22-gauge and 25-gauge needles. Gastrointest Endosc 2009;70:1093–7.

91. Yang MJ, Yim H, Hwang JC, et al. Endoscopic ultrasound-guided sampling of solid pancreatic masses: 22-gauge aspiration versus 25-gauge biopsy needles. BMC Gastroenterol 2015;15:122.

92. Storch I, Jorda M, Thurer R, et al. Advantage of EUS Trucut biopsy combined with fine-needle aspiration without immediate on-site cytopathologic examination. Gastrointest Endosc 2006;64:505–11.

93. Krishnan K, Dalal S, Nayar R, et al. Rapid on-site evaluation of endoscopic ultrasound core biopsy specimens has excellent specificity and positive predictive value for gastrointestinal lesions. Dig Dis Sci 2013;58:2007–12.

94. Keswani RN, Krishnan K, Wani S, et al. Addition of endoscopic ultrasound (EUS)-guided fine needle aspiration and on-site cytology to EUS-guided fine needle biopsy increases procedure time but not diagnostic accuracy. Clin Endosc 2014;47:242–7.

95. Aadam AA, Wani S, Amick A, et al. A randomized controlled cross-over trial and cost analysis comparing endoscopic ultrasound fine needle aspiration and fine needle biopsy. Endosc Int open 2016;4:E497–505.

96. Bang JY, Hebert-Magee S, Trevino J, et al. Randomized trial comparing the 22-gauge aspiration and 22-gauge biopsy needles for EUS-guided sampling of solid pancreatic mass lesions. Gastrointest Endosc 2012;76:321–7.

97. Strand DS, Jeffus SK, Sauer BG, et al. EUS-guided 22-gauge fine-needle aspiration versus core biopsy needle in the evaluation of solid pancreatic neoplasms. Diagn Cytopathol 2014;42:751–8.

98. Bang JY, Hawes R, Varadarajulu S. A meta-analysis comparing ProCore and standard fine-needle aspiration needles for endoscopic ultrasound-guided tissue acquisition. Endoscopy 2016;48:339–49.

99. Wani S, Muthusamy VR, Komanduri S. EUS-guided tissue acquisition: an evidence-based approach (with videos). Gastrointest Endosc 2014;80:939–59.e7.

100. Ma X, Zhu L, Wu X, et al. Cell-free DNA provides a good representation of the tumor genome despite its biased fragmentation patterns. PLoS One 2017;12: e0169231.

101. Ma M, Zhu H, Zhang C, et al. "Liquid biopsy"-ctDNA detection with great potential and challenges. Ann Transl Med 2015;3:235.
102. Allard WJ, Matera J, Miller MC, et al. Tumor cells circulate in the peripheral blood of all major carcinomas but not in healthy subjects or patients with nonmalignant diseases. Clin Cancer Res 2004;10:6897–904.
103. Hyun KA, Jung HI. Advances and critical concerns with the microfluidic enrichments of circulating tumor cells. Lab Chip 2014;14:45–56.
104. Khoja L, Backen A, Sloane R, et al. A pilot study to explore circulating tumour cells in pancreatic cancer as a novel biomarker. Br J Cancer 2012;106:508–16.
105. Catenacci DV, Chapman CG, Xu P, et al. Acquisition of portal venous circulating tumor cells from patients with pancreaticobiliary cancers by endoscopic ultrasound. Gastroenterology 2015;149:1794–803.e4.
106. Al-Haddad M, Gill KR, Raimondo M, et al. Safety and efficacy of cytology brushings versus standard fine-needle aspiration in evaluating cystic pancreatic lesions: a controlled study. Endoscopy 2010;42:127–32.
107. Nakai Y, Iwashita T, Park DH, et al. Diagnosis of pancreatic cysts: EUS-guided, through-the-needle confocal laser-induced endomicroscopy and cystoscopy trial: DETECT study. Gastrointestinal endoscopy 2015;81:1204–14.
108. Stavropoulos SN, Friedel D, Grendell JH, et al. Direct visualization of the wall of pancreatic cysts using the SPYGLASS optical probe: feasibility and preliminary results. 2009:AB377.
109. Nakai Y, Iwashita T, Park DH, et al. Diagnosis of pancreatic cysts: EUS-guided, through-the-needle confocal laser-induced endomicroscopy and cystoscopy trial: DETECT study. Gastrointest Endosc 2015;81:1204–14.
110. Konda VJ, Meining A, Jamil LH, et al. A pilot study of in vivo identification of pancreatic cystic neoplasms with needle-based confocal laser endomicroscopy under endosonographic guidance. Endoscopy 2013;45:1006–13.
111. Lozano MD, Subtil JC, Miravalles TL, et al. EchoBrush may be superior to standard EUS-guided FNA in the evaluation of cystic lesions of the pancreas: preliminary experience. Cancer Cytopathol 2011;119:209–14.
112. Nakai Y, Isayama H, Chang KJ, et al. A pilot study of EUS-guided through-the-needle forceps biopsy (with video). Gastrointest Endosc 2016;84:158–62.
113. Samarasena JB, Nakai Y, Shinoura S, et al. EUS-guided, through-the-needle forceps biopsy: a novel tissue acquisition technique. Gastrointest Endosc 2015;81:225–6.
114. Coman RM, Schlachterman A, Esnakula AK, et al. EUS-guided, through-the-needle forceps: clenching down the diagnosis. Gastrointest Endosc 2016;84:372–3.
115. Shakhatreh MH, Naini SR, Brijbassie AA, et al. Use of a novel through-the-needle biopsy forceps in endoscopic ultrasound. Endosc Int open 2016;4:E439–42.

Endoscopic Ultrasonography with Fine-needle Aspiration

New Techniques for Interpretation of Endoscopic Ultrasonography Cytology and Histology Specimens

Mehrvash Haghighi, MD[a], Christopher Packey, MD, PhD[b],
Tamas A. Gonda, MD[c],*

KEYWORDS

- Endoscopic ultrasonography • Fine-needle aspiration • Cytology • Histology

KEY POINTS

- Diagnostic accuracy of gastrointestinal lesions by EUS depends on multiple factors such as acquiring adequate tissue, proper histocytologic triage and selecting appropriate ancillary testing.
- The adequate tissue acquisition is impacted by the location of lesion, the size of needle and employment of rapid on-site evaluation by cytology expert.
- The proper triage and preparation of FNA sample for histocytologic evaluation is imperative. The combination of cytology and histology preparation can enhance the diagnostic accuracy.
- Utilization of ancillary testing such as immunohistochemistry, flowcytometry and molecular testing is crucial for determination of diagnosis, prognosis and therapeutic plan.
- Needle core biopsies have been introduced for tissue acquisition in certain clinical scenarios. Different studies have compared the advantages and disadvantages of the current core biopsy needles.

[a] Department of Pathology, Columbia University Medical Center, 161, Fort Washington Avenue, New York, NY 10023, USA; [b] Department of Medicine, Columbia University Medical Center, 161, Fort Washington Avenue, New York, NY 10023, USA; [c] Division of Digestive and Liver Diseases, Department of Medicine, Columbia University, 161, Fort Washington Avenue, New York, NY 10023, USA
* Corresponding author.
E-mail address: tg2214@cumc.columbia.edu

Gastrointest Endoscopy Clin N Am 27 (2017) 601–614
http://dx.doi.org/10.1016/j.giec.2017.06.003
1052-5157/17/© 2017 Elsevier Inc. All rights reserved.

INTRODUCTION: BRIEF OVERVIEW OF TISSUE ACQUISITION BY ENDOSCOPIC ULTRASONOGRAPHY

Endoscopic ultrasonography (EUS) with fine-needle aspiration (FNA) is an established method for sampling and diagnosing gastrointestinal cancers. It has been shown to be a safe and effective technique that is superior in the assessment of smaller lesions and superior to and safer than computed tomography–guided or ultrasonography-guided percutaneous tissue acquisition for tumors that are accessible.[1,2] Parallel to many of the technical advances that have allowed the procedure to be performed with greater safety and increasing ease, there has been significant success in understanding the biology of many tumors that are biopsied. This success has led to an increasing demand to not only provide highly accurate diagnoses but also obtain specimens that can be used to classify tumors or understand their responsiveness to different therapies. This article provide a highly practical approach to choosing biopsy sites and needle types, and how to process the material to ensure diagnostic accuracy and availability for downstream testing.

TARGETED TISSUE ACQUISITION

Performing high-quality EUS/FNA first involves locating the target tissue and determining the ideal needle approach. A single-center retrospective study showed that use of general anesthesia (GA) is associated with increased diagnostic yield (83% with GA compared with 73% without GA) when performing EUS/FNA of pancreatic masses.[3] Despite these results, current practice in most institutions is to perform the procedure using moderate sedation or monitored anesthesia care. Notably, recent studies have shown much higher diagnostic yield than either group in the previously noted study.

Limitations in approaching a pancreatic mass include small size, necrosis, vascularity, and difficult location. The mass is ideally located at the 6 o'clock position with the ultrasonography transducer applied to the luminal wall with suction. A transgastric approach is simplest when possible. This approach avoids angulation of the scope, which can make passage of the needle through the biopsy channel more challenging. However, the gastric wall is thick, which can make it more difficult to pass the needle through the wall. Acute angulation of the scope is often required when performing transduodenal FNA. A site with minimal intervening vasculature should be chosen using Doppler imaging to avoid bleeding.

The impact of needle size on the diagnostic yield of EUS/FNA for pancreatic lesions is controversial. Needles range from the small and highly flexible 25-gauge needles, to the most commonly used 22-gauge needle, to even larger 19-gauge needles. A meta-analysis comparing 25-gauge needles and 22-gauge needles for FNA of pancreatic masses found that sensitivity was higher (93% vs 85%; $P = .0003$) with 25-gauge needles.[4] The 25-gauge needle may be superior to the 22-gauge needle for accessing head and uncinate process lesions.[5,6] However, several studies have found comparable diagnostic yields when using the 22-gauge needle versus the 25-gauge needle.[6–9] A standard 19-gauge needle or a 19-gauge ProCore can provide good samples in more than 90% cases, although transduodenal puncture can be challenging.[10,11] The literature has consistently shown that smaller gauge needles should be chosen when performing transduodenal FNA of the head and uncinate process of the pancreas given the bend and tension on the distal scope that limits needle movement. One prospective study suggests that a 22-gauge or 25-gauge needle should be used for a transduodenal approach, whereas a 19-gauge needle should be used for a transgastric approach, or if more tissue is desired.[12]

Commercially available FNA needles vary in appearance and echogenicity. Quality FNA depends on visualization of the needle tip. In an attempt to approve visibility, needle tips have been tailored by sandblasting, mechanical dimpling, and laser etching. One large multicenter study evaluated and ranked 10 different EUS needles based on sharpness of distinction and echogenicity. A prototype needle with polymeric coating had the highest ranking, suggesting that the coating may improve visualization.[13]

EUS/FNA needles have stylets that are preloaded to prevent sample contamination from other tissues. Prospective, randomized controlled studies have suggested that use of stylets does not affect the likelihood of achieving a diagnosis with EUS/FNA.[14–16] Some endoscopists choose to remove the stylet and not replace it. Suction may increase the target tissue yield and/or increase sensitivity but may also contribute to bleeding, and hence its use is also variable.[17,18] Suction should be used sparingly or not at all if cytology samples are bloody.

The fanning technique is used to vary the trajectory of the needle using the dials on the echoendoscope or the elevator, and samples different areas of the mass by advancing and then retracting the needle, repeatedly. One randomized study found that fanning during EUS/FNA has 86% sensitivity compared with only 58% with standard techniques.[19,20]

Rapid on-site evaluation (ROSE) by a cytopathologist can increase diagnostic accuracy to more than 90% according to meta-analyses and systematic reviews.[21,22] The pathologist can evaluate the samples for diagnostic yield in real time after the endoscopist makes 1 or 2 passes. ROSE has been shown to decrease the need for repeat EUS and decrease the number of nondiagnostic samples. Based on several prospective, randomized studies, it is generally recommended that, if ROSE is unavailable, 7 passes should be performed during the FNA of a mass in the pancreas.[23,24]

TRIAGE OF FINE-NEEDLE ASPIRATION SAMPLES FOR HISTOCYTOLOGIC EVALUATION

EUS/FNA with a standard needle provides adequate tissue for diagnosis of most pancreatic tumors. It is recommended to combine cytology and histology preparation to improve the diagnostic yields and increase the sensitivity for cancer detection in certain specimens, such as pancreatic solid tumors, metastatic lymph nodes, liver lesions, and most gastrointestinal subepithelial masses.

SPECIMEN PROCESSING

Preparation techniques of aspirated material include cytology and histology processing, such as smears, liquid-based samples, and cell block.

1. Cytology:
   a. Direct smears[25]:
      - Use clean slides.
      - Visually identify the aspirate with tissue floaters if possible.
      - Transfer small amount of tissue-rich aspirate fluid to slide. The goal is to make a thin layer of cells without flowing over the edge.
      - Apply very little pressure to avoid crush artifact.
      - Make 2 mirror-image smears per pass: 1 for alcohol Pap stain and 1 air-dried for Diff-Quick.
         1. First, the Pap stain should be placed in alcohol immediately. Do not let the slide dry out. Air-drying alters the morphology by degrading chromatin material and enlarging or shrinking cells. In our institution, we rehydrate the air-dried slides by covering them with normal saline for 30 seconds. The

quality of the rehydrated smears is optimal if the smears are not dried for longer than 30 minutes.[26]

2. Second, the Diff-Quick stain could be stained and reviewed on site as part of ROSE evaluation.

b. Liquid-based cytology (ThinPrep processing): the FNA needle should be rinsed in CytoLyt solution at the end of procedure for ThinPrep and/or cell block preparation. There are no adequate studies comparing direct smear preparation versus ThinPrep preparations. The decision to prepare a ThinPrep slide and/or cell block should be left to the discretion of clinician and cytology experts. It depends on their level of confidence with different methods of preparation. Other important factors are clinical history, type of suspected tumor, and required ancillary testing for diagnosis or clinical management. Nevertheless, cell block should be used as a supplement to, rather than a replacement for, direct smears or ThinPrep.[27]

2. Histology:

a. Cell block: a cell block consists of mostly small tissue fragments and blood clot along with trapped cellular material. Tissue is usually whitish; however, red clots may also contain tissue. Collecting tissue fragments for histology does not seem to impede cytologic evaluation of the remaining specimen.[1,2] The aspirated tissue fragments should be placed in a fixative. Two types of fixative are most commonly used: formalin and alcohol. **Table 1**[27] compares the fixatives and their effects on morphology, immunohistochemistry (IHC), and molecular studies. In many scenarios, biopsy tissue is not available and prepared cell block from FNA rinse is the only source for molecular testing.

- Formalin fixation: formalin has been used to fix the material from FNA rinses. Although formalin is universally used for IHC, it can result in less reliable molecular studies by diminishing the DNA extractions because of denaturation of nucleic acids.[28]

- Alcohol: ThinPrep liquid-based cytology (CytoLyt) uses methanol as the fixative (approximately 50%). Although CytoLyt-fixed samples can be used for immunostains and molecular studies, the laboratory should perform proper validation to avoid false-negative and false-positive results in IHC stains.

The collected material in fixative is centrifuged, and embedded in paraffin, sectioned, and stained. Using hematoxylin-eosin stains in combination with cytology

Table 1
Comparison of fixatives and their effects on morphology, immunohistochemistry, and molecular studies

Fixative	Histology	Immunohistochemistry	Cytogenetic and Molecular Testing
CytoLyt	Good cytologic preservation, but cell shrinkage and increased nuclear-cytoplasmic holes	Inhibition of S100[a] and hormone receptors	Superior nucleic acid quality
Formalin	Poor discrimination of nuclear and cytologic details	Higher frequency of positivity for hormone receptors and other nuclear antigens, such as ki67 and p53	• DNA fragmentation and denaturation • Sequence artifact • Potential false-positives • Poor yield of RNA

Abbreviations: DNA, deoxyribonucleic acid; RNA, ribonucleic acid.
[a] S100 is commonly used for differential diagnosis of submucosal tumors.

preparations increases diagnostic accuracy by providing architectural pattern, which is valuable for the diagnosis of certain diseases such as submucosal masses, lymphomas, and autoimmune pancreatitis.[29] Cell block sections are also widely used for other ancillary tests, such as IHC stains, special stains, and molecular analysis.

DIAGNOSTIC ANCILLARY TESTING
Immunohistochemistry

IHC studies are instrumental for diagnosis of some specific lesions, such as submucosal tumors, endocrine tumors, acinar cell carcinoma, serous cystadenoma and metastatic lymph node, and liver lesions with unknown primary. Placing aspirated material into proper fixative is essential for cell preservation and retention of antigen specificity for an accurate stain result. Most immunohistochemical protocols are optimized for formalin-fixed paraffin-embedded tissue. **Tables 2** and **3** list immunohistochemical profiles for pancreatic neoplasm and subepithelial lesions, respectively.

Flow Cytometry

Flow cytometry is a laser-based or impedance-based technology used in cell counting, cell sorting, and immunophenotyping. It is an integral part of the diagnostic panel for hematopoietic malignancies such as lymphoma and leukemia. Some advantages of flow cytometry are rapid turnaround time (1–2 working days) and high flexibility and sensitivity of assays. Flow cytometry can detect aberrant cells at frequency of 1 in 1000 to 1 in 10,000 cells and also detects multiple markers on a single cell simultaneously. The marker panel can be customized based on clinical history and morphologic features. The combination of FNA with flow cytometry is a fundamental tool in diagnosis and classification of non-Hodgkin lymphoma. Many studies have shown the high sensitivity and specificity of a combination of FNA and flow cytometry approaches in the diagnosis of B-cell non-Hodgkin lymphoma by incorporating cytologic features and immunophenotypic profile. However, occasionally flow cytometric evaluation of aspirated material fails to detect lymphoma. Major factors in this failure are sampling error such as poor viability, scant cellularity, and peripheral blood contamination.[30] At a minimum, approximately 50,000 cells per tube are needed to analyze 10,000 events. If a sample contains a pure neoplastic population, even fewer

---

Table 2
Immunohistochemical profile of common pancreatic neoplasms

Label	Neuroendocrine	Serous Cystadenoma	ACC	SPT	Ductal[a] Neoplasms
CK19	+	+	−	−	++
Trypsin/chymotrypsin	−	−	++	−	−
Chromogranin	++	−	F	−	F
Synaptophysin	++	−	F	+	F
Inhibin	−	+	−	−	−
CD10	−	−	−	++	+
B-catenin	−	−	+	++	−

Abbreviations: ++, usually positive; +, may be positive; −, usually negative; F, may be focally positive.
[a] Ductal neoplasms include infiltrating ductal adenocarcinoma, mucinous cystic neoplasm, intraductal papillary mucinous neoplasm.
Data partially from Bosman FT, Carneiro F, Hruban RH, et al. WHO classification of tumours of the digestive system. 4th edition. Lyon (France): International Agency for Research on Cancer (IARC); 2010. p. 335.

Table 3 Immunohistochemical profile of intramural gastrointestinal lesions				
Label	GIST	Leiomyoma	Schwannoma	IFP
CD117	+	–	–	–
CD34	+ in 80%	–	Focal (+) in some	+
S100	–	–	+	–
Actin	–	+	–	–

Abbreviations: GIST, gastrointestinal stromal tumor; IFP, inflammatory fibroid polyp.
Data from Bardales RH, Stelow EB, Mallery S, et al. Review of endoscopic ultrasound-guided fine-needle aspiration cytology. Diagn Cytopathol 2006:34(2):140–75.

cells may be sufficient for diagnosis. It is recommended to at least rinse 2 to 3 passes into RPMI (Roswell Park Memorial Institute) medium for a short panel.[29] Some of other disadvantages of the FNA/flow cytometry method are limited success in diagnosis of T-cell lymphoma and Hodgkin lymphoma. For definite diagnosis of T-cell lymphomas a surgical biopsy and gene rearrangement test may be required. The Hodgkin lymphomas also do not show monoclonality by flow cytometric evaluation and some experts think that the diagnosis should not be made without surgical biopsy.[31]

- Indications of submitting aspirated material for flow cytometry (**Fig. 1**)[31]:
    1. Presence of atypical lymphoid cells or blasts on smears.
    2. Organomegaly and superficial mass lesions, including lymphadenopathy (when ROSE confirms the presence of atypical lymphocytes).
    3. Plasmacytosis or monoclonal gammopathy.
    4. Monocytosis.
    5. Staging of a previously diagnosed lymphoma.

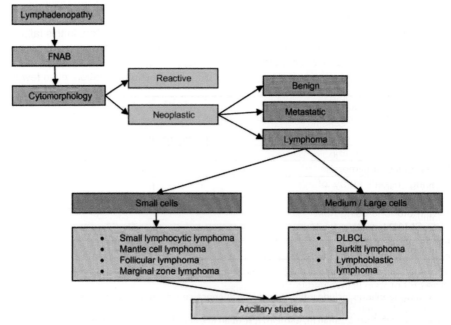

Fig. 1. Flow cytometry algorithm. FNAB, fine-needle aspiration biopsy; DLBCL, diffuse large B-cell lymphoma.

6. Monitoring treatment response by:
    a. Detection of minimal residual disease
    b. Diagnosis of relapse or progression
    c. Diagnosis of intercurrent hematologic disorders, such as therapy-related myelodysplastic syndrome
- Collecting material:
    ○ If any lymphoproliferative disorder is suspected, the tissue or fluid should immediately be placed in RPMI medium.
    ○ If RPMI is unavailable, the specimen should be kept fresh and immediately picked up by the laboratory. If there is a delayed transfer to the laboratory, the RPMI medium should be kept in a refrigerator.
    ○ If the quick pick-up is not feasible and no RPMI is available, then the specimen should be placed in a sterile container with a small amount of sterile saline added.

PROGNOSTIC AND THERAPEUTIC MARKERS IN PANCREATIC CANCER

Pancreatic adenocarcinoma is the result of multistep accumulation of genetic alterations and has been shown to be one of the malignancies to harbor the highest number of genetic alterations. Precursor lesion such as intraductal papillary mucinous neoplasm (IPMN), pancreatic intraepithelial neoplasia (PanIN), or mucinous cystic neoplasm, may progress to malignancy.[32] Whole-genome sequencing and whole-exome sequencing analyses have confirmed that mutations in 4 genes are most commonly seen in pancreatic adenocarcinoma: KRAS, SMAD4, TP53, and CDKN2A/p16.[33,34]

KRAS is a key protein in signaling pathways and KRAS gene mutations inhibit guanosine triphosphate (GTP) hydrolysis with the protein constitutively active.[35] Next-generation sequencing has been shown to improve the accuracy of KRAS mutation analysis in EUS/FNA pancreatic lesions,[36] and KRAS is mutated in more than 90% of low-grade PanINs[37] and is frequently mutated in IPMNs.[36] Several studies have suggested that combining cytopathology and KRAS analysis may improve the diagnostic accuracy between inflammatory processes (ie, chronic pancreatitis) versus neoplasms (mucinous neoplasms and cancers).[38–45] However, the presence of Kras mutation should not be interpreted to suggest invasive carcinoma but should be used to solidify a neoplastic diagnosis with uncertain malignant potential.[6,46]

Sequencing is the main technique for detecting KRAS mutations. Sanger sequencing has low sensitivity, detecting ∼10% to 20% of alleles. In direct EUS/FNA, a more sensitive sequencing technique such as next-generation sequencing or pyrosequencing should be used. Next-generation sequencing outperformed allele-specific polymerase chain reaction (PCR), Sanger sequencing, and pyrosequencing in one study of routine KRAS mutation analysis of 454 formalin-fixed, paraffin-embedded samples. From 5 to 10 ng of DNA are necessary to detect KRAS mutations using next-generation sequencing.[36,47]

The SMAD4 protein facilitates gene transcription and tumor suppression and the gene is inactivated in approximately 50% of pancreatic cancers.[48] In EUS/FNA specimens, the allelic loss of the SMAD4 gene at chromosome 18q shows a sensitivity and specificity of 78% and 57%, respectively.[49]

The p53 protein is involved in cell-cycle regulation, apoptosis, and genomic stability maintenance. TP53 gene mutations are common in almost all human cancers, including 49% of pancreatic cancers in the catalog of somatic mutations in cancer database.[50] Evaluating the presence of TP53 improves the sensitivity of pancreatic cancer diagnosis with EUS/FNA.[51–53] Combining p53 evaluation and histologic examination improved sensitivity up to 90% with 91% specificity in one study.[52] Combining p53 analysis and cytology improved sensitivity to 51%, and staining for both p53 and Ki67 improved EUS/FNA diagnosis of pancreatic adenocarcinoma to 57% with 100% specificity in a separate study.[51] Combining p53 and CA (cancer antigen) 19-9 evaluation increased sensitivity of cytology to 78% but decreased specificity from 100% to 80%.[53] Loss of p53 protein correlated with poor prognosis in one study of 106 patients with pancreatic adenocarcinoma, particularly if combined with loss of SMAD4 and p16.[54] Immunohistochemistry is most commonly used to detect p53 protein accumulation when the TP53 gene is mutated.[52,55,56] Sequencing can also detect TP53 mutations.

The CDKN2A gene negatively controls cell proliferation through activation of p53 and p16^{INK4A}, a cyclin-dependent kinase inhibitor. The gene is localized on chromosome 9p21 and encodes p14^{ARF}. CDKN2A gene mutations are associated with increased risk of many cancers and the gene is inactivated in 95% of sporadic pancreatic cancers.[57–59] The CDKN2A gene is causative in familial pancreatic cancer.[60] p16 loss correlates with a worse prognosis in patients with pancreatic adenocarcinoma, as for p53.[54] Allelic loss of the CDKN2A gene in 101 consecutive pancreatic EUS/FNA samples increased sensitivity and specificity to 85% and 64% respectively in the diagnosis of patients with resectable pancreatic cancer in one study.[49] Detection of p16 inactivation is mainly accomplished using IHC, although loss of heterozygosity at chromosome 9p is another preferred technique. Mutational analysis by PCR, single-strand conformation polymorphism reaction, or sequencing have also been used with success.[61]

MicroRNAs (miRNAs) are a promising class of diagnostic and prognostic biomarkers for human cancer. Unlike most messenger RNAs, miRNAs show significant stability both in vitro and in vivo, allowing their profiling in pancreatic FNA samples, as well as in blood, pancreatic juice, and cyst fluid. Several independent studies have shown miRNA expression profiling in pancreas cytology specimens to be diagnostically reliable.[62–64] Cell-free cyst-fluid miRNAs discriminate among high-risk pancreatic cysts and are promising biomarkers for early diagnosis of pancreatic adenocarcinoma.[65] There are several methods that can be used for miRNA expression profiling, including miRNA, microarray, quantitative reverse transcription PCR, and in-situ hybridization (which permits miRNA visualization at a cellular/subcellular level in histology/cytology specimens).[66]

Unlike in many other solid malignancies, the use of treatment-predictive or theranostic markers is still in early stages, partly because of the heterogeneity of pancreatic cancer and the modest number of treatment regimens. In 1997, gemcitabine was established as the standard of care for treatment of advanced pancreatic adenocarcinoma. However, gemcitabine resistance has been described via limited intracellular uptake of gemcitabine through a decrease in hENT1 expression.[15] In the Radiation Therapy Oncology Group (RTOG) trial 9704, 538 patients were randomly assigned to either gemcitabine or 5-fluorouracil (5FU) following pancreatic resection with postoperative concurrent chemoradiation. Immunohistochemistry for hENT1 was performed on a tissue microarray of 229 resected pancreatic tumors. hENT1 expression was associated with increased overall and disease-free survival in patients receiving gemcitabine, but not in those receiving 5FU.[30] Similar findings have been reproduced by other studies that have analyzed surgically resected specimens and have concluded that high levels of expression of hENT1 are associated with significantly longer survival after adjuvant gemcitabine.[29,31,67–69] Because expression of hENT1 is epithelial it is potentially detectable in biopsies containing malignant epithelial cells. No study has yet shown the reliability of this assessment in either FNA or core biopsy samples.

The importance of targeting the pancreatic tumor stroma in providing effective therapy in pancreatic cancer has also been shown. The hypovascular dense stromal matrix, which is a hallmark of pancreatic adenocarcinoma, is thought to lead to poor delivery of chemotherapeutic agents. Both prognostic and therapeutic markers expressed in the stroma have been identified and several of these markers are associated with stroma-targeted therapy. Collagen and hyaluronan expression in the stroma, as well as the density of alpha smooth muscle actin expression, has been correlated with prognosis. One of these stromal markers, SPARC, may predict response to Nab-paclitaxel, which is an active component of pancreatic cancer chemotherapy. Ongoing clinical studies targeting the stroma, such as the use of PEGPH20, may also show significantly better responses in hyaluronan-expressing tumors.

Most current pancreatic samples are not analyzed for stromal markers and it is unknown whether the lack of architectural preservation impedes evaluation of epithelial markers. Our goal is to use several stroma-specific markers (alpha-SMA, hyaluronan, and SPARC) and understand what biopsy method provides the greatest correlation between the expression pattern seen in the resected tumor and the biopsy.

Perhaps the most exciting development of cancer therapy in the last few years has been the remarkable progress of the use of immunotherapy. Despite the success seen in several solid malignancies (melanoma, lung cancer, urologic cancers), response rates have been minimal in pancreatic cancer. However, an immune response is present in pancreatic cancer and emerging strategies to turn on this immune response or identify tumors with an immune-sensitive phenotype are promising. It is therefore critical to be able to characterize the infiltrating immune cells in pancreatic cancer and this analysis is particularly challenging in biopsies because tumor-adjacent inflammation cannot histologically be distinguished from tumor-associated inflammatory cells.

FINE-NEEDLE CORE BIOPSIES

In most clinical settings EUS/FNA is the standard of care and the cytology preparations and cell block from aspirated materials are sufficient for diagnosis. However, FNA has certain limitations. First, the diagnosis of some specific disease requires preserved architectural pattern, such as subepithelial and intramural lesions, lymphomas, well-differentiated adenocarcinomas, autoimmune pancreatitis, and pancreatic adenocarcinomas surrounded by chronic pancreatitis. Second, certain tumors are routinely evaluated with immunohistochemical markers and molecular testing for diagnostic or therapeutic purposes. Third, dense tissue, such as highly desmoplastic pancreatic neoplasm, is better sampled with needle biopsy.

To overcome some of these limitations, fine-needle biopsy (FNB) was introduced as an adjunct or alternative to FNA. Most studies showed no significant statistical difference between the diagnostic accuracy of FNA versus FNB. However, the combination of FNA and FNB has shown higher diagnostic yield than either technique alone.

The first generation of biopsy needle was a spring-loaded 19-true cut biopsy (TCB) needle (Quick-core; Cook Medical, Winston-Salem, NC) that was used to procure larger quantities of histologic tissue. Early studies showed no significant difference in diagnostic accuracy with TCB; however, the number of passes for obtaining an adequate sample was much lower. The main disadvantage of TCB was the high failure rate of transduodenal biopsies. The routine use of TruCut is recommended because prior studies showed better diagnostic results compared with FNA, such as for lymphoma and autoimmune pancreatitis.[68]

The next generation of biopsy needles have been introduced (ProCore, Cook Endoscopy, Winston-Salem, NC) with reverse-bevel technology to overcome technical failure associated with TruCut needles. Current studies showed no statistical difference in diagnostic accuracy or sample adequacy but did show a higher cellular yield. The main consideration in using the ProCore needle is the cost-effectiveness. The next-generation needles are more expensive and are an estimated 1.5 times the cost of their predecessors.[69]

One randomized controlled crossover trial showed a 90% diagnostic yield with FNB compared with 67% with FNA.[70] A meta-analysis of the ProCore needle found no difference between the ProCore and FNA needles with regard to diagnostic yield, although, to achieve a diagnosis, more passes had to be performed with the FNA needles.[71] SharkCore FNB needles obtained better (95%) yield of tissue compared with 59% yield with FNA needles in one retrospective study.[72] More studies comparing the efficacy of FNB and FNA needles are needed to determine whether practices should be adjusted for increased use of FNB, particularly in places were ROSE is unavailable.

Comparison of needle aspirate versus needle biopsies			
	FNA	**FNB/TruCut**	**FNB/Core Needles**
Diagnostic Accuracy	Same	Same	Same
Number of Passes	High	Low	Low
Cellular Yield		Higher	Higher
Disadvantage	Higher rate of inadequate sample	High failure rate with transduodenal approach	Cost of needle

SUMMARY

Significant advances have been made in the last few years in the technologies available to sample pancreatic masses. Parallel to these developments, understanding of the biology of pancreatic cancer has evolved and there is an increasing sense that better and more targeted treatments will be available. Because most pancreatic cancers are likely to remain unresectable at diagnosis, the importance of high-quality, high-cellularity specimens cannot be understated. A tailored approach that considers indication, location, and treatment possibilities needs to be taken before embarking on a pancreatic biopsy. Because the demand from oncologists and patients for increasingly personalized therapy is likely to grow, optimal sampling beyond diagnostic accuracy is likely to become increasingly critical.

REFERENCES

1. Moller K, Papanikolaou IS, Toermer T, et al. Role of endoscopic ultrasound-guided fine-needle aspiration (EUS-FNA) of solid pancreatic masses: high yield of 2 passes with combined histology-cytology analysis. Gastrointest Endosc 2009;70:60–9.
2. Papanikolaou IS, Asler A, Wegener K, et al. Prospective pilot evaluation of a new needle prototype for endoscopic ultrasonography-guided fine-needle aspiration: comparison of cytology and histology yield. Eur J Gastroenterol Hepatol 2008;20: 342–8.
3. Ootaki C, Stevens T, Vargo J, et al. Does general anesthesia increase the diagnostic yield of endoscopic ultrasound-guided fine needle aspiration of pancreatic masses? Anesthesiology 2012;117:1044–50.
4. Madhoun MF, Wani SB, Rastogi A, et al. The diagnostic accuracy of 22-gauge and 25-gauge needles in endoscopic ultrasound-guided fine needle aspiration of solid pancreatic lesions: a meta-analysis. Endoscopy 2013;45:86–92.

5. Fabbri C, Polifemo AM, Luigiano C, et al. Endoscopic ultrasound-guided fine needle aspiration with 22-gauge and 25-gauge needles in solid pancreatic masses: a prospective comparative study with randomization of needle sequence. Dig Liver Dis 2011;43:647–52.
6. Siddiqui UD, Rossi F, Rosenthal LS, et al. EUS-guided FNA of solid pancreatic masses: a prospective, randomized trial comparing 22-gauge and 25-gauge needles. Gastrointest Endosc 2009;70:1093–7.
7. Brugge WR. EUS. Gastrointest Endosc 2013;78:414–20.
8. Affolter KE, Schmidt RL, Matynia AP, et al. Needle size has only a limited effect on outcomes in EUS-guided fine needle aspiration: a systematic review and meta-analysis. Dig Dis Sci 2013;58:1026–34.
9. Lee JH, Stewart J, Ross WA, et al. Blinded prospective comparison of the performance of 22-gauge and 25-gauge needles in endoscopic ultrasound-guided fine needle aspiration of the pancreas and peri-pancreatic lesions. Dig Dis Sci 2009; 54:2274–81.
10. Imazu H, Uchiyama Y, Kakutani H, et al. A prospective comparison of EUS-guided FNA using 25-gauge and 22-gauge needles. Gastroenterol Res Pract 2009;2009:546390.
11. Petrone MC, Poley JW, Bonzini M, et al. Interobserver agreement among pathologists regarding core tissue specimens obtained with a new endoscopic ultrasound histology needle; a prospective multicenter study in 50 cases. Histopathology 2013;62:602–8.
12. Bang JY, Hawes RH, Varadarajulu S. Objective evaluation of a new endoscopic ultrasound processor. Dig Endosc 2013;25:554–5.
13. Tang SJ, Vilmann AS, Saftoiu A, et al. EUS needle identification comparison and evaluation study (with videos). Gastrointest Endosc 2016;84:424–33.
14. Wani S, Early D, Kunkel J, et al. Diagnostic yield of malignancy during EUS-guided FNA of solid lesions with and without a stylet: a prospective, single blind, randomized, controlled trial. Gastrointest Endosc 2012;76:328–35.
15. Rastogi A, Wani S, Gupta N, et al. A prospective, single-blind, randomized, controlled trial of EUS-guided FNA with and without a stylet. Gastrointest Endosc 2011;74(1):58–64.
16. Sahai AV, Paquin SC, Gariépy G. A prospective comparison of endoscopic ultrasound-guided fine needle aspiration results obtained in the same lesion, with and without the needle stylet. Endoscopy 2010;42:900–3.
17. Bang JY, Ramesh J, Trevino J, et al. Objective assessment of an algorithmic approach to EUS-guided FNA and interventions. Gastrointest Endosc 2013;77: 739–44.
18. Puri R, Vilmann P, Săftoiu A, et al. Randomized controlled trial of endoscopic ultrasound-guided fine-needle sampling with or without suction for better cytological diagnosis. Scand J Gastroenterol 2009;44:499–504.
19. Storm AC, Lee LS. Endoscopic ultrasound-guided techniques for diagnosing pancreatic mass lesions: can we do better? World J Gastroenterol 2016;22: 8658–69.
20. Bang JY, Magee SH, Ramesh J, et al. Randomized trial comparing fanning with standard technique for endoscopic ultrasound-guided fine-needle aspiration of solid pancreatic mass lesions. Endoscopy 2013;45:445–50.
21. Hebert-Magee S, Bae S, Varadarajulu S, et al. The presence of a cytopathologist increases the diagnostic accuracy of endoscopic ultrasound-guided fine needle aspiration cytology for pancreatic adenocarcinoma: a meta-analysis. Cytopathology 2013;24:159–71.

22. Chen J, Yang R, Lu Y, et al. Diagnostic accuracy of endoscopic ultrasound-guided fine-needle aspiration for solid pancreatic lesion: a systematic review. J Cancer Res Clin Oncol 2012;138:1433–41.

23. Wani S, Mullady D, Early DS, et al. The clinical impact of immediate on-site cytopathology evaluation during endoscopic ultrasound-guided fine needle aspiration of pancreatic masses: a prospective multicenter randomized controlled trial. Am J Gastroenterol 2015;110:1429–39.

24. Lee LS, Nieto J, Watson RR, et al. Randomized noninferiority trial comparing diagnostic yield of cytopathologist-guided versus 7 passes for EUS-FNA of pancreatic masses. Dig Endo 2016;28:469–75.

25. Gill GW. Slide preparation. In: Gill GW, editor. Cytopreparation. Essentials in Cytopathology series. New York: (Springer); 2013. p. 56–8.

26. Chan JK, Kung IT. Rehydration of air-dried smears with normal saline. Application in fine-needle aspiration cytologic examination. Am J Clin Pathol 1998;89(1): 30–4.

27. Jain D, Mathur SR, Iyer VK. Cell blocks in cytopathology: a review of preparative methods, utility in diagnosis and role in ancillary studies. Cytopathol 2014;25: 356–71.

28. Serth J, Kuczyk MA, Paeslack U, et al. Quantitation of DNA extracted after micropreparation of cells from frozen and formalin-fixed tissue sections. Am J Pathol 2000;156:1189–96.

29. Jorgensen JL. State of the Art Symposium: flow cytometry in the diagnosis of lymphoproliferative disorders by fine needle aspiration. Cancer Cytopathol 2005; 105:443–51.

30. Meda BA, Geisinger KR, Buss DH, et al. Diagnosis and subclassification of primary and recurrent lymphoma: the usefulness and limitations of combined fine-needle aspiration cytomorphology and flow cytometry. Am J Clin Pathol 2000;113:688–99.

31. Swart GJ, Wright CA. The utilization of fine needle aspiration biopsy (FNAB) and flow cytometry (FC) in the diagnosis and classification of non-Hodgkin B-cell and T-cell lymphomas. Transfus Apher Sci 2010;42:199–207.

32. Fassan M, Baffa R, Kiss A. Advanced precancerous lesions within the GI tract: the molecular background. Best Pract Res Clin Gastroenterol 2013;27:159–69.

33. Waddell N, Pajic M, Patch AM, et al. Whole genomes redefine the mutational landscape of pancreatic cancer. Nature 2015;518:495–501.

34. Biankin AV, Waddell N, Kassahn KS, et al. Pancreatic cancer genomes reveal aberrations in axon guidance pathway genes. Nature 2012;491:399–405.

35. Pylayeva-Gupta Y, Grabocka E, Bar-Sagi D. RAS oncogenes: weaving a tumorigenic web. Nat Rev Cancer 2011;11:761–74.

36. De Biase D, Visani M, Baccarini P, et al. Next generation sequencing improves the accuracy of KRAS mutation analysis in endoscopic ultrasound fine needle aspiration pancreatic lesions. PLoS One 2014;9:e87651.

37. Kanda M, Matthaei H, Wu J, et al. Presence of somatic mutations in most early-stage pancreatic intraepithelial neoplasia. Gastroenterology 2012;142:730–3.

38. Bournet B, Selves J, Grand D, et al. Endoscopic ultrasound-guided fine-needle aspiration biopsy coupled with a KRAS mutation assay using allelic discrimination improves the diagnosis of pancreatic cancer. J Clin Gastroenterol 2015;49:50–6.

39. Ginesta MM, Mora J, Mayor R, et al. Genetic and epigenetic markers in the evaluation of pancreatic masses. J Clin Pathol 2013;66:192–7.

40. Ogura T, Yamao K, Sawaki A, et al. Clinical impact of K-ras mutation analysis in EUS-guided FNA specimens from pancreatic masses. Gastrointest Endosc 2012;75:769–74.
41. Bournet B, Souque A, Senesse P, et al. Endoscopic ultrasound-guided fine-needle aspiration biopsy coupled with KRAS mutation assay to distinguish pancreatic cancer from pseudotumoral chronic pancreatitis. Endoscopy 2009;41:552–7.
42. Maluf-Filho F, Kumar A, Gerhardt R, et al. Kras mutation analysis of fine needle aspirate under EUS guidance facilitates risk stratification of patients with pancreatic mass. J Clin Gastroenterol 2007;41:906–10.
43. Takahashi K, Yamao K, Okubo K, et al. Differential diagnosis of pancreatic cancer and focal pancreatitis by using EUS-guided FNA. Gastrointest Endosc 2005;61:76–9.
44. Pellise M, Castells A, Gines A, et al. Clinical usefulness of KRAS mutational analysis in the diagnosis of pancreatic adenocarcinoma by means of endosonography-guided fine-needle aspiration biopsy. Aliment Pharmacol Ther 2003;17:1299–307.
45. Tada M, Komatsu Y, Kawabe T, et al. Quantitative analysis of K-ras gene mutation in pancreatic tissue obtained by endoscopic ultrasonography-guided fine needle aspiration: clinical utility for diagnosis of pancreatic tumor. Am J Gastroenterol 2002;97:2263–70.
46. Bournet B, Gayral M, Torrisani J, et al. Role of endoscopic ultrasound in the molecular diagnosis of pancreatic cancer. World J Gastroenterol 2014;20:10758–68.
47. Altimari A, de Biase D, De Maglio G, et al. 454 next generation-sequencing outperforms allele-specific PCR, Sanger sequencing, and pyrosequencing for routine KRAS mutation analysis of formalin-fixed, paraffin-embedded samples. Onco Targets Ther 2013;6:1057–64.
48. Maitra A, Hruban RH. Pancreatic cancer. Ann Rev Pathol 2008;3:157–88.
49. Salek C, Benesova L, Zavoral M, et al. Evaluation of clinical relevance of examining KRAS, p16 and p53 mutations along with allelic losses at 9p and 18q in EUS-guided fine needle aspiration samples of patients with chronic pancreatitis and pancreatic cancer. World J Gastroenterol 2007;13:3714–20.
50. Forbes SA, Beare D, Gunasekaran P, et al. COSMIC: exploring the world's knowledge of somatic mutations in human cancer. Nucleic Acids Res 2015;43:D805–11.
51. Jahng AW, Reicher S, Chung D, et al. Staining for p53 and Ki-67 increases the sensitivity of EUS/FNA to detect pancreatic malignancy. World J Gastrointest Endosc 2010;2:362–8.
52. Itoi T, Takei K, Sofuni A, et al. Immunohistochemical analysis of p53 and MIB-1 in tissue specimens obtained from endoscopic ultrasonography-guided fine needle aspiration biopsy for the diagnosis of solid pancreatic masses. Oncol Rep 2005;13:229–34.
53. Mu DQ, Wang GF, Peng SY. p53 protein expression and Ca 19.9 values in differential cytological diagnosis of pancreatic cancer complicated with chronic pancreatitis and chronic pancreatitis. World J Gastroenterol 2003;9:1815–8.
54. Oshima M, Okano K, Muraki S, et al. Immunohistochemically detected expression of 3 major genes (CDKN2A/p16, TP53, and SMAD4/DPC4) strongly predicts survival in patients with resectable pancreatic cancer. Ann Surg 2013;258:336–46.
55. Redston MS, Caldas C, Seymour AB, et al. p53 mutations in pancreatic carcinoma and evidence of common involvement of homocopolymer tracts in DNA microdeletions. Cancer Res 1994;54:3025–33.
56. Barton CM, Staddon SL, Hughes CM, et al. Abnormalities of the p53 tumour suppressor gene in human pancreatic cancer. Br J Cancer 1991;64:1076–82.

57. Rozenblum E, Schutte M, Goggins M, et al. Tumor-suppressive pathways in pancreatic carcinoma. Cancer Res 1997;57:1731–4.
58. Bartsch D, Shevlin DW, Tung WS, et al. Frequent mutations of CDKN2 in primary pancreatic adenocarcinoma. Genes Chromosomes Cancer 1995;14:189–95.
59. Caldas C, Hahn SA, da Costa LT, et al. Frequent somatic mutations and homozygous deletions of the p16 (MTS1) gene in pancreatic adenocarcinoma. Nat Genet 1994;8:27–32.
60. Bartsch DK, Sina-Frey M, Lang S, et al. CDKN2A germline mutations in familial pancreatic cancer. Ann Surg 2002;236:730–7.
61. Singh P, Srinivasan R, Wig JD. SMAD4 genetic alterations predict a worse prognosis in patients with pancreatic ductal adenocarcinoma. Pancreas 2012;41:541–6.
62. Szafanska AE, Doleshal M, Edmunds HS, et al. Analysis of microRNAs in pancreatic fine-needle aspirates can classify benign and malignant tissues. Clin Chem 2008;54:1716–24.
63. Hernandez YG, Lucas AL. MicroRNA in pancreatic ductal adenocarcinoma and its precursor lesions. World J Gastrointest Oncol 2016;8:18–29.
64. Visani M, Acquaviva G, Fiorino S, et al. Contribution of microRNA analysis to characterization of pancreatic lesions: a review. J Clin Pathol 2015;68:859–69.
65. Farrell JJ, Toste P, Wu N, et al. Endoscopically acquired pancreatic cyst fluid microRNA 21 and 221 are associated with invasive cancer. Am J Gastroenterol 2013;108:1352–9.
66. Hewitt MJ, McPhail MJ, Possamai L, et al. EUS-guided FNA for diagnosis of solid pancreatic neoplasms: a meta-analysis. Gastrointest Endosc 2012;75:319–31.
67. Bardales RH, Stelow EB, Mallery S, et al. Review of endoscopic ultrasound-guided fine-needle aspiration cytology. Diagn Cytopathol 2006;34(2):140–75.
68. Levy MJ, Reddy RP, Wiersem MJ, et al. EUS-guided TruCut biopsy in establishing autoimmune pancreatitis as the cause of obstructive jaundice. Gastrointest Endosc 2005;61:467–72.
69. Dwyer J, Pantanowitz L, Ohori NP, et al. Endoscopic ultrasound-guided FNA and ProCore biopsy in sampling pancreatitis and intra-abdominal masses. Cancer Cytopathol 2016;41(12):1069–74.
70. Aadam AA, Wani S, Amick A, et al. A randomized controlled cross-over trial and cost analysis comparing endoscopic ultrasound fine needle aspiration and fine needle biopsy. Endosc Int Open 2016;4:E497–505.
71. Bang JY, Hawes R, Varadarajulu S, et al. A meta-analysis comparing ProCore and standard fine-needle aspiration needles for endoscopic ultrasound-guided tissue acquisition. Endoscopy 2016;48:339–49.
72. Kandel P, Tranesh G, Nassar A, et al. EUS-guided fine needle biopsy sampling using a novel fork-tip needle: a case-control study. Gastrointest Endosc 2016;84:1034–9.

Endoscopic Ultrasound Imaging for Diagnosing and Treating Pancreatic Cysts

Wiriyaporn Ridtitid, MD[a], Mohammad A. Al-Haddad, MD, MSc[b],*

KEYWORDS

- Pancreatic cysts • Intraductal papillary mucinous neoplasm
- Mucinous cystic neoplasm • Serous cystic neoplasm
- Endosonographic characteristics of pancreatic cysts • Fine needle aspiration
- Endosonographic-guided pancreas cyst ablation

KEY POINTS

- Pancreatic cysts are increasingly detected owing to wide spread use of cross-sectional imaging.
- Imaging alone is inadequate to appropriately classify pancreatic cysts from a pathologic perspective.
- Endoscopic ultrasound-guided fine needle aspiration provides valuable information including cytology, tumor and molecular markers that help to classify pancreatic cysts appropriately.
- Mucinous pancreatic cysts with high-risk features for malignancy should be resected in surgically fit patients.
- Low-risk mucinous pancreatic cysts can be managed conservatively with periodic imaging surveillance.

 Video content accompanies this article at http://www.giendo.theclinics.com.

INTRODUCTION

In recent years, the diagnosis of cystic lesions of the pancreas (CLPs) has significantly increased owing to the widespread use of cross-sectional radiologic imaging technologies.[1] In the radiologic literature, the prevalence of CLPs on computed tomography (CT) and MRI examination is estimated to range between 2.4% to 14%.[2–4] One population-based study demonstrated that the overall frequency of detecting

[a] Division of Gastroenterology and Hepatology, Chulalongkorn University, King Chulalongkorn Memorial Hospital, Thai Red Cross Society, Bangkok 10330, Thailand; [b] Division of Gastroenterology and Hepatology, Indiana University School of Medicine, 550 North University Boulevard, Suite 4100, Indianapolis, IN 46202, USA
* Corresponding author.
E-mail address: moalhadd@iu.edu

Gastrointest Endoscopy Clin N Am 27 (2017) 615–642
http://dx.doi.org/10.1016/j.giec.2017.06.004
1052-5157/17/© 2017 Elsevier Inc. All rights reserved.

malignant in CLPs at 2.9% in patient surveyed for known pancreatic cysts, with an annual incidence of 0.4% per year.[5] Based on the presence of epithelial tissue, the World Health Organization classifies CLPs into epithelial and nonepithelial lesions.[6] Inflammatory pancreatic fluid collections (pancreatitis-associated pseudocysts) are not considered true cysts owing to the absence of epithelial component.

A combination of clinical and imaging findings in addition to cyst fluid markers can help to classify CLPs appropriately and guide management. Although some lesions require surgical resection, the majority of CLPs can be surveyed safely by imaging over the long term. In this review, we expand on each of the main types of epithelial CLPs and discuss the role of endoscopic ultrasound (EUS) examination in the diagnosis and management of the commonly encountered types in clinical practice.

DIAGNOSIS OF CYSTIC LESIONS OF THE PANCREAS
Mucinous Cystic Pancreatic Tumors

Mucinous CLPs are mucin-producing neoplasms, which are composed of 2 distinct groups: intraductal papillary mucinous neoplasms (IPMNs) and mucinous cystic neoplasms (MCNs). Although mucinous CLPs are considered "premalignant," many of them remain indolent and do not exhibit an aggressive biological behavior when observed over time. Because of this malignant potential, however, mucinous CLPs require baseline investigation to assess risk of malignant transformation and interval follow-up. Therefore, it is necessary to distinguish between mucinous and nonmucinous CLPs before making final management recommendations.

Intraductal Papillary Mucinous Neoplasms

Histopathologic features
IPMNs are mucinous tumors that arise in the main pancreatic duct or its major branches.[6] Based on the World Health Organization classification, IPMNs are classified histologically into benign, borderline, and malignant; the malignant ones encompass noninvasive and invasive lesions.[6] According to the consensus on the pathologic classification,[7] IPMNs are categorized based on the presence or absence of invasive adenocarcinoma in the resected specimen owing to the negative impact of any invasive component on local recurrence and overall patient survival. In addition, the consensus suggested classifying noninvasive IPMN into low-grade dysplasia (adenomas in previous classification), moderate dysplasia (borderline tumors in previous classification), or high-grade dysplasia (carcinoma in situ), based on the maximal degree of dysplasia in the lining epithelium. From a pathologic and morphologic perspective, IPMNs can be classified as main duct (MD-IPMN), branched duct (BD-IPMN), or mixed IPMN.[8]

Clinical characteristics
MD-IPMN and mixed-type IPMN are slightly more prevalent in men,[8,9] with a peak age of incidence in the 6th to 7th decades (**Table 1**).[9,10] The majority of patients are asymptomatic and most BD-IPMNs are diagnosed incidentally on imaging studies.[9,11] However, IPMNs can present with symptoms such as abdominal pain, jaundice, weight loss, diabetes, steatorrhea, and pancreatitis.[11,12] The overall malignancy risk in MD-IPMN has been reported to be between 40% and 50%,[13-17] although in BD-IPMN, this risk varied significantly in surgical literature but is believed to be 20% or less.[13,15,17,18] Nevertheless, many experts believe that these reported risks are inflated, citing selection bias in these mostly surgical series.

It is believed that IPMN lesions grow slowly and follow and adenoma to carcinoma sequence.[19] Clinical factors associated with invasive cancer in IPMN include jaundice,

Table 1
Endoscopic ultrasound examination morphology and pathologic features of the various types of cystic pancreatic neoplasms

	IPMNs	MCNs	Serous Cystic Neoplasms	cPNETs	SPTPs
Age range	60s–70s	50s–70s	60s–70s	50s–60s	30s
Gender	Male > female	Female > male	Female > male	Male = female	Female > male
Presentation	Mostly asymptomatic with BD-IPMNs	Asymptomatic if small Pain/weight loss if larger	Frequently asymptomatic	Nonfunctioning lesions and often asymptomatic	Asymptomatic or abdominal pain
Macroscopic findings	Various degrees of ductal dilatation in MD-IPMNs; mucin-filled cystic cavity in BD-IPMNs	A smooth surface and a fibrous pseudocapsule with variable thickness septations	A few or numerous small cysts filled with serous fluid around a central fibronodular core	A single locule, surrounded by a rim of neoplastic parenchyma, filled with clear to straw-colored fluid	Cystic areas of hemorrhage and necrosis with a well-defined fibrous pseudocapsule
Microscopic findings	Intraductal proliferation of columnar mucin-producing cells	Benign: no mitosis Malignant: changes of high-grade intraepithelial neoplasia or invasive adenocarcinoma	A single layer of cuboidal or flattened epithelial cells with clear cytoplasm; positive PAS staining	Monotonous cells with granular chromatin and plasmacytoid morphology, positive synaptophysin and chromogranin A stains	Pseudopapillary structures composed of tumor cells surrounding small central vessels
Location	Head > body, tail	Body, tail > head	Body, tail ≥ head	Body, tail > head	Throughout the pancreas

Abbreviations: cPNETs, cystic neuroendocrine tumors of the pancreas; MD-IPMN, main duct intraductal papillary mucinous neoplasm; PAS, periodic acid Schiff; SB-IPMN, side branch intraductal papillary mucinous neoplasm; SPTPs, solid pseudopapillary tumors of the pancreas.

weight loss, intramural nodules, progressive dilation of the main duct, and malignant cytology on fine needle aspiration (FNA).[20,21] Although BD-IPMN is associated with a lower risk of malignancy, pancreatic ductal adenocarcinoma has been reported concomitantly in patients with BD-IPMN[22–24] in a location distant from the IPMN lesion. During follow-up, the 3- and 5-year rates of IPMN-concomitant pancreatic ductal adenocarcinoma occurrence were 4.0% and 8.8%, respectively, according to 1 report[22]; therefore, surveillance is recommended for all lesions.[25–27]

Radiologic and endoscopic ultrasound-guided fine needle aspiration features

On CT imaging, MD-IPMN demonstrates diffuse or focal dilatation of the main pancreatic duct with possible intraductal heterogeneous densities, representing mucin or intraductal tumor growth (**Table 2**).[28] BD-IPMN can be either unifocal or multifocal.[11,29] MRI technology is better suited to outline the morphology of the main duct and its side branches, as well as determine the presence of septations, mural nodules, or mass.[28,30] MCNs and BD-IPMNs may be difficult to differentiate on imaging alone because both can appear as simple unilocular cystic lesions, with variable cystic wall thickness. Intramural filling defects seen on imaging of BD-IPMNs can be either mucin or mural nodules. Based on earlier studies,[30–34] CT or MRI features associated with malignancy in IPMNs include lesion size of greater than 3 cm, main duct dilation of greater than 6 mm, irregularly thickened wall, mural nodule larger than 5 mm, ductal wall enhancement, and common bile duct dilation. A metaanalysis evaluating imaging features to distinguish malignant from benign BD-IPMNs[35] found that the presence of mural nodules was the most suggestive finding for malignancy (odds ratio [OR], 6.0), followed by main pancreatic duct dilatation (OR, 3.4), thick septum or cyst wall (OR, 2.3), and cyst size greater than 3 cm (OR, 2.3).

The classic endoscopic finding of fish-mouth appearance of the papilla, which is characterized by the presence of mucin exuding from a patulous major or minor papilla with or without papillary tissue protrusion (fish egg appearance) is diagnostic of MD-IPMN (**Fig. 1**). EUS characteristics include a macrocystic morphology of the cyst, with or without septations, which could communicate with a dilated main pancreatic duct (Video 1) or a side branch (**Fig. 2**).[36] However, in the absence of duct communication, BD-IPMN may be morphologically indistinguishable from MCNs. A mucin nodule may be seen with a hypoechoic core and a hyperechoic rim (**Fig. 3**) and should be differentiated from real tissue nodules (**Fig. 4**). The differential diagnosis of a unilocular pancreatic cyst on EUS imaging includes commonly macrocystic serous cystic neoplasm, MCN, and inflammatory cyst.[37] Previous studies reported a strong association between the presence of mural nodule (height >10 mm, lateral spread >15 mm) and malignancy in BD-IPMN.[38,39] FNA is generally recommended for cyst fluid acquisition, mainly owing to the limitations of relying on EUS morphology alone to classify the lesion appropriately. A large, prospective, multicenter US study found that the accuracy of EUS imaging features alone for the diagnosis of mucinous lesions was only 51%.[40]

CYST FLUID EVALUATION
Cytology and Tumor Markers

Cytologic aspirates from IPMNs are typically viscous and cytology may reveal columnar epithelial cells and thick extracellular mucin although often are hypocellular.[41–43] Columnar mucinous cells from IPMNs may be arranged in a papillary configuration. The sensitivity of EUS-FNA for invasive malignancy in IPMNs is reportedly as low as 44%, but can be enhanced with cytology brushings and recent microforceps.[41,44–46]

Table 2
General and endoscopic ultrasound examination-specific morphology of cystic tumors of the pancreas and corresponding cyst fluid analysis features

	IPMNs	MCNs	SCNs	cPNETs	SPTPs
Typical features	Fish mouth appearance on endoscopy. Macrocystic, septated cyst with dilated PD (main or side branch)	Macrocystic cyst with a visible wall	A well-demarcated lesions with multiple small fluid filled cavities, with or without central calcified scar	Unilocular or multilocular lesion with a visible wall	Well-defined, mixed echogenicity lesion, with or without internal or peripheral calcifications
Echogenicity	Anechoic	Anechoic	Usually anechoic. Hypoechoic if solid variant	Anechoic, hypoechoic, or mixed	Anechoic, hypoechoic, or mixed
Wall thickness	Thin	Mostly thick	Thin	Mostly thick	Mostly thick
Septation	Yes	Yes	Yes	Yes	No
Nodule	Mucin aggregation; with or without true soft tissue mural nodule	With or without mural nodule	Rare	With or without mural nodule	With or without mural nodule
Communication with the pancreatic duct	Usually seen	Rarely seen	Not seen	Not seen	Not seen
Cyst fluid viscosity	High	High	Low	Low	Low
Cyst fluid cytology	Acellular with background of mucin. Mucinous epithelial cells with papillary projections and variable atypia may be seen	Hypocellular with background mucin. Occasional mucinous epithelium and variable atypia	Mostly bloody and acellular aspirate. Rarely shows glycogen staining cuboidal cells	Small homogenous population of cells with round nuclei that stain positive for chromogranin and synaptophysin	Branching papillae with myxoid stroma that reacts to Vimentin on cell block
Cyst fluid CEA	Moderate elevation	Usually high	Undetectable to low	Undetectable to low	NA
Cyst fluid amylase	Usually high	Variable	Low	Low	NA
Molecular Markers	K-ras mutation; GNAS mutation	K-ras mutation; p53 mutation; SMAD4 mutation	Von Hippel-Lindau gene mutation		CTNNB1 mutation

Abbreviations: CEA, carcinoembryonic antigen; cPNETs, Cystic neuroendocrine tumors of the pancreas; MD-IPMN, main duct intraductal papillary mucinous neoplasm; NA, not applicable; PAS, periodic acid Schiff; PD, pancreatic duct; SB-IPMN, side branch intraductal papillary mucinous neoplasm; SCN, serous cystic neoplasm; SPTPs, solid pseudopapillary tumors of the pancreas.

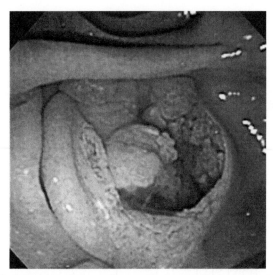

Fig. 1. Fish mouth deformity of the major papilla in a patient with main duct intraductal papillary mucinous neoplasm with polypoid, fish egg–appearing epithelium protruding through the gaping papilla.

Multiple tumor markers present in IPMNs such as carcinoembryonic antigen (CEA), carbohydrate antigen (CA) 19-9, CA 72-4, and CA 125 have been evaluated to improve diagnostic yield. CEA, the most commonly used marker, is generally higher in mucinous lesions and lower in pseudocysts and nonmucinous tumors (see **Table 2**). Early studies using percutaneous FNA reported that a CEA of less than 5 ng/mL provided 100% sensitivity and 86% specificity for distinguishing mucinous neoplasms from other cystic lesions.[47] A large, prospective study[40] using EUS-FNA determined that a cyst fluid CEA cutoff of 192 ng/mL provided a sensitivity of 73% and specificity of 84% for differentiating mucinous from nonmucinous CLPs. Furthermore, no other combination of factors, including cytology, morphology, and CEA levels, was found

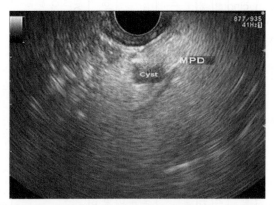

Fig. 2. A small side branch intraductal papillary mucinous neoplasm incidentally detected on endoscopic ultrasound examination performed for an unrelated reason. The communication with the undilated main pancreatic duct is clear.

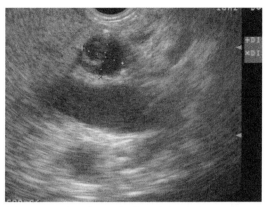

Fig. 3. A mucin nodule attached to the wall of a side branch intraductal papillary mucinous neoplasm with a hyperechoic rim and hypoechoic core.

to be more accurate than CEA levels alone in diagnosing mucinous cysts according to this study. Cyst fluid amylase is usually elevated in IPMN owing to communication with the main pancreatic duct.

Recent advances in the diagnosis of CLPs include the identification of specific genetic changes associated with various tumors and premalignant potential (**Table 3**). The increasing knowledge about common genetic alterations leading to pancreatic adenocarcinoma, like p53 and K-ras mutations, increased interest in the evaluation of similar changes in CLPs. In malignant transformation of CLPs,[48] K-ras mutations seem to occur early in the malignant transformation process.[49] In IPMN, this occurrence is reported to be a result of tumor suppressor gene inactivation, which is represented by loss of heterozygosity at 9p12(p16) and 17p13(p53).[50] The use of these markers has been evaluated in pancreatic juice and cyst fluid.[51–53] K-ras mutation is a very specific for mucinous cysts and specific mutation acquisition sequences we found to be associated with malignancy. CEA alone had the highest sensitivity (82%) compared with 11% for K-ras mutation and 70% for allelic imbalance.[54] Al-Haddad and colleagues[55] demonstrated in a prospective study including mainly IPMNs that molecular markers had a sensitivity of 50% and a specificity of 80% in identifying cystic mucinous lesions with an overall accuracy of 56%. The combination of molecular analysis with cyst fluid CEA and cytology resulted in higher diagnostic

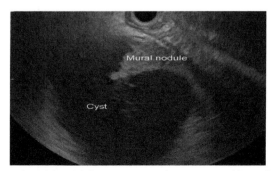

Fig. 4. A "true" mural nodule with homogenous echotexture and irregular contour seen in a side branch lesion.

Table 3
Studies assessing DNA-based markers for the diagnosis of benign and malignant mucinous lesions of the pancreas

Study (Year) (Ref)	Study Design	N[a]	Malignant Cysts (%)	Mucinous vs Nonmucinous Cysts				Malignant vs Nonmalignant Cysts			
				K-ras		LOH		K-ras		LOH	
				Sensitivity (%)	Specificity (%)	Sensitivity (%)	Specificity (%)	Sensitivity (%)	Specificity (%)	Sensitivity (%)	Specificity (%)
Khalid et al,[155] 2005	Prospective	36	31	—	—	—	—	91	86	—	—
Schoedel et al,[156] 2006	Retrospective	16	25	25	—	44	—	50	83	75	58
Khalid et al,[157] 2009	Prospective	113	35	45	96	67	66	53	71	92	36
Sawhney et al,[54] 2009	Retrospective	100	26	11	100	70	100	29	93	100	50
Shen et al,[158] 2009	Retrospective	35	17	57	100	43	93	83	76	83	83
Sreenarasimhaiah et al,[159] 2009	Retrospective	20	45	33	93	50	71	33	—	50	—
Nikiforova et al,[160] 2013	Retrospective	142	8	54	100	—	—	—	—	—	—
Al-Haddad et al,[55] 2014	Prospective	48	16	42	90	11	100	—	—	—	—
Winner et al,[161] 2015	Retrospective	40	20	48	89	31	67	44	56	88	62

Using surgical pathology reference standard whenever available.
Abbreviation: LOH, loss of heterozygosity.
[a] Number of patients included with confirmed diagnosis; retrospective.

performance than either one of its individual components. GNAS is another oncogene mutation that is almost exclusively found in IPMNs and has not been observed in MCNs or in solid pancreatic adenocarcinoma of a non-IPMN origin.[56,57] The combination of KRAS and GNAS mutation testing are highly sensitive and specific for IPMNs.

Despite the expanding role of genetic markers, they are best reserved for pancreatic cysts in which cytology and CEA testing is inconclusive for classifying the lesion as mucinous or nonmucinous, or in cases when the volume of fluid obtained is insufficient for CEA. Additional studies are needed to further elucidate the role of molecular markers in the diagnostic and management algorithms of IPMN.

MUCINOUS CYSTIC NEOPLASMS
Histopathologic Features

MCNs are defined as cystic epithelial neoplasms with no communication with the pancreatic ductal system and is composed of columnar, mucin-producing epithelium, supported by ovarian-type stroma, which is the pathologic hallmark and is required to differentiate this tumor from IPMN.[6] Similar to IPMNs, MCNs are classified as noninvasive (low-grade dysplasia, moderate dysplasia, and high-grade dysplasia) and invasive lesions. Histologically, MCNs exhibit columnar epithelium with basally located nuclei and the absent or minimal mitosis, whereas mucinous cystadenocarcinomas show changes of high-grade intraepithelial neoplasia (nuclear stratification, severe nuclear atypia, and frequent mitoses), which are usually focal.[6]

Clinical Characteristics

Females are more frequently affected with MCNs, particularly in their 5th to 7th decades (see **Table 1**).[58–60] The tumors occur most frequently in the pancreatic body and tail.[10] MCNs can be found incidentally,[61] however, and can present with abdominal pain, palpable mass, and weight loss, particularly in association with large lesions.[8,10] Pancreatitis is infrequent with MCNs but can be seen in up to 10% to 20% of cases.[58,62,63] A recent study demonstrated factors predictive of high-grade dysplasia and or invasive carcinoma in MCNs, which included the presence of symptoms, obstructive jaundice, and elevated serum CEA and CA 19-9.[64] Although MCNs have malignant potential, they carry a lower overall risk of malignancy in comparison with MD-IPMNs.[61] In a study of 163 patients undergoing surgery, the prevalence of malignancy in such tumors was found to be 17.5% (5.5% with carcinoma in situ and 12% with invasive cancer).[62] Nevertheless, surgical resection is recommended for all surgically fit patients with MCNs owing to the long-term risk of cancer in this predominantly younger cohort of patients.[21]

Radiologic and Endoscopic Ultrasound-Guided Fine Needle Aspiration Findings

CT typically shows a unilocular cystic lesion in pancreatic body or tail, with or without septations and a thick enhancing wall (see **Table 2**). Peripheral calcifications can be present in 15% to 23% of cases, and occasionally can be linear taking the shape of an egg shell.[58,63] MCNs appear as round and homogenous, with high signal intensity on T2-weighted MRI, with regular rim enhancement on delayed T1-weighted images.[28,65] On EUS, MCNs present as macrocystic lesions with a visible wall and septations of variable thickness (**Fig. 5**).[36] Solid component or mural nodule may be seen. Peripheral calcifications can be present focally or as a rim but is only seen in up to 15% of lesions.[58] Mucinous cystadenocarcinoma are more likely to appear as a hypoechoic cystic or solid mass, or a complex cyst, and are frequently associated with a dilated main pancreatic duct upstream from the lesion and regional adenopathy.[66] Cyst fluid

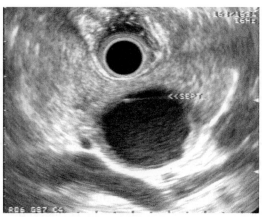

Fig. 5. A 2.5-cm mucinous cystic neoplasm with a thin wall and a single septum incidentally diagnosed on a computed tomography scan in a 45-year-old woman.

amylase is usually low in MCN (see **Table 2**). In a pooled analysis from 12 studies, a cyst fluid amylase of less than 250 U/L supported a diagnosis of serous cysts or MCNs (sensitivity 44%, specificity 98%) and thus virtually excluded pseudocysts.[41] In the same analysis, cyst fluid CEA of less than 5 ng/mL suggested a serous cyst or pseudocyst (sensitivity 50%, specificity 95%) and a CEA of greater than 800 ng/mL strongly suggested MCN (sensitivity 48%, specificity 98%). Cytologic analysis from FNA of MCNs could reveal mucinous epithelium, but this can be difficult to differentiate IPMN based on cytology alone because ovarian stroma is rarely present on FNA specimens. Molecular analysis can assist in the diagnosis of MCNs with similar findings to IPMN lesions (see **Table 3**).[55] Kim and colleagues[67] found that one-third of MCN were associated with K-ras mutations and further changes in tumor suppressor genes like p16 and p53, but were not observed in any serous cystic lesions.

NONMUCINOUS CYSTIC LESIONS OF THE PANCREAS

Nonmucinous CLPs vary greatly in their clinical, radiologic, and EUS characteristics owing to variable underlying pathology. Serous cystadenomas (SCAs) are the most commonly encountered nonmucinous true cystic tumors of the pancreas. Other nonmucinous pure cystic or mixed solid cystic tumors such as pancreatic neuroendocrine tumors (PNETs) and solid pseudopapillary tumors of the pancreas (SPTPs) are discussed elsewhere in this article.

SEROUS CYSTADENOMAS
Histopathologic Features

SCAs are defined as cystic epithelial neoplasms composed of glycogen-rich, ductular-type epithelial cells that produce a watery fluid similar to serum.[6] Gross pathology often demonstrates a few or numerous small cysts filled with serous fluid around a central fibrous core with fine septations (central scars).[6] By histology, the cysts are lined by a single layer of cuboidal or flattened epithelial cells with clear cytoplasm. The periodic acid-Schiff stain is positive owing to their intracytoplasmic glycogen.[6,68] Morphologically, microcystic SCAs (typically with individual cysts measuring <5 mm in size) are more common, whereas the macrocystic variant (>2 cm in size) is relatively infrequent. Microcystic tumors are usually well-delineated with multiple small fluid-filled cavities that are separated by thin septae and lined by cuboidal epithelial cells.[11] Macrocystic SCAs may be difficult to differentiate from MCNs or BD-IPMNs based on morphology alone. The presence of any intramural nodules, cyst wall thickening, floating debris, mucin, or associated pancreatic duct dilation or communication often indicates a mucinous lesion.[66,69]

Clinical Characteristics

SCAs frequently occur in females around the 6th to 7th decades of life,[8,10,70] and are believed to be predominantly located in the pancreatic body and tail[8,9] (see **Table 1**). However, a multicenter study from Japan reported similar distribution in the pancreas head (39%), body (35%), and tail (22%).[70] Patients are usually asymptomatic, with SCAs being an incidental finding on imaging studies.[10,70] Among symptomatic patients, abdominal pain is the most common presentation (12%),[70] but other symptoms include back pain, jaundice, or pancreatitis.[8,9,70] Malignant SCAs of the pancreas are extremely rare; therefore, these tumors are considered to have a negligible malignant potential.[71,72] An observational study showed a steady rate of growth of pancreatic SCA over time, with an estimated doubling in size time of 12 years.[73]

Radiologic and Endoscopic Ultrasound-Guided Fine Needle Aspiration Characteristics

SCAs can appear as polycystic (70%), honeycomb (20%), or oligocystic (<10%) on imaging (see **Table 2**),[74] with a central scar in some cases.[75] The honeycomb appearance is described as numerous subcentimeter cysts, separated by fibrous septa[28,74]; however, this may appear as a well-delineated mass with mixed attenuation and a sharp interface with vascular structures on CT scan.[74] The oligocystic pattern is recognized by fewer large cysts measuring greater than 2 cm, which may appear like MCNs or BD-IPMNs.[74] Magnetic resonance cholangiopancreatography usually shows no communication with the pancreatic duct.

The typical SCA is a well-demarcated lesion on EUS studies with multiple small, fluid-filled cavities separated by thin septations (**Fig. 6**, Video 2).[10,37] The honeycomb

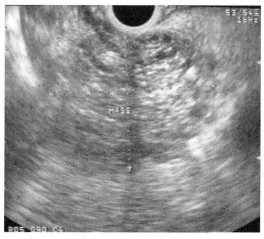

Fig. 6. A serous cystic neoplasm (SCN) in a patient referred for suspicion of a solid mass on a computed tomography scan. Microcystic variants of SCN can be mistaken for solid tumors in imaging.

pattern is noted in most of the microcystic lesions by EUS.[70] A central calcified scar may exhibit a "sunburst" appearance.[10,37] The solid variant of SCAs has been rarely reported, but can lead to misdiagnosis as a solid tumor.[37,70,74,76,77] Nevertheless, the presence of mural nodule, wall thickening, ductal dilatation, or a mucin-filled cavity is an atypical manifestation for SCAs and should raise the suspicion of a mucinous lesion.[37,74]

Owing to the distinctive endosonographic appearance of microcystic SCA, cyst sampling is generally not needed. Furthermore, the diagnostic yield of EUS-FNA for SCA is usually poor owing to the small size of the cystic compartments and the relatively vascular intercystic septa, leading to typically very bloody aspirates. Cyst fluid from SCA is usually thin, nonviscous, and colorless if no blood contamination occurred. Cellularity from cyst fluid is usually very low, but when present may contain cuboidal epithelial cells that stain positive for glycogen but not mucin (see **Table 2**).[78] The macrocystic variant of SCA should be sampled for cytology and tumor markers because morphology alone cannot differentiate these from mucinous lesions. In a pooled analysis from 12 studies, a cyst fluid amylase of less than 250 U/L supported the diagnosis of SCA (sensitivity 44%, specificity 98%) and virtually excluded pseudocysts.[41] In the same analysis, cyst fluid CEA of less than 5 ng/mL suggested an SCA or pseudocyst (sensitivity 50%, specificity 95%). Molecular analysis in SCAs is less studied compared with mucinous lesions. Moore and colleagues[79] described allelic losses on chromosome 10q in 50% and on chromosome 3p in 40% of cases, in addition to von Hippel-Lindau (VHL) gene mutations in 22% of patients. The same study reported the complete absence of K-ras or p53 mutations in these tumors. In 1 small study, 4 of 8 lesions included contained mutations of the VHL gene.[80]

CYSTIC PANCREATIC NEUROENDOCRINE TUMORS
Histopathologic Features

PNETs pathology typically shows small or medium-sized monotonous cells with granular chromatin and plasmacytoid morphology.[81] Tumor cells may be difficult to detect in the cystic fluid.[82] However, the diagnosis can be confirmed by synaptophysin and chromogranin A staining, which are practically diagnostic of these lesions.[82,83] In comparison with ductal adenocarcinomas, tumor necrosis, perineural invasion, vascular invasion, and regional lymph node metastasis are less likely to be seen in cystic PNETs.[84,85]

Clinical Characteristics

PNETs make up as much as 1% to 2% of all pancreatic neoplasms, which typically occur in the body and tail of the pancreas and could have a cystic component less than 10% of the time.[1,6,82,86,87] The majority of cases are detected incidentally on imaging studies.[8] Compared with solid neuroendocrine tumors, cystic PNETs tend to be larger, are more likely to be nonfunctional, and are associated less frequently with multiple endocrine neoplasia type 1.[88,89] Furthermore, cystic PNETs have been reported in 4% to 15% of patients with VHL disease.[90,91] Similar to solid tumors, they occur nearly equally among males and females who are 50 to 60 years of age at diagnosis (see **Table 1**).[8,84] Patients may present with abdominal pain, pancreatitis, or symptoms related to the functioning cystic PNETs.[82,83,87]

Radiologic and Endoscopic Ultrasound-Guided Fine Needle Aspiration Characteristics

CT scanning usually demonstrates a cystic lesion with peripheral arterial enhancement (see **Table 2**).[28,92] Septations or solid components are occasionally identified.[93]

Compared with solid pancreatic neoplasms, cystic PNETs are less likely to be associated with lymph node or liver metastases.[89] MRI shows homogenous unilocular lesion on T2-weighted imaging with thick wall enhancement.[65] On EUS, cystic PNETs can appear as a unilocular or multilocular, anechoic, mixed solid cystic, or hypoechoic lesion.[82,83,87,94] Wall thickening and nodule may be present in 60% of cases (**Fig. 7**).[83] Cystic neuroendocrine tumors vary in size and morphology; therefore, FNA is recommended.[87] Cytology shows a small, homogenous small cell population with round nuclei that should stain positive for chromogranin and synaptophysin (see **Table 2**). Routine cell block preparation is therefore recommended in these patients.

SOLID PSEUDOPAPILLARY TUMORS OF THE PANCREAS
Histopathology and Clinical Features

SPTPs are uncommon neoplasms, composed of monomorphic cells forming solid and pseudopapillary structures, frequently undergoing hemorrhagic–cystic changes.[6,95] Microscopically, SPTPs are composed of solid nests of uniform neuroendocrine-looking epithelial cells around delicate fibrovascular stalks.[95] SPTPs predominantly affect young women in their third decade of life (see **Table 1**).[8,9] Patients may be asymptomatic, presenting with such lesion incidentally on imaging studies. Abdominal pain is the most common presenting symptom, followed by abdominal mass, pancreatitis, and weight loss.[95,96] The tumors can occur throughout the pancreas. SPTPs are usually of low-grade pathology, but high-grade carcinomas have been rarely reported.[97–101]

Radiologic and Endoscopic Ultrasound-Guided Fine Needle Aspiration Characteristics

SPTPs are typically of mixed density on imaging, with a solid part in the periphery and cystic component in the center on CT scan (see **Table 2**).[95] Large tumors have a well-defined capsule and often demonstrate peripheral or central calcifications.[65,95,100] Magnetic resonance cholangiopancreatography does not show communication with pancreatic duct, and pancreatic duct dilation, vessel encasement and metastasis may be used to differentiate solid pseudopapillary carcinomas from benign SPTPs.[101] SPTPs are endosonographically well-defined, echo-poor lesions[96] and can be solid, mixed solid cystic, or cystic in nature (**Fig. 8**). Internal or peripheral calcifications may be seen with postacoustic shadowing. EUS-FNA is useful for definitive preoperative diagnosis of SPTPs.[102] The largest series of EUS-FNA (with or without

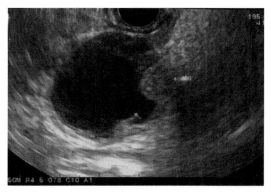

Fig. 7. A cystic neuroendocrine tumors of the pancreas incidentally diagnosed in a 55-year-old man. The lesions exhibits a thick wall that is nodular.

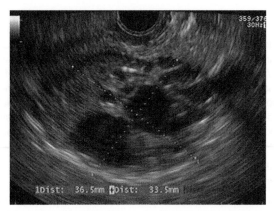

Fig. 8. A 28-year-old woman presents with a mixed solid-cystic mass on a computed tomography scan performed for abdominal pain. The mixed solid-cystic morphology is clear on endoscopic ultrasound examination and fine need aspiration biopsy was diagnostic for solid pseudopapillary tumors of the pancreas.

immunochemistry) for the preoperative diagnosis of SPTPs demonstrated a diagnostic accuracy of 75%.[96] FNA usually shows branching papillae with myxoid stroma, which is best seen on cell block slides (see **Table 2**).

OTHER CYSTIC LESIONS OF THE PANCREAS

Lymphoepithelial cysts (LECs) of the pancreas are rare lesions composed mainly of keratinous material and can occur throughout the pancreas. Histologically, the cysts are lined by stratified squamous epithelium and surrounded by dense epithelial lymphoid tissue containing lymphoid follicles.[103] Since the first case was reported in 1985,[104] more than 110 patients with LECs have been described in the literature.[105] Such lesions are predominantly seen in middle-aged men.[106] Although the most common presentation is abdominal pain, nausea, vomiting, anorexia, and back pain may occur or patients could be asymptomatic. LECs exhibit a benign behavior and are not considered a risk factor for the development of pancreatic cancer.[105,107] The imaging characteristics of LECs on CT can be similar to those of a pseudocyst or an MCN.[105] EUS typically shows a hypoechoic, uniloculated, or multiloculated lesion with fine or coarse hyperechoic debris within the cyst (**Fig. 9**).[103,108,109] Thick milky, creamy, or

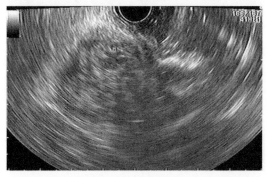

Fig. 9. Lymphoepithelial cyst lesion appears as a uniloculated lesion with coarse hyperechoic debris within the cyst cavity on endoscopic ultrasound examination.

frothy aspirate may be seen during EUS-FNA.[107,109] Cyst fluid CEA and amylase levels were highly variable and therefore are not useful markers.[107,109,110]

VHL disease is a rare autosomal-dominant hereditary disorder resulting from a germline mutation in the VHL gene.[111] Pancreatic cysts can occur in approximately 70% of patients with VHL disease[112,113] and include simple cysts (47%) and SCAs (11%), which are benign lesions.[91] In addition, cystic PNETs have been reported in 4% to 15% of patients with VHL disease, which have malignant potential,[91] but are believed to be of lower metastatic risk.[114] Most pancreatic lesions in VHL disease are asymptomatic; however, abdominal pain and jaundice may be present.[111] Pancreatic involvement in previous series of VHL detected by CT and MRI has varied from 20% to 80%.[115–117] Simple cysts appear as unilocular, homogenous, fluid-attenuation or fluid signal lesions with a thin wall and no calcification or enhancement.[116] SCAs and PNETs in this context have similar morphology to those identified without VHL and, as described elsewhere in this review, EUS can be helpful to better characterize the cystic lesions and may influence on clinical management.

MANAGEMENT OF PANCREATIC CYSTS

The management of CLPs continues to evolve as our knowledge of their natural history and biological behavior increases. Nevertheless, significant variability exists among practitioners despite the multiple existing guidelines endorsed by various medical societies.[20,21,118] Practically, the decision to resect a lesion should take into consideration surgical morbidity and mortality associated with surgery, which should be examined against the risk of malignant transformation of the lesion. Additional factors that directly impact a surgical decision should include patient age, comorbidities, and life expectancy. The next section of this review discusses available management options.

Surgery

Surgery is the only radical treatment for malignant and premalignant CLPs and is recommended for all malignant lesions or those mucinous lesions suspected to harbor minimally invasive disease or advanced dysplasia. Mortality and morbidity associated with pancreatic surgery continue to decrease in centers of expertise and are currently estimated to be less than 3% and 22%, respectively.[119–121] Enucleation has emerged as a less invasive alternative to resection, with reported reduced operative times and blood loss without increasing postoperative morbidity.[122,123] However, this approach remains limited to certain tertiary care centers and to a selective population of patients.

Owing to their malignant potential, published guidelines[20] recommend surgical resection in all fit patients with MCNs. These patients are often younger than those with IPMNs and MCNs in the body or tail are often amenable to distal pancreatectomy. Patients with a unifocal MCN who have a complete resection with pathologically negative margins are not considered at risk for the development of new tumors in the remnant pancreas. Therefore, after surgical resection, postoperative surveillance for MCN recurrence or new tumor formation is not required.[62] The 5-year survival for mucinous cystadenocarcinomas after resection exceeds 60%,[68,124] which far exceeds that of standard pancreatic ductal adenocarcinoma (<10%). Similarly, the prognosis after resection of noninvasive MCN is excellent.

The International Consensus Guidelines for the Management of IPMN published in 2006 and updated in 2012[20,21] recommend resection of all MD-IMPNs and mixed variant IPMN regardless of the presence or absence of referable symptoms owing to the high risk of malignancy in this group.[16,17] Resection is also recommended for symptomatic SB-IPMN in surgically fit patients with a reasonable life expectancy. Any IPMN lesion with intracystic mural nodules, extracystic masses (indicative of possible malignancy), or cytopathology demonstrating high-grade dysplasia or malignancy should be resected when possible, regardless of the presence of symptoms.

Asymptomatic BD-IPMNs pose a particular management dilemma owing to the increase in the diagnosis of these lesions in recent years and the overall low risk of malignant transformation. It widely agreed, however, that SB-IPMNs in general have a malignancy progression rate of 5% or less over the short and intermediate terms. Studies that have reported higher rates of malignancy were surgical series that likely overestimate this risk owing to selecting patients with symptoms and those with high-risk criteria. Despite the expanding knowledge about the natural history of SB-IPMNs, controversies about the management of these patients continue to exist. The previous consensus guidelines, including the recently published American Gastroenterological Association (AGA) Guidelines,[118] attempt to refine surgical resection criteria to avoid unnecessary operations in patients with benign disease, which according to one study of 147 patients with pure BD-IPMNs was as high as 88% of resected patients.[125] For example, cyst size alone exceeding 3 cm has been abandoned as the sole criterion for resection in asymptomatic patients in the International Consensus Guidelines of 2012 and endorsed by the AGA guidelines. What complicates decision making in this group of patients is the conflicting data on the true incidence of malignancy in larger side branch lesions, described to be as high as 46% in some studies,[14,18] including invasive cancer detected in lesions less than 3 cm in size.[126–128] Most literature and experts, however, endorse that size alone is not an independent criterion for the development of malignancy and should not be the sole criterion for resection.[17,125]

Resection is recommended for all symptomatic SCAs. Clinical and radiologic observation are usually sufficient for low risk, asymptomatic SCAs less than 4 cm in size because these lesions seldom undergo malignant transformation or experience rapid growth rates.[129] Natural history studies, however, suggest that lesions greater than 4 cm may experience faster growth rates (and therefore symptoms) than small tumors and thus should be resected in fit patients.[130,131]

Cystic PNETs seem to exhibit less aggressive biological behavior compared with their solid counterparts, but should be considered for resection in fit patients owing to the risk of growth and metastasis.[89] Surgery is recommended for SPTs owing to the risk of malignant transformation (up to 15%) and the relatively young age of the patients. Overall prognosis after surgical resection is excellent.[132]

Expectant Management and Imaging Surveillance

Published practice guidelines and recent data take into consideration the balance between the risk of malignancy and the benefit of pancreatic resection or periodic imaging surveillance and its cost and impact on the quality of life.[133] A cost-effective analysis for asymptomatic incidental solitary CLPs demonstrated risk stratification of malignant potential by EUS-guided FNA and cyst fluid analysis was most effective.[134] Literature overall supports the expectant observation of small and asymptomatic mucinous CLPs lacking high-risk features like mural nodules and solid components and with benign cytology on FNA. In a study of 539 patients with various CLPs, the risk of progression to malignancy among lesions less than 3 cm in size without a solid component was found to be 3%,[121] which is similar to the mortality associated with surgical resection of the pancreas.[119,120] Other studies[27,135–140] reported that asymptomatic BD-IPMN less than 3 cm in size can be safely surveyed by annual imaging alone. However, factors associated with progression of SB-IPMN lesions remain to be fully elucidated, resulting in significant heterogeneity in the management styles of these lesions. This issue is further complicated by the paucity of long-term follow-up data beyond 5 years, and concerns among clinicians about adherence to the consensus guidelines or the lack of awareness of the guidelines.[141–143] There are limited data on the nonoperative management of small MCNs, but recent systematic review indicates that only 0.03% of resected lesions less than 4 cm in size harbored invasive adenocarcinoma.[144] Therefore, expectant management may be considered in unfit patients or older patients with multiple comorbidities and limited life expectancy.

Imaging surveillance is generally unnecessary in MCNs and SCAs after surgical resection. In contrast, IPMN are often multifocal and are thought to have a 'field defect' that considers all pancreatic duct epithelium at risk for neoplasia.[145] Thus, after resection (whether or not radiographic IPMN remains present), follow-up imaging is recommended for the possible development of new lesions in the remnant pancreas. It is estimated that approximately 20% of patients will develop new IPMN lesions during surveillance imaging after surgical resection.[146] Patients with invasive IPMNs are much more likely to develop recurrence after resection compared with those with noninvasive disease.[147,148] Nevertheless, patients with invasive IPMN have a longer survival over "traditional" pancreatic adenocarcinoma after surgical resection.[149] All guidelines endorse postresection imaging surveillance of the pancreatic remnant in patients with invasive cancer or dysplasia in a cyst that has been surgically resected every 1 to 2 years. The AGA guidelines suggest against routine postoperative surveillance of pancreatic cysts without high-grade dysplasia or malignancy at surgical resection. This is supported by recent data on postoperative recurrence of pure SB-IPMN where only benign recurrent lesions were observed up to 8 years after resection.[148]

The question of how long IPMN lesions need to be surveyed by imaging and if there is a safe period of time after which it can be discontinued remains to be answered. The recent AGA guidelines recommend terminating surveillance when no significant change in the characteristics of the cyst has occurred after 5 years of surveillance or if the patient is no longer a surgical candidate. The remains one of the most controversial aspects of these guidelines and further data are needed to support implementing this recommendation in all patients.

Minimally Invasive Management

Alternative nonoperative therapies for CLPs have been described in the last decade. Since the initial pilot study of EUS-guided cyst ablation with ethanol demonstrated cyst resolution in one-third of patients,[150] multiple other trials have demonstrated variables degrees of ablation success (**Table 4**). A multicenter, randomized, double-blind study reported that ethanol lavage of pancreatic cysts decreased cyst surface area greater than saline lavage alone.[151] Overall, 33% of patients in this series had complete cyst resolution on follow-up imaging. The chemotherapeutic agent paclitaxel has been added to ethanol lavage to improve response rates. According to Oh and colleagues,[152] this protocol of ablation resulted in 62% complete response rates. Because it is believed that the pancreatitis described after ablation can be mainly attributed to alcohol, its role in ablation was tested in a study of 10 patients randomized to alcohol or saline in addition to a chemotherapy cocktail of paclitaxel and gemcitabine. Complete ablation was achieved in 67% of patients in the alcohol-free arm compared with 75% in the alcohol arm at 12 months.[153]

Long-term follow-up (>1 year) after successful cyst ablation seems to be associated with persistent cyst resolution by follow-up imaging according to earlier studies.[87] However, in a recent study by Gomez and colleagues[154] using alcohol for ablation, initial response rates at 6 months ranged from 34% to 100% reduction in cyst volume

Table 4
Summary of published studies of endoscopic ultrasound-guided ablation of pancreatic cysts

Study (Year)	No. of Patients	Ablative Agent	FU Period, Median, mo (Range)	Resolution Rate
Gan et al,[150] 2005	25	5%–80% EtOH	6–12	35% CR (8/23) 7% PR (2/23)
Oh et al,[162] 2008	14	80%/90% EtOH + paclitaxel	9 (6–23)	79% CR (11/14) 14% PR (2/14)
Oh et al,[163] 2009	10	99% EtOH + paclitaxel	8.5 (6–18)	60% CR (6/10) 20% PR (2/10)
DeWitt et al,[151] 2009	42	80% EtOH	3–4	33% CR (12/36)
Oh et al,[152] 2011	47	99% EtOH + paclitaxel	20 (12–44)	62% CR (29/47) 13% PR (6/47)
DiMaio et al,[164] 2011	13	80% EtOH	13	38% CR (5/13)
DeWitt et al,[165] 2014	22	100% EtOH + paclitaxel	27 (17–42)	50% CR (10/20) 25% PR (5/20)
Gomez et al,[154] 2016	23	80% EtOH	40	9% CR (2/23) 44% PR (10/23)
Moyer et al,[153] 2016	10	Paclitaxel and gemcitabine +80% EtOH	12	75% (3/4) CR

Abbreviations: CR, complete response; EtOH, ethanol; FU, follow-up; PR, partial response.

in 20 patients. When this cohort was followed for 12 months and then yearly, an increase in cyst volume was demonstrated in 9 patients.

Lesions suitable for ablation are typically less than 4 cm in size, ideally with 5 locules or fewer in multiseptated lesions, with no imaging evidence of communication with the main pancreatic duct. Factors associated with increased ablation response rates include smaller size of the cyst, multiple ablation sessions, and combining alcohol with chemotherapeutic agents like paclitaxel (see **Table 4**). Although the body of data supporting EUS-guided cyst lavage continues to grow, adoption of this technique remains limited owing to associated adverse events, and a limited ability to achieve complete ablation. A cumulative adverse events rate of 10% to 15%, including pancreatitis, peritonitis, and splenic or portal venous thrombosis, has been reported. Additionally, the persistence of neoplastic epithelium after ablation leaves a theoretic risk of progression of malignancy and therefore requires long-term surveillance.

SUMMARY

Practitioners are faced with the task of managing a rapidly increasing number of patients with CLPs detected by various imaging studies. Depending on the pathologic type of the cyst, clinical features, radiologic characteristics, and EUS morphology vary significantly. In combination with minimally invasive investigations like EUS-FNA, clinical and imaging findings are essential to provide an accurate diagnosis of CLPs and improving early detection of cancer in the potentially malignant ones. FNA can guide further management by providing valuable information like tumor and molecular markers to appropriately classify the lesion. Ongoing cyst fluid biomarker research can provide reliable information about biological behavior and allow risk stratification in the near future. Until then, patients with CLPs are best managed by a team of experts in a multidisciplinary approach.

SUPPLEMENTARY DATA

Supplementary data related to this article can be found online at http://dx.doi.org/10.1016/j.giec.2017.06.004.

REFERENCES

1. Valsangkar NP, Morales-Oyarvide V, Thayer SP, et al. 851 resected cystic tumors of the pancreas: a 33-year experience at the Massachusetts General Hospital. Surgery 2012;152:S4–12.
2. Laffan TA, Horton KM, Klein AP, et al. Prevalence of unsuspected pancreatic cysts on MDCT. AJR Am J Roentgenol 2008;191:802–7.
3. Lee KS, Sekhar A, Rofsky NM, et al. Prevalence of incidental pancreatic cysts in the adult population on MR imaging. Am J Gastroenterol 2010;105:2079–84.
4. de Jong K, Nio CY, Hermans JJ, et al. High prevalence of pancreatic cysts detected by screening magnetic resonance imaging examinations. Clin Gastroenterol Hepatol 2010;8:806–11.
5. Wu BU, Sampath K, Berberian CE, et al. Prediction of malignancy in cystic neoplasms of the pancreas: a population-based cohort study. Am J Gastroenterol 2014;109:121–9 [quiz: 130].
6. Bosman FT, World Health Organization, International Agency for Research on Cancer. WHO classification of tumours of the digestive system. Lyon (France): IARC Press; 2010.
7. Hruban RH, Takaori K, Klimstra DS, et al. An illustrated consensus on the classification of pancreatic intraepithelial neoplasia and intraductal papillary mucinous neoplasms. Am J Surg Pathol 2004;28:977–87.
8. Farrell JJ, Fernandez-del Castillo C. Pancreatic cystic neoplasms: management and unanswered questions. Gastroenterology 2013;144:1303–15.
9. Yoon WJ, Brugge WR. Pancreatic cystic neoplasms: diagnosis and management. Gastroenterol Clin North Am 2012;41:103–18.
10. Al-Haddad M, El H II, Eloubeidi MA. Endoscopic ultrasound for the evaluation of cystic lesions of the pancreas. JOP 2010;11:299–309.
11. Al-Haddad M, Schmidt MC, Sandrasegaran K, et al. Diagnosis and treatment of cystic pancreatic tumors. Clin Gastroenterol Hepatol 2011;9:635–48.
12. Capurso G, Boccia S, Salvia R, et al. Risk factors for intraductal papillary mucinous neoplasm (IPMN) of the pancreas: a multicentre case-control study. Am J Gastroenterol 2013;108:1003–9.
13. Kobari M, Egawa S, Shibuya K, et al. Intraductal papillary mucinous tumors of the pancreas comprise 2 clinical subtypes: differences in clinical characteristics and surgical management. Arch Surg 1999;134:1131–6.
14. Doi R, Fujimoto K, Wada M, et al. Surgical management of intraductal papillary mucinous tumor of the pancreas. Surgery 2002;132:80–5.
15. Sugiyama M, Izumisato Y, Abe N, et al. Predictive factors for malignancy in intraductal papillary-mucinous tumours of the pancreas. Br J Surg 2003;90:1244–9.
16. Salvia R, Fernandez-del Castillo C, Bassi C, et al. Main-duct intraductal papillary mucinous neoplasms of the pancreas: clinical predictors of malignancy and long-term survival following resection. Ann Surg 2004;239:678–85 [discussion: 685–7].
17. Schmidt CM, White PB, Waters JA, et al. Intraductal papillary mucinous neoplasms: predictors of malignant and invasive pathology. Ann Surg 2007;246:644–51 [discussion: 651–4].

18. Matsumoto T, Aramaki M, Yada K, et al. Optimal management of the branch duct type intraductal papillary mucinous neoplasms of the pancreas. J Clin Gastroenterol 2003;36:261–5.

19. Sohn TA, Yeo CJ, Cameron JL, et al. Intraductal papillary mucinous neoplasms of the pancreas: an updated experience. Ann Surg 2004;239:788–97 [discussion: 797–9].

20. Tanaka M, Chari S, Adsay V, et al. International consensus guidelines for management of intraductal papillary mucinous neoplasms and mucinous cystic neoplasms of the pancreas. Pancreatology 2006;6:17–32.

21. Tanaka M, Fernandez-del Castillo C, Adsay V, et al. International consensus guidelines 2012 for the management of IPMN and MCN of the pancreas. Pancreatology 2012;12:183–97.

22. Kamata K, Kitano M, Kudo M, et al. Value of EUS in early detection of pancreatic ductal adenocarcinomas in patients with intraductal papillary mucinous neoplasms. Endoscopy 2014;46:22–9.

23. Yamaguchi K, Ohuchida J, Ohtsuka T, et al. Intraductal papillary-mucinous tumor of the pancreas concomitant with ductal carcinoma of the pancreas. Pancreatology 2002;2:484–90.

24. Uehara H, Nakaizumi A, Ishikawa O, et al. Development of ductal carcinoma of the pancreas during follow-up of branch duct intraductal papillary mucinous neoplasm of the pancreas. Gut 2008;57:1561–5.

25. Kobayashi G, Fujita N, Maguchi H, et al. Natural history of branch duct intraductal papillary mucinous neoplasm with mural nodules: a Japan pancreas society multicenter study. Pancreas 2014;43:532–8.

26. Maguchi H, Tanno S, Mizuno N, et al. Natural history of branch duct intraductal papillary mucinous neoplasms of the pancreas: a multicenter study in Japan. Pancreas 2011;40:364–70.

27. Tanno S, Nakano Y, Nishikawa T, et al. Natural history of branch duct intraductal papillary-mucinous neoplasms of the pancreas without mural nodules: long-term follow-up results. Gut 2008;57:339–43.

28. Kucera JN, Kucera S, Perrin SD, et al. Cystic lesions of the pancreas: radiologic-endosonographic correlation. Radiographics 2012;32:E283–301.

29. Rodriguez JR, Salvia R, Crippa S, et al. Branch-duct intraductal papillary mucinous neoplasms: observations in 145 patients who underwent resection. Gastroenterology 2007;133:72–9 [quiz: 309–10].

30. Ku YM, Shin SS, Lee CH, et al. Magnetic resonance imaging of cystic and endocrine pancreatic neoplasms. Top Magn Reson Imaging 2009;20:11–8.

31. Ogawa H, Itoh S, Ikeda M, et al. Intraductal papillary mucinous neoplasm of the pancreas: assessment of the likelihood of invasiveness with multisection CT. Radiology 2008;248:876–86.

32. Sahani DV, Kadavigere R, Blake M, et al. Intraductal papillary mucinous neoplasm of pancreas: multi-detector row CT with 2D curved reformations–correlation with MRCP. Radiology 2006;238:560–9.

33. Lee CJ, Scheiman J, Anderson MA, et al. Risk of malignancy in resected cystic tumors of the pancreas < or =3 cm in size: is it safe to observe asymptomatic patients? A multi-institutional report. J Gastrointest Surg 2008;12:234–42.

34. Manfredi R, Graziani R, Motton M, et al. Main pancreatic duct intraductal papillary mucinous neoplasms: accuracy of MR imaging in differentiation between benign and malignant tumors compared with histopathologic analysis. Radiology 2009;253:106–15.

35. Kim KW, Park SH, Pyo J, et al. Imaging features to distinguish malignant and benign branch-duct type intraductal papillary mucinous neoplasms of the pancreas: a meta-analysis. Ann Surg 2014;259:72–81.
36. Nakai Y, Isayama H, Itoi T, et al. Role of endoscopic ultrasonography in pancreatic cystic neoplasms: where do we stand and where will we go? Dig Endosc 2014;26(2):135–43.
37. Levy MJ. Pancreatic cysts. Gastrointest Endosc 2009;69:S110–6.
38. Kobayashi N, Sugimori K, Shimamura T, et al. Endoscopic ultrasonographic findings predict the risk of carcinoma in branch duct intraductal papillary mucinous neoplasms of the pancreas. Pancreatology 2012;12:141–5.
39. Zhong N, Zhang L, Takahashi N, et al. Histologic and imaging features of mural nodules in mucinous pancreatic cysts. Clin Gastroenterol Hepatol 2012;10: 192–8, 198.e1–2.
40. Brugge WR, Lewandrowski K, Lee-Lewandrowski E, et al. Diagnosis of pancreatic cystic neoplasms: a report of the cooperative pancreatic cyst study. Gastroenterology 2004;126:1330–6.
41. van der Waaij LA, van Dullemen HM, Porte RJ. Cyst fluid analysis in the differential diagnosis of pancreatic cystic lesions: a pooled analysis. Gastrointest Endosc 2005;62:383–9.
42. Sperti C, Pasquali C, Pedrazzoli S, et al. Expression of mucin-like carcinoma-associated antigen in the cyst fluid differentiates mucinous from nonmucinous pancreatic cysts. Am J Gastroenterol 1997;92:672–5.
43. Stelow EB, Stanley MW, Bardales RH, et al. Intraductal papillary-mucinous neoplasm of the pancreas. The findings and limitations of cytologic samples obtained by endoscopic ultrasound-guided fine-needle aspiration. Am J Clin Pathol 2003;120:398–404.
44. Maire F, Couvelard A, Hammel P, et al. Intraductal papillary mucinous tumors of the pancreas: the preoperative value of cytologic and histopathologic diagnosis. Gastrointest Endosc 2003;58:701–6.
45. Al-Haddad M, Raimondo M, Woodward T, et al. Safety and efficacy of cytology brushings versus standard FNA in evaluating cystic lesions of the pancreas: a pilot study. Gastrointest Endosc 2007;65:894–8.
46. Al-Haddad M, Bonatti H, Pungpapong S, et al. Intraductal papillary mucinous neoplasm: is it safe to watch and wait? Gastrointest Endosc 2006;63:AB273.
47. Hammel P, Levy P, Voitot H, et al. Preoperative cyst fluid analysis is useful for the differential diagnosis of cystic lesions of the pancreas. Gastroenterology 1995; 108:1230–5.
48. Yan L, McFaul C, Howes N, et al. Molecular analysis to detect pancreatic ductal adenocarcinoma in high-risk groups. Gastroenterology 2005;128:2124–30.
49. Gerdes B, Wild A, Wittenberg J, et al. Tumor-suppressing pathways in cystic pancreatic tumors. Pancreas 2003;26:42–8.
50. Wada K, Takada T, Yasuda H, et al. Does "clonal progression" relate to the development of intraductal papillary mucinous tumors of the pancreas? J Gastrointest Surg 2004;8:289–96.
51. Berthelemy P, Bouisson M, Escourrou J, et al. Identification of K-ras mutations in pancreatic juice in the early diagnosis of pancreatic cancer. Ann Intern Med 1995;123:188–91.
52. Tada M, Teratani T, Komatsu Y, et al. Quantitative analysis of ras gene mutation in pancreatic juice for diagnosis of pancreatic adenocarcinoma. Dig Dis Sci 1998;43:15–20.

53. Tateishi K, Tada M, Yamagata M, et al. High proportion of mutant K-ras gene in pancreatic juice of patients with pancreatic cystic lesions. Gut 1999;45:737–40.

54. Sawhney MS, Devarajan S, O'Farrel P, et al. Comparison of carcinoembryonic antigen and molecular analysis in pancreatic cyst fluid. Gastrointest Endosc 2009;69:1106–10.

55. Al-Haddad M, DeWitt J, Sherman S, et al. Performance characteristics of molecular (DNA) analysis for the diagnosis of mucinous pancreatic cysts. Gastrointest Endosc 2014;79:79–87.

56. Komatsu H, Tanji E, Sakata N, et al. A GNAS mutation found in pancreatic intraductal papillary mucinous neoplasms induces drastic alterations of gene expression profiles with upregulation of mucin genes. PLoS One 2014;9:e87875.

57. Furukawa T, Kuboki Y, Tanji E, et al. Whole-exome sequencing uncovers frequent GNAS mutations in intraductal papillary mucinous neoplasms of the pancreas. Sci Rep 2011;1:161.

58. Sarr MG, Carpenter HA, Prabhakar LP, et al. Clinical and pathologic correlation of 84 mucinous cystic neoplasms of the pancreas: can one reliably differentiate benign from malignant (or premalignant) neoplasms? Ann Surg 2000;231: 205–12.

59. Zamboni G, Scarpa A, Bogina G, et al. Mucinous cystic tumors of the pancreas: clinicopathological features, prognosis, and relationship to other mucinous cystic tumors. Am J Surg Pathol 1999;23:410–22.

60. Khalid A, Brugge W. ACG practice guidelines for the diagnosis and management of neoplastic pancreatic cysts. Am J Gastroenterol 2007;102:2339–49.

61. Reddy RP, Smyrk TC, Zapiach M, et al. Pancreatic mucinous cystic neoplasm defined by ovarian stroma: demographics, clinical features, and prevalence of cancer. Clin Gastroenterol Hepatol 2004;2:1026–31.

62. Crippa S, Salvia R, Warshaw AL, et al. Mucinous cystic neoplasm of the pancreas is not an aggressive entity: lessons from 163 resected patients. Ann Surg 2008;247:571–9.

63. Le Baleur Y, Couvelard A, Vullierme MP, et al. Mucinous cystic neoplasms of the pancreas: definition of preoperative imaging criteria for high-risk lesions. Pancreatology 2011;11:495–9.

64. Goh BK, Thng CH, Tan DM, et al. Evaluation of the Sendai and 2012 International Consensus Guidelines based on cross-sectional imaging findings performed for the initial triage of mucinous cystic lesions of the pancreas: a single institution experience with 114 surgically treated patients. Am J Surg 2014;208(2):202–9.

65. Barral M, Soyer P, Dohan A, et al. Magnetic resonance imaging of cystic pancreatic lesions in adults: an update in current diagnostic features and management. Abdom Imaging 2014;39:48–65.

66. Gress F, Gottlieb K, Cummings O, et al. Endoscopic ultrasound characteristics of mucinous cystic neoplasms of the pancreas. Am J Gastroenterol 2000;95: 961–5.

67. Kim SG, Wu TT, Lee JH, et al. Comparison of epigenetic and genetic alterations in mucinous cystic neoplasm and serous microcystic adenoma of pancreas. Mod Pathol 2003;16:1086–94.

68. Warshaw AL, Compton CC, Lewandrowski K, et al. Cystic tumors of the pancreas. New clinical, radiologic, and pathologic observations in 67 patients. Ann Surg 1990;212:432–43 [discussion: 444–5].

69. Song MH, Lee SK, Kim MH, et al. EUS in the evaluation of pancreatic cystic lesions. Gastrointest Endosc 2003;57:891–6.

70. Kimura W, Moriya T, Hirai I, et al. Multicenter study of serous cystic neoplasm of the Japan pancreas society. Pancreas 2012;41:380–7.
71. Bramis K, Petrou A, Papalambros A, et al. Serous cystadenocarcinoma of the pancreas: report of a case and management reflections. World J Surg Oncol 2012;10:51.
72. Bano S, Upreti L, Puri SK, et al. Imaging of pancreatic serous cystadenocarcinoma. Jpn J Radiol 2011;29:730–4.
73. El-Hayek KM, Brown N, O'Rourke C, et al. Rate of growth of pancreatic serous cystadenoma as an indication for resection. Surgery 2013;154:794–800 [discussion: 800–2].
74. Choi JY, Kim MJ, Lee JY, et al. Typical and atypical manifestations of serous cystadenoma of the pancreas: imaging findings with pathologic correlation. AJR Am J Roentgenol 2009;193:136–42.
75. Sarr MG, Kendrick ML, Nagorney DM, et al. Cystic neoplasms of the pancreas: benign to malignant epithelial neoplasms. Surg Clin North Am 2001;81:497–509.
76. Sanaka MR, Kowalski TE, Brotz C, et al. Solid serous adenoma of the pancreas: a rare form of serous cystadenoma. Dig Dis Sci 2007;52:3154–6.
77. Yamaguchi M. Solid serous adenoma of the pancreas: a solid variant of serous cystadenoma or a separate disease entity? J Gastroenterol 2006;41:178–9.
78. Carlson SK, Johnson CD, Brandt KR, et al. Pancreatic cystic neoplasms: the role and sensitivity of needle aspiration and biopsy. Abdom Imaging 1998;23: 387–93.
79. Moore PS, Zamboni G, Brighenti A, et al. Molecular characterization of pancreatic serous microcystic adenomas: evidence for a tumor suppressor gene on chromosome 10q. Am J Pathol 2001;158:317–21.
80. Wu J, Jiao Y, Dal Molin M, et al. Whole-exome sequencing of neoplastic cysts of the pancreas reveals recurrent mutations in components of ubiquitin-dependent pathways. Proc Natl Acad Sci U S A 2011;108:21188–93.
81. Chatzipantelis P, Salla C, Konstantinou P, et al. Endoscopic ultrasound-guided fine-needle aspiration cytology of pancreatic neuroendocrine tumors: a study of 48 cases. Cancer 2008;114:255–62.
82. Yoon WJ, Daglilar ES, Pitman MB, et al. Cystic pancreatic neuroendocrine tumors: endoscopic ultrasound and fine-needle aspiration characteristics. Endoscopy 2013;45:189–94.
83. Ho HC, Eloubeidi MA, Siddiqui UD, et al. Endosonographic and cyst fluid characteristics of cystic pancreatic neuroendocrine tumours: a multicentre case series. Dig Liver Dis 2013;45:750–3.
84. Singhi AD, Chu LC, Tatsas AD, et al. Cystic pancreatic neuroendocrine tumors: a clinicopathologic study. Am J Surg Pathol 2012;36:1666–73.
85. Boninsegna L, Partelli S, D'Innocenzio MM, et al. Pancreatic cystic endocrine tumors: a different morphological entity associated with a less aggressive behavior. Neuroendocrinology 2010;92:246–51.
86. Brugge WR, Lauwers GY, Sahani D, et al. Cystic neoplasms of the pancreas. N Engl J Med 2004;351:1218–26.
87. Kongkam P, Al-Haddad M, Attasaranya S, et al. EUS and clinical characteristics of cystic pancreatic neuroendocrine tumors. Endoscopy 2008;40:602–5.
88. Bordeianou L, Vagefi PA, Sahani D, et al. Cystic pancreatic endocrine neoplasms: a distinct tumor type? J Am Coll Surg 2008;206:1154–8.
89. Ridtitid W, Halawi H, DeWitt JM, et al. Cystic pancreatic neuroendocrine tumors: outcomes of preoperative endosonography-guided fine needle aspiration, and recurrence during long-term follow-up. Endoscopy 2015;47:617–25.

90. Graziani R, Mautone S, Vigo M, et al. Spectrum of magnetic resonance imaging findings in pancreatic and other abdominal manifestations of Von Hippel-Lindau disease in a series of 23 patients: a pictorial review. JOP 2014;15:1–18.

91. Charlesworth M, Verbeke CS, Falk GA, et al. Pancreatic lesions in von Hippel-Lindau disease? A systematic review and meta-synthesis of the literature. J Gastrointest Surg 2012;16:1422–8.

92. Kawamoto S, Johnson PT, Shi C, et al. Pancreatic neuroendocrine tumor with cystlike changes: evaluation with MDCT. AJR Am J Roentgenol 2013;200: W283–90.

93. Gaujoux S, Tang L, Klimstra D, et al. The outcome of resected cystic pancreatic endocrine neoplasms: a case-matched analysis. Surgery 2012;151:518–25.

94. Morales-Oyarvide V, Yoon WJ, Ingkakul T, et al. Cystic pancreatic neuroendocrine tumors: the value of cytology in preoperative diagnosis. Cancer Cytopathol 2014;122(6):435–44.

95. Sunkara S, Williams TR, Myers DT, et al. Solid pseudopapillary tumours of the pancreas: spectrum of imaging findings with histopathological correlation. Br J Radiol 2012;85:e1140–4.

96. Jani N, Dewitt J, Eloubeidi M, et al. Endoscopic ultrasound-guided fine-needle aspiration for diagnosis of solid pseudopapillary tumors of the pancreas: a multi-center experience. Endoscopy 2008;40:200–3.

97. Nishihara K, Tsuneyoshi M. Papillary cystic tumours of the pancreas: an analysis by nuclear morphometry. Virchows Arch A Pathol Anat Histopathol 1993;422: 211–7.

98. Das G, Bhuyan C, Das BK, et al. Spleen-preserving distal pancreatectomy following neoadjuvant chemotherapy for papillary solid and cystic neoplasm of pancreas. Indian J Gastroenterol 2004;23:188–9.

99. Tang LH, Aydin H, Brennan MF, et al. Clinically aggressive solid pseudopapillary tumors of the pancreas: a report of two cases with components of undifferentiated carcinoma and a comparative clinicopathologic analysis of 34 conventional cases. Am J Surg Pathol 2005;29:512–9.

100. Raman SP, Kawamoto S, Law JK, et al. Institutional experience with solid pseudopapillary neoplasms: focus on computed tomography, magnetic resonance imaging, conventional ultrasound, endoscopic ultrasound, and predictors of aggressive histology. J Comput Assist Tomogr 2013;37:824–33.

101. Lee JH, Yu JS, Kim H, et al. Solid pseudopapillary carcinoma of the pancreas: differentiation from benign solid pseudopapillary tumour using CT and MRI. Clin Radiol 2008;63:1006–14.

102. Hosokawa I, Shimizu H, Ohtsuka M, et al. Preoperative diagnosis and surgical management for solid pseudopapillary neoplasm of the pancreas. J Hepatobiliary Pancreat Sci 2014;21(8):573–8.

103. Foley KG, Christian A, Roberts SA. EUS-FNA diagnosis of a pancreatic lymphoepithelial cyst: three-year imaging follow-up. JOP 2012;13:681–3.

104. Luchtrath H, Schriefers KH. A pancreatic cyst with features of a so-called branchiogenic cyst. Pathologe 1985;6:217–9 [in German].

105. Kavuturu S, Sarwani NE, Ruggeiro FM, et al. Lymphoepithelial cysts of the pancreas. Can preoperative imaging distinguish this benign lesion from malignant or pre-malignant cystic pancreatic lesions? JOP 2013;14:250–5.

106. Adsay NV, Hasteh F, Cheng JD, et al. Lymphoepithelial cysts of the pancreas: a report of 12 cases and a review of the literature. Mod Pathol 2002;15:492–501.

107. Nasr J, Sanders M, Fasanella K, et al. Lymphoepithelial cysts of the pancreas: an EUS case series. Gastrointest Endosc 2008;68:170–3.

108. Ahlawat SK. Lymphoepithelial cyst of pancreas. Role of endoscopic ultrasound guided fine needle aspiration. JOP 2008;9:230–4.

109. Dalal KS, DeWitt JM, Sherman S, et al. Endoscopic ultrasound characteristics of pancreatic lymphoepithelial cysts: a case series from a large referral center. Endosc Ultrasound 2016;5:248–53.

110. Centeno BA, Stockwell JW, Lewandrowski KB. Cyst fluid cytology and chemical features in a case of lymphoepithelial cyst of the pancreas: a rare and difficult preoperative diagnosis. Diagn Cytopathol 1999;21:328–30.

111. van Asselt SJ, de Vries EG, van Dullemen HM, et al. Pancreatic cyst development: insights from von Hippel-Lindau disease. Cilia 2013;2:3.

112. Hammel PR, Vilgrain V, Terris B, et al. Pancreatic involvement in von Hippel-Lindau disease. The Groupe Francophone d'Etude de la Maladie de von Hippel-Lindau. Gastroenterology 2000;119:1087–95.

113. Horton WA, Wong V, Eldridge R. Von Hippel-Lindau disease: clinical and pathological manifestations in nine families with 50 affected members. Arch Intern Med 1976;136:769–77.

114. Tamura K, Nishimori I, Ito T, et al. Diagnosis and management of pancreatic neuroendocrine tumor in von Hippel-Lindau disease. World J Gastroenterol 2010;16:4515–8.

115. Mukhopadhyay B, Sahdev A, Monson JP, et al. Pancreatic lesions in von Hippel-Lindau disease. Clin Endocrinol (Oxf) 2002;57:603–8.

116. Davenport MS, Caoili EM, Cohan RH, et al. Pancreatic manifestations of von Hippel-Lindau disease-effect of imaging on clinical management. J Comput Assist Tomogr 2010;34:517–22.

117. Kobayashi N, Sato T, Kato S, et al. Imaging findings of pancreatic cystic lesions in von Hippel-Lindau disease. Intern Med 2012;51:1301–7.

118. Vege SS, Ziring B, Jain R, et al. American gastroenterological association institute guideline on the diagnosis and management of asymptomatic neoplastic pancreatic cysts. Gastroenterology 2015;148:819–22 [quiz: 12–3].

119. Lillemoe KD, Kaushal S, Cameron JL, et al. Distal pancreatectomy: indications and outcomes in 235 patients. Ann Surg 1999;229:693–8 [discussion: 698–700].

120. Yeo CJ, Cameron JL. Improving results of pancreaticoduodenectomy for pancreatic cancer. World J Surg 1999;23:907–12.

121. Allen PJ, D'Angelica M, Gonen M, et al. A selective approach to the resection of cystic lesions of the pancreas: results from 539 consecutive patients. Ann Surg 2006;244:572–82.

122. Madura JA, Yum MN, Lehman GA, et al. Mucin secreting cystic lesions of the pancreas: treatment by enucleation. Am Surg 2004;70:106–12 [discussion: 113].

123. Kiely JM, Nakeeb A, Komorowski RA, et al. Cystic pancreatic neoplasms: enucleate or resect? J Gastrointest Surg 2003;7:890–7.

124. Le Borgne J, de Calan L, Partensky C. Cystadenomas and cystadenocarcinomas of the pancreas: a multiinstitutional retrospective study of 398 cases. French Surgical Association. Ann Surg 1999;230:152–61.

125. Pelaez-Luna M, Chari ST, Smyrk TC, et al. Do consensus indications for resection in branch duct intraductal papillary mucinous neoplasm predict malignancy? A study of 147 patients. Am J Gastroenterol 2007;102:1759–64.

126. Kubo H, Chijiiwa Y, Akahoshi K, et al. Intraductal papillary-mucinous tumors of the pancreas: differential diagnosis between benign and malignant tumors by endoscopic ultrasonography. Am J Gastroenterol 2001;96:1429–34.

127. Serikawa M, Sasaki T, Fujimoto Y, et al. Management of intraductal papillary-mucinous neoplasm of the pancreas: treatment strategy based on morphologic classification. J Clin Gastroenterol 2006;40:856–62.

128. Kawamoto S, Lawler LP, Horton KM, et al. MDCT of intraductal papillary mucinous neoplasm of the pancreas: evaluation of features predictive of invasive carcinoma. AJR Am J Roentgenol 2006;186:687–95.

129. Matsumoto T, Hirano S, Yada K, et al. Malignant serous cystic neoplasm of the pancreas: report of a case and review of the literature. J Clin Gastroenterol 2005;39:253–6.

130. Tseng JF, Warshaw AL, Sahani DV, et al. Serous cystadenoma of the pancreas: tumor growth rates and recommendations for treatment. Ann Surg 2005;242:413–9 [discussion: 419–21].

131. Wargo JA, Fernandez-del-Castillo C, Warshaw AL. Management of pancreatic serous cystadenomas. Adv Surg 2009;43:23–34.

132. Alexandrescu DT, O'Boyle K, Feliz A, et al. Metastatic solid-pseudopapillary tumour of the pancreas: clinico-biological correlates and management. Clin Oncol (R Coll Radiol) 2005;17:358–63.

133. Weinberg BM, Spiegel BM, Tomlinson JS, et al. Asymptomatic pancreatic cystic neoplasms: maximizing survival and quality of life using Markov-based clinical nomograms. Gastroenterology 2010;138:531–40.

134. Das A, Ngamruengphong S, Nagendra S, et al. Asymptomatic pancreatic cystic neoplasm: a cost-effectiveness analysis of different strategies of management. Gastrointest Endosc 2009;70:690–9.e6.

135. Carbognin G, Zamboni G, Pinali L, et al. Branch duct IPMTs: value of cross-sectional imaging in the assessment of biological behavior and follow-up. Abdom Imaging 2006;31:320–5.

136. Lee DH. Natural history of branch-duct type intraductal papillary mucinous neoplasm of the pancreas. Korean J Gastroenterol 2007;49:50–2 [in Korean].

137. Pausawasdi N, Heidt D, Kwon R, et al. Long-term follow-up of patients with incidentally discovered pancreatic cystic neoplasms evaluated by endoscopic ultrasound. Surgery 2010;147:13–20.

138. Rautou PE, Levy P, Vullierme MP, et al. Morphologic changes in branch duct intraductal papillary mucinous neoplasms of the pancreas: a midterm follow-up study. Clin Gastroenterol Hepatol 2008;6:807–14.

139. Salvia R, Crippa S, Falconi M, et al. Branch-duct intraductal papillary mucinous neoplasms of the pancreas: to operate or not to operate? Gut 2007;56:1086–90.

140. Salvia R, Partelli S, Crippa S, et al. Intraductal papillary mucinous neoplasms of the pancreas with multifocal involvement of branch ducts. Am J Surg 2009;198:709–14.

141. Buscaglia JM, Shin EJ, Giday SA, et al. Awareness of guidelines and trends in the management of suspected pancreatic cystic neoplasms: survey results among general gastroenterologists and EUS specialists. Gastrointest Endosc 2009;69:813–20 [quiz: 820.e1–17].

142. Nagai K, Doi R, Ito T, et al. Single-institution validation of the international consensus guidelines for treatment of branch duct intraductal papillary mucinous neoplasms of the pancreas. J Hepatobiliary Pancreat Surg 2009;16:353–8.

143. Sawhney MS, Al-Bashir S, Cury MS, et al. International consensus guidelines for surgical resection of mucinous neoplasms cannot be applied to all cystic lesions of the pancreas. Clin Gastroenterol Hepatol 2009;7:1373–6.

144. Nilsson LN, Keane MG, Shamali A, et al. Nature and management of pancreatic mucinous cystic neoplasm (MCN): a systematic review of the literature. Pancreatology 2016;16:1028–36.
145. Izawa T, Obara T, Tanno S, et al. Clonality and field cancerization in intraductal papillary-mucinous tumors of the pancreas. Cancer 2001;92:1807–17.
146. Landa J, Allen P, D'Angelica M, et al. Recurrence patterns of intraductal papillary mucinous neoplasms of the pancreas on enhanced computed tomography. J Comput Assist Tomogr 2009;33:838–43.
147. Chari ST, Yadav D, Smyrk TC, et al. Study of recurrence after surgical resection of intraductal papillary mucinous neoplasm of the pancreas. Gastroenterology 2002;123:1500–7.
148. Ridtitid W, DeWitt JM, Schmidt CM, et al. Management of branch-duct intraductal papillary mucinous neoplasms: a large single-center study to assess predictors of malignancy and long-term outcomes. Gastrointest Endosc 2016;84: 436–45.
149. Niedergethmann M, Grutzmann R, Hildenbrand R, et al. Outcome of invasive and noninvasive intraductal papillary-mucinous neoplasms of the pancreas (IPMN): a 10-year experience. World J Surg 2008;32:2253–60.
150. Gan SI, Thompson CC, Lauwers GY, et al. Ethanol lavage of pancreatic cystic lesions: initial pilot study. Gastrointest Endosc 2005;61:746–52.
151. DeWitt J, McGreevy K, Schmidt CM, et al. EUS-guided ethanol versus saline solution lavage for pancreatic cysts: a randomized, double-blind study. Gastrointest Endosc 2009;70:710–23.
152. Oh HC, Seo DW, Song TJ, et al. Endoscopic ultrasonography-guided ethanol lavage with paclitaxel injection treats patients with pancreatic cysts. Gastroenterology 2011;140:172–9.
153. Moyer MT, Dye CE, Sharzehi S, et al. Is alcohol required for effective pancreatic cyst ablation? The prospective randomized CHARM trial pilot study. Endosc Int Open 2016;4:E603–7.
154. Gomez V, Takahashi N, Levy MJ, et al. EUS-guided ethanol lavage does not reliably ablate pancreatic cystic neoplasms (with video). Gastrointest Endosc 2016;83:914–20.
155. Khalid A, McGrath KM, Zahid M, et al. The role of pancreatic cyst fluid molecular analysis in predicting cyst pathology. Clin Gastroenterol Hepatol 2005;3:967–73.
156. Schoedel KE, Finkelstein SD, Ohori NP. K-Ras and microsatellite marker analysis of fine-needle aspirates from intraductal papillary mucinous neoplasms of the pancreas. Diagn Cytopathol 2006;34:605–8.
157. Khalid A, Zahid M, Finkelstein SD, et al. Pancreatic cyst fluid DNA analysis in evaluating pancreatic cysts: a report of the PANDA study. Gastrointest Endosc 2009;69:1095–102.
158. Shen J, Brugge WR, Dimaio CJ, et al. Molecular analysis of pancreatic cyst fluid: a comparative analysis with current practice of diagnosis. Cancer 2009;117: 217–27.
159. Sreenarasimhaiah J, Lara LF, Jazrawi SF, et al. A comparative analysis of pancreas cyst fluid CEA and histology with DNA mutational analysis in the detection of mucin producing or malignant cysts. JOP 2009;10:163–8.
160. Nikiforova MN, Khalid A, Fasanella KE, et al. Integration of KRAS testing in the diagnosis of pancreatic cystic lesions: a clinical experience of 618 pancreatic cysts. Mod Pathol 2013;26:1478–87.
161. Winner M, Sethi A, Poneros JM, et al. The role of molecular analysis in the diagnosis and surveillance of pancreatic cystic neoplasms. JOP 2015;16:143–9.

162. Oh HC, Seo DW, Lee TY, et al. New treatment for cystic tumors of the pancreas: EUS-guided ethanol lavage with paclitaxel injection. Gastrointest Endosc 2008; 67:636–42.

163. Oh HC, Seo DW, Kim SC, et al. Septated cystic tumors of the pancreas: is it possible to treat them by endoscopic ultrasonography-guided intervention? Scand J Gastroenterol 2009;44:242–7.

164. DiMaio CJ, DeWitt JM, Brugge WR. Ablation of pancreatic cystic lesions: the use of multiple endoscopic ultrasound-guided ethanol lavage sessions. Pancreas 2011;40:664–8.

165. DeWitt JM, Al-Haddad M, Sherman S, et al. Alterations in cyst fluid genetics following endoscopic ultrasound-guided pancreatic cyst ablation with ethanol and paclitaxel. Endoscopy 2014;46:457–64.

The Role of Endoscopic Ultrasound in the Diagnosis of Autoimmune Pancreatitis

Larissa L. Fujii-Lau, MD[a], Michael J. Levy, MD[b],*

KEYWORDS

- Steroid responsive pancreatitis • Immunoglobulin G4 • Fine needle aspiration
- Fine needle biopsy • Pancreatic mass

KEY POINTS

- Type 1 autoimmune pancreatitis (AIP) is the classical presentation with elevated Immuno-globulin G4 and other organ involvement, while type I AIP is limited to the pancreas and requires histology for diagnosis.
- The presence of chronic, severe pain or weight loss should suggest an alternative diagnosis.
- The role of imaging enhancing techniques employed during endoscopic ultrasound (EUS) in assisting the differentiation between AIP and pancreatic cancer is unknown and currently experimental.
- There may be an increasing role for EUS guided core biopsies in the diagnosis of AIP.

INTRODUCTION

Autoimmune pancreatitis (AIP) has historically been considered a rare disease, but it is increasingly recognized due to an improved understanding of its diverse nature and clearer criteria for its diagnosis. Current international consensus diagnostic criteria (ICDC) for the diagnosis of AIP incorporate 5 categories: characteristic imaging findings of the pancreatic parenchyma and duct, serology, other organ involvement, pancreatic histopathology, and response to steroids.[1] Despite consensus diagnostic criteria, the diagnosis of AIP often remains elusive.[2–4] Although the current diagnostic criteria rely on the use of imaging modalities such as computed tomography (CT), MRI and cholangiopancreatography (MRCP), and endoscopic retrograde cholangiopancreatography (ERCP), endoscopic ultrasound (EUS) findings are not included.

[a] The Queen's Medical Center, Honolulu, HI, USA; [b] Division of Gastroenterology and Hepatology, Mayo Clinic, 200 1st Street Southwest, Rochester, MN 55902, USA
* Corresponding author.
E-mail address: levy.michael@mayo.edu

Gastrointest Endoscopy Clin N Am 27 (2017) 643–655
http://dx.doi.org/10.1016/j.giec.2017.06.005
1052-5157/17/© 2017 Elsevier Inc. All rights reserved.

Nevertheless, studies have clearly demonstrated the utility of EUS in this setting, with the ability to obtain tissue by either fine needle aspiration (FNA) or fine needle biopsy (FNB), allowing a definitive diagnosis in many patients. This article will review the diagnostic challenges of AIP and the current role of EUS in the diagnosis of this disorder.

CLASSIFICATION OF AUTOIMMUNE PANCREATITIS

Two distinct subtypes of AIP have been established, type 1 and type 2 AIP. Type 1 AIP is also referred to as lymphoplasmacytic sclerosing pancreatitis (LPSP) and is the pancreatic manifestation of the systemic disease process referred to as Immunoglobulin G4 (IgG$_4$)-related disease (IgG$_4$-RD). Type 2 AIP is also known as idiopathic duct-centric pancreatitis (IDCP). Worldwide, type 1 AIP is more common and is the predominant subtype found in Asian countries.[5] The 2 subtypes have differing epidemiologic factors, clinical presentations, histopathologic features, and outcomes as outlined in **Table 1**.

As type 1 AIP has historically been associated with the initially described classical AIP, some suggest that the term AIP apply solely to type 1 AIP, while the term IDCP be used for type 2 AIP.[6] This shift in nomenclature and has not been broadly adopted. In this article, the authors will continue to refer to the 2 distinct subtypes as type 1 and type 2 AIP.

CLINICAL PRESENTATION OF AUTOIMMUNE PANCREATITIS

Most patients with AIP present with either obstructive jaundice and/or a pancreatic mass that often mimics pancreatic adenocarcinoma (PaC). Less often, patients with AIP present with typical acute pancreatitis or abdominal pain, which are more often

Table 1 Type 1 versus Type 2 Autoimmune Pancreatitis		
	Type 1 AIP	**Type 2 AIP**
Other names	Lymphoplasmacytic sclerosing pancreatitis (LPSP) IgG$_4$-related pancreatitis	Idiopathic duct-centric pancreatitis (IDCP) AIP with granulocyte epithelial lesion (GEL)
Patient population	Older (7th decade) Male predilection (3:1) Asian >>> Western countries	4th-5th decade No gender predilection Western >>> Asian countries
Clinical presentation	Obstructive jaundice - 75% Pancreatic mass - 40% Abdominal pain - 41% Acute pancreatitis - 5%	Obstructive jaundice - 47% Pancreatic mass - 30% Abdominal pain - 68% Acute pancreatitis - 34%
Other organ involvement	Common- 60%	None (pancreas-specific)
IBD present	2%–6%	30%
IgG$_4$	Elevated in serum (typically ≥2x ULN) Stains positive in tissues (≥10 cells per high power field)	Usually normal
Diagnosis	Does not require histology	Requires histology
Histology	Lymphoplasmacytic infiltration, storiform fibrosis	Granulocyte epithelial lesions (GEL)
Natural history	Frequent relapses (up to 60%)	Rare (<10%)

associated with type 2 AIP.[5] Patients presenting with acute pancreatitis commonly also have obstructive jaundice.[7] Those presenting with abdominal pain alone typically suffer from only mild and intermittent pain. The presence of severe, narcotic-requiring, or chronic pain raises doubt regarding the presence of AIP. Likewise, the presence of anorexia and particularly significant unexplained weight loss is quite uncommon and seldom explained by AIP.[1]

DIAGNOSIS OF AUTOIMMUNE PANCREATITIS
Diagnosis of Type 1 Autoimmune Pancreatitis

The ICDC incorporates 5 cardinal criteria for the diagnosis of type I AIP: imaging of the pancreatic parenchyma (P) or pancreatic duct (D), serology (S), other organ involvement (OOI), pancreatic histology (H), and response to steroid therapy (Rt).[1]

The classic cross-sectional imaging feature of the pancreatic parenchyma (P) is the presence of diffuse pancreatic enlargement with delayed or rim-like enhancement. Less common findings include segmental or focal enlargement with delayed enhancement or a low-density mass. Cholangiography, via MRCP or ERCP, demonstrates the pancreatic duct (D) characteristically containing a long more than one-third the length of the duct stricture or the presence of multiple strictures in the absence of marked upstream dilation (duct diameter <5 mm).

Serum IgG_4, the best serologic marker for type 1 AIP, is elevated in 80% of patients, and is the only serum test utilized in the ICDC.[8] A positive serologic (S) result for IgG_4 requires a twofold or greater elevation above the upper limit of normal (ULN), although values between 1 to 2 times the ULN are considered level 2 evidence for AIP. In a recent meta-analysis, the sensitivity and specificity of serum IgG_4 in AIP were 75% (95% confidence interval [CI] 70%–77%) and 94% (95% CI 93%–95%), respectively.[9]

As the pancreatic manifestation of IgG_4-RD, type 1 AIP commonly coexists with extrapancreatic involvement (OOI), including biliary strictures (resembling primary sclerosing cholangitis), parotid or lacrimal gland involvement (resembling Sjogren syndrome), mediastinal lymphadenopathy, retroperitoneal fibrosis, and tubulointerstitial nephritis.[10,11] Excluding lymph node and kidney involvement, biopsy of the extrapancreatic sites of involvement typically manifest the histologic triad of lymphoplasmacytic infiltration, storiform fibrosis, and obliterative phlebitis seen in AIP. In addition, tissue from OOI usually contains increased numbers of IgG_4-positive plasma cells.

Pancreatic biopsies are not required to establish the diagnosis of type 1 AIP; if other classic diagnostic criteria (P, D, S, or OOI) are present, a noninvasive diagnosis is possible. However, if pancreatic biopsies are obtained, histopathology (H) requires at least 1 of the 3 triad features, and in addition demonstration of increased number of tissue IgG_4 plasma cells (**Figs. 1** and **2**).

For patients requiring a diagnostic steroid trial (Rt), a rapid ($\leq$2 weeks) radiologic response manifested by a marked improvement in both the pancreatic and extrapancreatic findings is required. Diagnostic steroid trials should be used with caution in order to minimize the risk of delaying treatment of other more common diagnoses including PaC. In only a select patient cohort who have the classic imaging characteristics, negative cancer work-up, and OOI should a steroid trial be considered in the diagnostic algorithm.[7]

Diagnosis of Type 2 Autoimmune Pancreatitis

The diagnosis of type 2 AIP using the ICDC criteria is similar to that of type I AIP with the following exceptions: (1) lack of serology (S) and other organ involvement

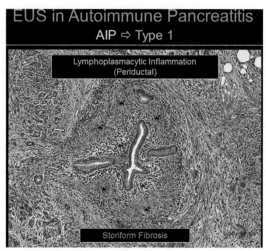

Fig. 1. Core biopsies from a patient with type 1 AIP reveals the classic lymphoplasmacytic inflammation (*green asterisks*), storiform fibrosis (*orange asterisks*).

(OOI), (2) requires core biopsy for confirmation, and (3) different histopathologic (H) findings. Although the histopathology findings may overlap with type 1, the storiform pattern in type 2 AIP is usually less pronounced, and obliterative phlebitis is rare. Most importantly, neutrophils are present in type 2 AIP, with the classic finding of granulocytic inflammation of the duct epithelium, referred to as a granulocyte epithelial lesion (GEL) (**Fig. 3**). The neutrophils also tend to be numerous in and around acini. Type 2 AIP usually has little or no tissue IgG_4 (<10 IgG_4-positive plasma cells per HPF).

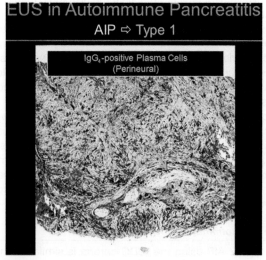

Fig. 2. IgG_4 staining further confirmed the diagnosis of type 1 AIP.

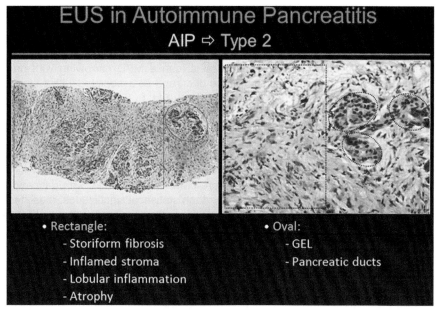

Fig. 3. Core biopsies from a patient with type 2 AIP demonstrate the diagnostic feature of granulocyte epithelial lesions (*blue oval*).

ENDOSCOPIC ULTRASOUND IMAGING FEATURES OF AUTOIMMUNE PANCREATITIS
Endoscopic Ultrasound Imaging of the Pancreas

There are no pathognomonic imaging characteristics on EUS for AIP; the pancreas may even appear normal endosonographically. However, there are classic EUS findings that include diffuse pancreatic enlargement with parenchyma that is hypoechoic, patchy, and heterogeneous.[12–14] (**Fig. 4**) In the authors' experience, a patient has a

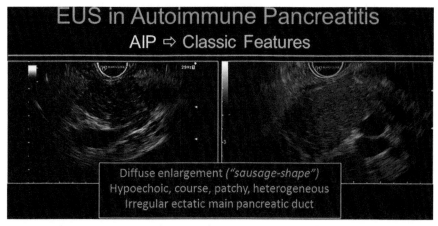

Fig. 4. EUS demonstrates classic features of AIP that include a diffusely enlarged (*sausage-shape*) gland, parenchyma that is hypoechoic, course, patchy, and heterogeneous, and an irregular ectatic main pancreatic duct.

high probability of AIP when all these EUS features are present, which may be seen in up to 57% of patients.[13,14]

EUS may also demonstrate a focal solitary mass, which typically is visualized as a hypoechoic lesion, commonly located in the pancreatic head. The mass may appear to involve peripancreatic vessels, cause MPD narrowing with duct wall thickening and upstream dilation of the duct, and be associated with enlarged peripancreatic lymph nodes, mimicking PaC.[12–14] (**Fig. 5**) Given the overlap in imaging features, but greatly disparate outcomes, it is important to accurately differentiate focal AIP from PaC. The presence of diffuse hypoechoic regions, diffuse pancreatic enlargement, a hypoechoic thickened bile duct wall, and peripancreatic hypoechoic margins has been seen more commonly in patients ultimately diagnosed with AIP rather than pancreatic cancer.[15] On the other hand, focal hyperechoic areas and focal enlargement are more common in patients with pancreatic cancer(**Fig. 6**). Although each criterion can reach statistical significance, these features (except peripancreatic hypoechoic margins) may be seen in both AIP and PaC.

EUS findings of the pancreatic parenchyma may also mimic typical chronic pancreatitis including the presence of hyperechoic foci, hyperechoic strands, and lobularity (**Fig. 7**). In a case series of AIP patients treated with corticosteroids, pancreatic parenchymal enlargement, lobularity, and lobular outer margins decreased with treatment, while the presence of hyperechoic foci and strands persisted despite therapy.[16] In the authors' experience, EUS often detects a clear line of demarcation between involved and uninvolved areas of AIP that is often not seen on CT or MRI (**Fig. 8**).

Endoscopic Ultrasound Imaging of Other Organs in Type 1 Autoimmune Pancreatitis

As the biliary tree is the most common site of extrapancreatic organ involvement in AIP, it is important to evaluate the bile ducts during EUS (**Fig. 9**). In 38% of patients who underwent EUS for AIP, the extrahepatic bile duct and gallbladder wall were thickened.[17] There were 2 types of bile duct wall thickening reported including: (1) a 3-layer type with a high-low-high echo appearance and (2) a parenchymal-echo type with a thickened wall throughout the entire bile lumen and a parenchymal echo present within the bile duct itself. A similar appearance to the 3-layer type with a regular homogenous thickening with a

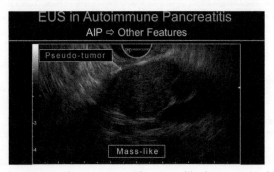

Fig. 5. Patients with AIP may also present with a mass-like lesion as in this patient who at the referring hospital was felt to represent pancreatic adenocarcinoma. EUS-guided core biopsies confirmed the presence of AIP instead.

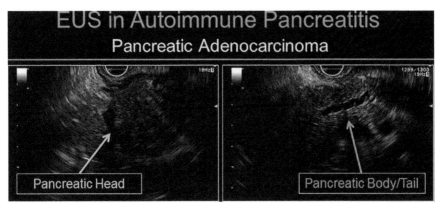

Fig. 6. EUS demonstrates findings more suggestive of usual nonspecific pancreatitis in a patient with biopsy-proven AIP.

hyper-hypo-hyperechoic series of layers of the ductal wall (termed sandwich pattern) was seen on EUS in a different series.[13] The authors also described bile duct dilatation in those with biliary involvement of AIP. This EUS appearance differs from what is typically seen with pancreaticobiliary malignancies, in which the biliary tree is often more irregular.

The authors similarly find that patients with IgG$_4$-SC most often demonstrate profound symmetric bile duct wall thickening that is homogenous, with smooth inner and outer margins. The bile duct wall involvement and strictures are typically segmental or long and often extend into the cystic duct and gallbladder. Although not excluding IgG$_4$-SC, the findings of short, band like strictures, beading, pruning, biliary diverticula, and proximal ductal dilatation, pancreatic duct dilation, pancreatic atrophy, or evidence of malignancy elsewhere suggest an alternate diagnosis. However, there may be considerable overlap of these findings for various disease processes, which may be impacted by the timing of imaging relative to disease onset, therapies provided, presence of an indwelling stent, and disease course.

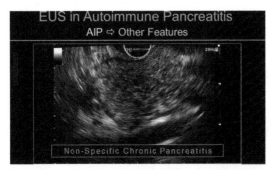

Fig. 7. In patients with AIP, there is often a fairly sharply demarcated transition zone that is not demonstrated at CT or MRI. This is a point where the gland abruptly transitions from normal appearing to the typical manifestations of AIP. It is important to carefully examine this area and to perform EUS-guided core biopsy in the appropriate region.

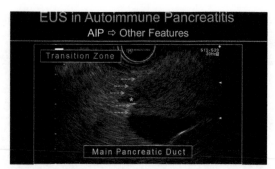

Fig. 8. EUS demonstrates findings that were indeterminate for AIP versus pancreatic adenocarcinoma, the latter of which was confirmed at EUS FNA.

Image-Enhancing Techniques in Endoscopic Ultrasound

Given the lack of pathognomonic features and the variety of EUS findings in patients with AIP, several imaging-enhancing techniques have been investigated to determine their diagnostic utility. The authors consider each of these image-enhancing techniques to be in their experimental phase and discourage routine clinical use in evaluating possible AIP. Furthermore, the results from the following studies must be interpreted with caution, as additional investigation is needed to confirm their findings.

While slightly compressing an area that encompasses both the abnormal and normal tissue, EUS elastography can distinguish tissues based on their stiffness by measuring tissue strain.[18] Five patients with focal AIP were found to have a homogenous stiff (blue) pattern in the mass and throughout the entire pancreas, which differed from the intermediate stiffness (green) of the pancreatic parenchyma seen in pancreatic cancer or normal pancreas.[19]

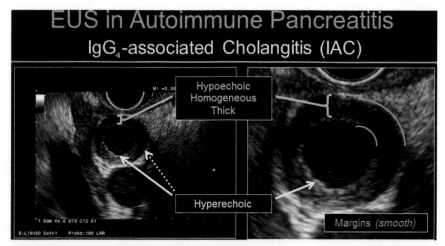

Fig. 9. A key feature and clue to the presence of AIP, when present, is the finding of IgG₄-associated cholangitis (IAC), which presents with a hypoechoic, uniformly thickened wall circumferentially, and is homogenous in echodensity and echopattern as shown.

Contrast-enhanced EUS uses intravenously administered ultrasound contrast agents (eg, Sonovue [sulfur hexafluoride MBs; Bracco Interventional BV, Amsterdam], Levovist [Bayer AG, Leverkusen, Germany], or Sonazoid [perfluorobutane; GE Healthcare, Little Chalfont, Buckinghamshire, United Kingdom]) to produce microbubbles that allow visualization of an organs vascular pattern.[18] In 10 patients who received Sonovue contrast during EUS imaging in the bicolor Doppler mode, AIP was associated with hypervascularity within the involved region of the pancreas and surrounding pancreatic parenchyma.[20] This was compared to pancreatic cancer in which the mass was hypovascular compared to its surrounding pancreatic parenchyma. Using contrast-enhanced EUS in the eFLOW color mode, another study found a dendritic vascular network in majority of patients with AIP (82%) as compared with a few feeder vessels seen in all patients with pancreatic cancer.[21]

Contrast-enhanced harmonic EUS uses ultrasound contrast agents while visualizing using a dedicated contrast harmonic mode. The use of contrast-enhanced harmonic imaging allows for decreased artifact (eg, ballooning and overpainting) produced by the Doppler.[18] In 1 study, 8 patients with focal AIP and 22 patients with pancreatic cancer were administered Sonazoid contrast.[22] The ultrasonographic contrast uptake and distribution was isoehanced and homogenous, respectively, in all patients with AIP compared with only 1 patient with pancreatic cancer. In comparison, the majority of patients with pancreatic cancer had a hypoenhanced uptake in a heterogenous pattern distribution. Furthermore, the optimal maximum intensity gain (MIG) cutoff value to differentiate between AIP and pancreatic cancer with a 100% specificity and sensitivity using a receiver operator characteristic (ROC) curve was 12.5. More data are needed to clarify the potential utility and role of each of these newer imaging modalities before their incorporation into the diagnostic algorithm.

ENDOSCOPIC ULTRASOUND-GUIDED TISSUE ACQUISITION
Endoscopic Ultrasound Fine Needle Aspiration

In addition to providing imaging clues to the diagnosis, EUS may confirm the diagnosis of AIP by EUS-guided biopsy. EUS-guided tissue acquisition is important, particularly in the diagnosis of type 2 AIP, since pancreatic histology is among the diagnostic criteria of the ICDC. FNA samples usually obtained with a 22-gauge needle usually yield small specimens for cytologic review, most of which have a loss of tissue architecture. Currently, there is no broadly accepted consensus as to the utility of cytology in diagnosing AIP, but most pathologists are reluctant to rely solely on FNA specimens.[23–27] Only 1 of the 4 diagnostic histopathologic criteria for the diagnosis of type I AIP can routinely be assessed cytologically (IgG$_4$+ plasma cells).[28] Although there are a few reports claiming the ability to diagnose AIP using FNA specimens alone, the studies report conflicting outcomes on the diagnostic usefulness of EUS FNA.[25–27,29–31]

Some suggest that the role of EUS FNA is predominately to exclude pancreatic cancer rather than diagnose AIP.[32–34] However, with a 10% to 40% false-negative rate, one cannot rely on a negative FNA result to exclude PaC.[35–39]

Endoscopic Ultrasound Tru-Cut Biopsy

To overcome some of the limitations associated with EUS FNA, larger caliber cutting biopsy needles were developed to preserve tissue architecture during tissue acquisition, allowing for histologic evaluation.[40–47] A 19-gauge EUS TCB device (Quick-Core, Wilson-Cook, Winston-Salem, North Carolina) with a tissue tray and sliding sheath was designed to capture a core biopsy. With the larger specimen size and the ability to preserve tissue architecture, TCB can reliably distinguish AIP from classic chronic pancreatitis and pancreatic cancer.[4,48] EUS TCB appears to be safe and may provide a sufficient histologic specimen to aid in the diagnosis of AIP, thereby guiding treatment and avoiding surgical intervention.

The diagnostic sensitivity and safety of EUS TCB was evaluated among 48 patients ultimately diagnosed with AIP at the Mayo Clinic, Rochester, Minnesota. Only 23% of these patients had a serum IgG_4 greater than 2x the ULN. Histologic examination of the EUS TCB specimens provided a diagnosis in 35 patients (73%). The diagnostic sensitivity varied among 5 endosonographers ranging from 33% to 90%. Nondiagnostic cases were ultimately diagnosed with chronic pancreatitis (n = 8), failed tissue acquisition (n = 3), or nondiagnostic histology (n = 2). Adverse events included mild transient abdominal pain (n = 3) and self-limited intraprocedural bleeding (n = 1); no patient required hospitalization or therapeutic intervention. Over a mean follow-up of 2.6 years, no false-negative diagnoses of PaC were identified in the patients diagnosed with AIP by EUS TCB. Prior to undergoing EUS, AIP was strongly suspected in only 14 patients based on clinical, laboratory, or imaging findings. Therefore, the potential utility of EUS imaging to the initial suspicion of AIP was seen in 12 patients, thereby initiating TCB. More recently, the use of EUS TCB in pediatric patients with a suspected diagnosis of AIP was studied.[49] The diagnostic yield of EUS TCB in this patient population was 87%; all patients who were eventually diagnosed with AIP had the type 2 subset.

Some suggest the use of EUS TCB as a rescue technique to obtain adequate tissue samples if EUS FNA fails.[26,50] The current ICDC guidelines recommend a pancreatic core biopsy in patients presenting with a focal mass and/or obstructive jaundice once cancer has been excluded and the diagnosis remains elusive.[1] The authors perform core biopsy in patients with a compatible clinical presentation, but the diagnosis remains uncertain, as does when the findings are likely to alter management. By performing EUS TCB, pancreatic cancer may be excluded, and unnecessary surgical intervention may be averted.

Other Endoscopic Ultrasound Fine Needle Biopsy

As TCB has fallen out of favor due to its lack of flexibility and failure of the spring-loading charging mechanism, other EUS fine needle biopsy (FNB) devices have emerged including but not limited to the ProCore (Cook Ireland, Limerick, Ireland), SharkCore (Covidien/Medtronic, Boston, Massachusetts), Acquire (Boston Scientific, Marlborough, Massachusetts). Most of the studies on these needles have not focused on EUS FNB in the setting of suspected AIP. Only 1 recent case report used the SharkCore needle, which is a fork-tipped needle, to diagnose type 1 AIP.[51] As more studies bring to light the capability of these needles to obtain core biopsy samples, there may be an increased role in the diagnostic utility of EUS FNB.

SUMMARY

As recognition and diagnosis of AIP continues to expand, the diagnostic criteria for both type 1 and type 2 AIP are likely to be refined. Although EUS is not currently in the diagnostic algorithm for AIP, with its ability to provide high-quality images and obtain tissue samples, EUS has a promising role in the diagnosis of this disorder. Furthermore, as new EUS tissue acquisition needles are being increasingly used in clinical practice, the ease of obtaining core biopsies may make EUS an important diagnostic tool for histologic confirmation of AIP.

REFERENCES

1. Shimosegawa T, Chari ST, Frulloni L, et al. International consensus diagnostic criteria for autoimmune pancreatitis: guidelines of the International Association of Pancreatology. Pancreas 2011;40:352–8.
2. Kamisawa T, Egawa N, Nakajima H, et al. Clinical difficulties in the differentiation of autoimmune pancreatitis and pancreatic carcinoma. Am J Gastroenterol 2003; 98:2694–9.
3. Taniguchi T, Tanio H, Seko S, et al. Autoimmune pancreatitis detected as a mass in the head of the pancreas without hypergammaglobulinemia, which relapsed after surgery: case report and review of the literature. Dig Dis Sci 2003;48: 1465–71.
4. Yadav D, Notahara K, Smyrk TC, et al. Idiopathic tumefactive chronic pancreatitis: clinical profile, histology, and natural history after resection. Clin Gastroenterol Hepatol 2003;1:129–35.
5. Kamisawa T, Chari ST, Giday SA, et al. Clinical profile of autoimmune pancreatitis and its histological subtypes: an international multicenter survey. Pancreas 2011; 40:809–14.
6. Sah RP, Chari ST. Recent developments in steroid-responsive pancreatititis (autoimmune pancreatitis). Curr Opin Gastroenterol 2015;31:387–94.
7. Sah RP, Chari ST. Autoimmune pancreatitis: an update on classification, diagnosis, natural history and management. Curr Gastroenterol Rep 2012;14:95–105.
8. Sah RP, Chari ST, Pannala R, et al. Differences in clinical profile and relapse rate of type 1 versus type 2 autoimmune pancreatitis. Gastroenterology 2010;139: 140–8 [quiz: e12–3].
9. Lian MJ, Liu S, Wu GY, et al. Serum IgG4 and IgG for the diagnosis of autoimmune pancreatitis: a systematic review with meta-analysis. Clin Res Hepatol Gastroenterol 2016;40:99–109.
10. Chari ST. Diagnosis of autoimmune pancreatitis using its five cardinal features: introducing the Mayo Clinic's HISORt criteria. J Gastroenterol 2007;42(Suppl 18):39–41.
11. Chari ST, Smyrk TC, Levy MJ, et al. Diagnosis of autoimmune pancreatitis: the Mayo Clinic experience. Clin Gastroenterol Hepatol 2006;4:1010–6 [quiz: 934].
12. Buscarini E, Lisi SD, Arcidiacono PG, et al. Endoscopic ultrasonography findings in autoimmune pancreatitis. World J Gastroenterol 2011;17:2080–5.
13. De Lisi S, Buscarini E, Arcidiacono PG, et al. Endoscopic ultrasonography findings in autoimmune pancreatitis: be aware of the ambiguous features and look for the pivotal ones. JOP 2010;11:78–84.
14. Farrell JJ, Garber J, Sahani D, et al. EUS findings in patients with autoimmune pancreatitis. Gastrointest Endosc 2004;60:927–36.
15. Hoki N, Mizuno N, Sawaki A, et al. Diagnosis of autoimmune pancreatitis using endoscopic ultrasonography. J Gastroenterol 2009;44:154–9.
16. Okabe Y, Ishida Y, Kaji R, et al. Endoscopic ultrasonographic study of autoimmune pancreatitis and the effect of steroid therapy. J Hepatobiliary Pancreat Sci 2012;19:266–73.
17. Koyama R, Imamura T, Okuda C, et al. Ultrasonographic imaging of bile duct lesions in autoimmune pancreatitis. Pancreas 2008;37:259–64.
18. Fusaroli P, Saftoiu A, Mancino MG, et al. Techniques of image enhancement in EUS (with videos). Gastrointest Endosc 2011;74:645–55.
19. Dietrich CF, Hirche TO, Ott M, et al. Real-time tissue elastography in the diagnosis of autoimmune pancreatitis. Endoscopy 2009;41:718–20.

20. Hocke M, Ignee A, Dietrich CF. Contrast-enhanced endoscopic ultrasound in the diagnosis of autoimmune pancreatitis. Endoscopy 2011;43:163–5.

21. Kobayashi G, Fujita N, Noda Y, et al. Vascular image in autoimmune pancreatitis by contrast-enhanced color-Doppler endoscopic ultrasonography: comparison with pancreatic cancer. Endosc Ultrasound 2014;3:S13.

22. Imazu H, Kanazawa K, Mori N, et al. Novel quantitative perfusion analysis with contrast-enhanced harmonic EUS for differentiation of autoimmune pancreatitis from pancreatic carcinoma. Scand J Gastroenterol 2012;47:853–60.

23. Chari ST, Kloeppel G, Zhang L, et al. Histopathologic and clinical subtypes of autoimmune pancreatitis: the Honolulu consensus document. Pancreas 2010; 39:549–54.

24. Deshpande V, Mino-Kenudson M, Brugge WR, et al. Endoscopic ultrasound guided fine needle aspiration biopsy of autoimmune pancreatitis: diagnostic criteria and pitfalls. Am J Surg Pathol 2005;29:1464–71.

25. Kanno A, Ishida K, Hamada S, et al. Diagnosis of autoimmune pancreatitis by EUS-FNA by using a 22-gauge needle based on the International Consensus Diagnostic Criteria. Gastrointest Endosc 2012;76:594–602.

26. Mizuno N, Bhatia V, Hosoda W, et al. Histological diagnosis of autoimmune pancreatitis using EUS-guided trucut biopsy: a comparison study with EUS-FNA. J Gastroenterol 2009;44:742–50.

27. Ishikawa T, Itoh A, Kawashima H, et al. Endoscopic ultrasound-guided fine needle aspiration in the differentiation of type 1 and type 2 autoimmune pancreatitis. World J Gastroenterol 2012;18:3883–8.

28. Majumder S, Chari ST. EUS-guided FNA for diagnosing autoimmune pancreatitis: does it enhance existing consensus criteria? Gastrointest Endosc 2016;84:805–7.

29. Iwashita T, Yasuda I, Doi S, et al. Use of samples from endoscopic ultrasound-guided 19-gauge fine-needle aspiration in diagnosis of autoimmune pancreatitis. Clin Gastroenterol Hepatol 2012;10:316–22.

30. Kanno A, Masamune A, Fujishima F, et al. Diagnosis of autoimmune pancreatitis by EUS-guided FNA using a 22-gauge needle: a prospective multicenter study. Gastrointest Endosc 2016;84:797–804.e1.

31. Morishima T, Kawashima H, Ohno E, et al. Prospective multicenter study on the usefulness of EUS-guided FNA biopsy for the diagnosis of autoimmune pancreatitis. Gastrointest Endosc 2016;84:241–8.

32. Moon SH, Kim MH. The role of endoscopy in the diagnosis of autoimmune pancreatitis. Gastrointest Endosc 2012;76:645–56.

33. Naitoh I, Nakazawa T, Hayashi K, et al. Clinical differences between mass-forming autoimmune pancreatitis and pancreatic cancer. Scand J Gastroenterol 2012;47:607–13.

34. Takuma K, Kamisawa T, Gopalakrishna R, et al. Strategy to differentiate autoimmune pancreatitis from pancreas cancer. World J Gastroenterol 2012;18:1015–20.

35. Chen J, Yang R, Lu Y, et al. Diagnostic accuracy of endoscopic ultrasound-guided fine-needle aspiration for solid pancreatic lesion: a systematic review. J Cancer Res Clin Oncol 2012;138:1433–41.

36. Eloubeidi MA, Tamhane A. EUS-guided FNA of solid pancreatic masses: a learning curve with 300 consecutive procedures. Gastrointest Endosc 2005;61:700–8.

37. Mitsuhashi T, Ghafari S, Chang CY, et al. Endoscopic ultrasound-guided fine needle aspiration of the pancreas: cytomorphological evaluation with emphasis on

adequacy assessment, diagnostic criteria and contamination from the gastrointestinal tract. Cytopathology 2006;17:34–41.
38. Turner BG, Cizginer S, Agarwal D, et al. Diagnosis of pancreatic neoplasia with EUS and FNA: a report of accuracy. Gastrointest Endosc 2010;71:91–8.
39. Voss M, Hammel P, Molas G, et al. Value of endoscopic ultrasound guided fine needle aspiration biopsy in the diagnosis of solid pancreatic masses. Gut 2000;46:244–9.
40. Ball AB, Fisher C, Pittam M, et al. Diagnosis of soft tissue tumours by Tru-Cut biopsy. Br J Surg 1990;77:756–8.
41. Brandt KR, Charboneau JW, Stephens DH, et al. CT- and US-guided biopsy of the pancreas. Radiology 1993;187:99–104.
42. Harrison BD, Thorpe RS, Kitchener PG, et al. Percutaneous Trucut lung biopsy in the diagnosis of localised pulmonary lesions. Thorax 1984;39:493–9.
43. Ingram DM, Sheiner HJ, Shilkin KB. Operative biopsy of the pancreas using the Trucut needle. Aust N Z J Surg 1978;48:203–6.
44. Kovalik EC, Schwab SJ, Gunnells JC, et al. No change in complication rate using spring-loaded gun compared to traditional percutaneous renal allograft biopsy techniques. Clin Nephrol 1996;45:383–5.
45. Lavelle MA, O'Toole A. Trucut biopsy of the prostate. Br J Urol 1994;73:600.
46. Piccinino F, Sagnelli E, Pasquale G, et al. Complications following percutaneous liver biopsy. A multicentre retrospective study on 68,276 biopsies. J Hepatol 1986;2:165–73.
47. Welch TJ, Sheedy PF 2nd, Johnson CD, et al. CT-guided biopsy: prospective analysis of 1,000 procedures. Radiology 1989;171:493–6.
48. Suda K, Takase M, Fukumura Y, et al. Histopathologic characteristics of autoimmune pancreatitis based on comparison with chronic pancreatitis. Pancreas 2005;30:355–8.
49. Fujii LL, Chari ST, El-Youssef M, et al. Pediatric pancreatic EUS-guided trucut biopsy for evaluation of autoimmune pancreatitis. Gastrointest Endosc 2013;77: 824–8.
50. Levy MJ, Reddy RP, Wiersema MJ, et al. EUS-guided trucut biopsy in establishing autoimmune pancreatitis as the cause of obstructive jaundice. Gastrointest Endosc 2005;61:467–72.
51. Kerdsirichairat T, Saini SD, Chamberlain PR, et al. Autoimmune pancreatitis diagnosed with core biopsy obtained from a novel fork-tip EUS needle. ACG Case Rep J 2017;4:e7.

Recent Advances in Therapeutic Endosonography for Cancer Treatment

Saurabh Mukewar, MD,
Venkataraman Raman Muthusamy, MD, MAS*

KEYWORDS

• EUS oncotherapy • Brachytherapy • Celiac plexus neurolysis • Tumor ablation

KEY POINTS

• Several novel EUS guided applications in cancer have emerged over the last three decades
• EUS guided fiducial marker placement is safe and can aid in stereotactic radiation therapy
• EUS guided tumor ablations has potential for palliation of locally advanced malignancies
• EUS guided anti-tumor injections are promising, however randomized trials have not shown survival benefit
• EUS guided CPN is safe and quite effective for pain control in cancer patients

INTRODUCTION

Traditionally, endosonography (EUS) has played an important role in evaluation of gastrointestinal malignancies such as esophageal, gastric, pancreatic, and rectal cancers. Although EUS-guided tissue acquisition via fine needle aspiration or fine needle biopsy is still essential in cancer diagnosis, the staging of gastrointestinal malignancies with EUS may become less relevant with the increased use of neoadjuvant chemoradiation therapy and advancements in radiologic imaging. Over the last 2 decades, some novel applications of therapeutic EUS in management of cancers have been demonstrated (**Table 1**). These include fiducial marker placement to aid in targeted radiation therapy; direct brachytherapy with placement of radioactive seeds in tumors; tumor ablation for palliation; intratumoral injection of modified viruses, immunogenic cells,

Disclosure: No commercial or financial conflict of interest (Dr S. Mukewar). Consultant for Boston Scientific and Medtronic (COVB2710467/ IRB#15-000626 / NCT02395471); Research Support from Medtronic (Dr V.R. Muthusamy).
The Vatche and Tamar Manoukian Division of Digestive Diseases, David Geffen School of Medicine at UCLA, 200 UCLA Medical Plaza, Room 330-37, Los Angeles, CA 90095, USA
* Corresponding author. 200 UCLA Medical Plaza, Room 330-37, Los Angeles, CA 90095.
E-mail address: raman@mednet.ucla.edu

Table 1
Summary of endosonography-guided interventions in oncology

Therapy	Types
Radiotherapy	Fiducial marker placement
	Brachytherapy
Tissue ablation	Radiofrequency ablation
	Photodynamic therapy
	Laser therapy
	Alcohol ablation
Antitumor injections	Immunotherapy
	Gene therapy
	Chemotherapy
Celiac plexus neurolysis	Celiac plexus injection
	Brachytherapy

and drugs; and chemical neurolysis of the celiac ganglion. The following review discusses each of these applications, highlighting key studies and relevant findings.

ENDOSONOGRAPHY-GUIDED FIDUCIAL MARKER PLACEMENT AND BRACHYTHERAPY
Endosonography-Guided Fiducial Marker Placement

Imaging-guided stereotactic radiotherapy has distinct advantages over traditional radiotherapy, with the ability to deliver large doses of radiation accurately at the site of malignancy while avoiding radiation to surrounding structures. To precisely localize the site of malignancy, fiducial markers are placed within the tumor. These markers are radiographically visible and can be tracked with respiratory movements during radiotherapy. Fiducial marker placement was traditionally performed via a surgical or percutaneous technique. However, surgery is highly invasive and has been associated with a variety of adverse events (AEs) and the percutaneous route, although safe, is limited to percutaneously accessible tumors. Pishvaian and colleagues[1] described a novel approach for placement of fiducial markers via EUS in a series of 13 patients with various intraabdominal and intrathoracic malignancies. Since this initial description, various centers have reported their experiences.[2–6]

Two types of markers are commercially available: (1) standard fiducials are gold seeds measuring 3 or 5 mm in length and 0.8 to 1.2 mm in diameter, and (2) Visicoil fiducials are gold coils measuring 10 mm in length and 0.35 mm in diameter (Core Oncology, Santa Barbara, CA). The standard fiducials require a 19-G needle for placement. This needle size can be challenging in anatomically difficult locations where the scope may need to be torqued, such as the uncinate process of the pancreas. Additionally, the larger 19-G needle may not be able to traverse a firm tumor mass. The newer Visicoil fiducials can be placed via a 22-G needle, which is technically less challenging compared with traditional fiducials placed via 19-G needles. However, a recent study[4] compared the 2 types of fiducials and interestingly found no difference in placement success rates or rates of migration. The visibility of standard fiducials was better than Visicoil fiducials.

Fiducials can be loaded on an EUS needle either by a "front-loading" or "back-loading" technique. The front-loading technique involves advancing the needle tip into the tumor, removing the stylet, manually loading the fiducials in the needle lumen, reinserting the stylet in the needle channel, and then advancing the stylet with deployment of fiducials in the target tissue (**Fig. 1**). One study[1] reported kinking or resistance while attempting to advance the stylet with fiducials, although another study did not.[2] The back-loading technique involves inserting the fiducials into the needle tip with the

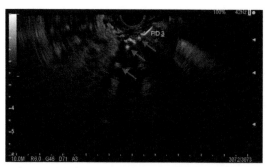

Fig. 1. Endosonography-guided fiducial placement. Three fiducials are seen (*red arrows*) within a hypoechoic mass previously determined to be pancreatic adenocarcinoma.

stylet slightly withdrawn followed by insertion of bone wax at the tip to keep them in place. The needle tip is then advanced into the tumor and the stylet advanced with deployment of markers. Although resistance is not encountered while placing these markers, there is a risk of needle tip injury while loading the fiducials onto an exposed needle tip. An alternative hydrostatic technique has been described by Park and colleagues,[5] in which saline is flushed in the needle lumen to deploy the fiducials instead of using a stylet, thus avoiding some of the difficulties encountered in stylet advancement owing to scope angulation. The number of fiducials placed depends on the endoscopists' preference as well as the size and location of the tumor. Generally, 2 to 6 markers are placed at the margins of the tumor (see **Fig. 1**). Other novel applications of EUS-guided marking include placement of fiducials in pancreatic neuroendocrine tumors and tattooing pancreas masses to aid in their resection.[7,8]

EUS-guided placement of fiducials is successful in 85% to 100% of cases.[1–6,9] Failures are typically owing to an inability to advance the scope to access the tumor,[1] lack of adequate lesion visualization,[6] the presence of intervening blood vessels,[6] and an inability to advance the needle into the tumor secondary to desmoplastic reaction with a firm tumor wall.[5] After successful fiducial placement, migration can occur owing to tumor treatment and inflammation in 0% to 16% of cases.[1,6,9] Fiducial placement is generally safe and AEs are rare. Out of nearly 850 cases reported in literature, fewer than 1% developed significant AEs such as cholangitis, pancreatitis, mediastinitis, or pneumothorax.[3] Minor bleeding is the most common complication and has been reported in about 1% of patients.[3]

Endosonography-Guided Brachytherapy

Interstitial brachytherapy is an effective method for the locoregional control of tumors. The procedure involves placement of radioactive seeds in the target tissue resulting in tissue exposure to gamma rays, which produce radiation over a short distance causing localized tissue injury and tumor ablation. The technique for seed placement is similar to that used for fiducial placement.

After initial demonstration of the feasibility and safety of EUS-guided brachytherapy in a porcine pancreas,[10] a few authors have studied its application in advanced unresectable cancer patients.[11–13] Nearly 60% to 80% patients had stable disease or partial clinical response after EUS-guided brachytherapy. Interestingly, response to pain was observed in 30% of patients in 1 study.[13] However, this was short lived. Few AEs were reported. In 1 study, pancreatitis (20%) and pseudocyst (14%) were observed, whereas in another study, postprocedure infection (50%) was seen, which resolved with antibiotics. Although these studies have shown promising results, they were limited by a small number of subjects and the lack of a control group. Larger controlled studies are needed to determine the precise role of EUS-guided brachytherapy in cancer management. In addition, EUS-guided brachytherapy has also shown to be effective for celiac plexus neurolysis (CPN) and ablation of metastatic lymph nodes.[14,15]

ENDOSONOGRAPHY-GUIDED TUMOR ABLATION

Various EUS-guided tumor ablation therapies have been demonstrated (**Table 2**).

Endosonography-Guided Radiofrequency Ablation

Radiofrequency ablation (RFA) involves local tissue injury secondary to heat generated from application of a medium frequency alternating current. In the first porcine study, a modified 19-G needle tip electrode was used to perform EUS-guided RFA. This resulted in smaller area of necrosis (8–12 mm). Although this study demonstrated feasibility of this technique, multiple AEs such as gastric and intestinal burns (31%) and pancreatic fluid collection (8%) were reported. Subsequent reports of RFA via laparotomy in humans for pancreatic tissue raised concerns of developing local AEs, such as portal vein thrombosis, duodenal bleeding, and necrotizing pancreatitis secondary to thermal injury to surrounding normal tissues.[16–18] To prevent such AEs, new applicator devices have been developed. First, a new flexible cryotherm probe was developed, which combines RFA with cryotherapy. The application of a probe led to successful coagulation necrosis in a porcine study, with fewer AEs.[19] In a subsequent human study, although successful coagulation was achieved in all the patients who underwent RFA, the probe could not be advanced into the tumor in almost one-third of patients owing to tumor stiffness.[20] None of the patients developed any AE. Second, a modified 19-G needle fitted with an umbrella-shaped monopolar electrode array at its tip was created. The large size and design of the electrode led to a large area of necrosis (>2 cm) and prevented gastric or intestinal burns in a porcine study.[21] In another recent study, a monopolar EUS-guided RFA catheter showed feasibility for ablation of pancreatic neuroendocrine tumors in 2 cases.[22]

Endosonography-Guided Photodynamic Therapy

Photodynamic therapy (PDT) involves systemic injection of a photosensitizing agent, which is taken up by various organs. Subsequently, when the desired tissues are exposed to light of the appropriate wavelength, the photosensitizer is activated and interacts with oxygen to form reactive oxygen species that lead to cell apoptosis. Studies have shown that pancreatic tissue avidly uptakes the photosensitizing agent, making the pancreas a potential target for ablation with PDT. A porcine study of EUS-guided PDT with porfimer sodium demonstrated complete necrosis in 100% of pancreas tissue compared with 22.5% of liver tissue.[23] Of note, porfimer sodium has a long half-life (21 days) and, therefore, a higher potential risk of photosensitivity. Recently Verteprofin, a photosensitizer with a shorter half-life (5 hours), was studied in a porcine model.[24] Six pigs underwent EUS-guided PDT of the tail of the pancreas. Tissue necrosis was seen in all the animals, which was greater with increasing light dosimetry. In the only human study of EUS-guided PDT, successful necrosis and stable tumor burden was seen in all 4 patients with advanced pancreaticobiliary malignancies (2 caudate lobe, 1 distal common bile duct, and 1 tail of pancreas).[25] A second generation photosensitizing agent (Photolon) with short half-life was used for this study. There were no procedure-related AEs. Tumor burden remained stable in all patients at a median follow-up of 5 months.

Table 2
Summary of studies describing endosonography-guided ablation

Study	Humans/Animals	Design	Tissue	n	Intervention	Additional Therapy	Outcome	Median Survival	Adverse Events
Brachytherapy									
	Pigs	Case series	Pancreas	6	Radioactive I-125 seeds	None	3.8-cm necrotic cavity with fibrosis	N/A	Hyperamylesemia (n = 1)
Sun et al,[10] 2005	Humans	Case series	Pancreas cancer	15	Radioactive I-125 seeds	None	Partial response (27%), minimal response (20%), stable disease (33%)	10.6 mo (range, 4.2–25)	Pancreatitis (n = 3), PFC (n = 2)
Jin et al,[11] 2008	Humans	Case series	Pancreas cancer	22	Radioactive I-125 seeds	Chemotherapy (gemcitabine)	Partial response (13%), stable disease (45%)	9 mo (range, 6.7–11.3)	Postprocedure infection (n = 11), resolved with antibiotics
Sun et al,[12] 2012	Humans	Case series	Pancreas cancer	8	Radioactive I-125 seeds	Chemotherapy (gemcitabine)	Partial response (12.5%), minimal response (25%), stable disease (37.5%)	8.3 mo (range, 5.2–11.4)	None
Radiofrequency ablation									
Goldberg et al,[80] 1999	Pigs	Case series	Pancreas	13	Modified 19-G needle electrode	None	8–12 mm necrotic cavity	N/A	Gastric or intestinal burns (n = 4), pancreatitis, PFC (n = 1)
Carrara et al,[19] 2008	Pigs	Case series	Pancreas	14	Cryotherm probe	None	Increasing size of necrosis with duration of application	N/A	Adhesions between pancreas and intestine (n = 4), pancreatitis (n = 1), gastric burn (n = 1)

(continued on next page)

Table 2
(continued)

Study	Humans/Animals	Design	Tissue	n	Intervention	Additional Therapy	Outcome	Median Survival	Adverse Events
Varadarajulu et al,[21] 2009	Pigs	Case series	Liver	5	Modified 19-G needle with an umbrella-shaped electrode array	None	A 2.6-cm focus of coagulation necrosis	N/A	None
Arcidiacono et al,[20] 2012	Humans	Case series	Pancreas cancer	22	Cryotherm probe	None	Necrosis, maximum diameter, range 20–54 mm	6 mo	PFC (n = 1)
Pai et al,[22] 2015	Humans	Case series	Pancreatic neuroendocrine tumor	2	Monopolar RF catheter	None	Change in vascularity (n = 1), necrosis (n = 1)	N/A	None
Photodynamic therapy									
Chan et al,[23] 2004	Pigs	Case series	Liver, pancreas, kidney, spleen	3	Photodynamic therapy (Porfimer sodium)	None	Extent of complete necrosis: liver (22.5%), kidney (31%), spleen (67%), pancreas (100%)	N/A	None
Yusuf et al,[24] 2008	Pigs	Case series	Pancreas	6	Photodynamic therapy (Verteprofin): increasing light dosimetry	None	Necrosis, mean diameter of 6.6 mm (10 min), 9.4 mm (15 min), 26.3 mm (20 min)	N/A	None
Choi et al,[25] 2015	Humans	Case series	Pancreaticobiliary malignancies	4	Photodynamic therapy (Photolon)	None	Necrosis, median volume: 4.0 cm^3 (range, 0.7–11.3)	Stable tumor burden at 6 mo	None

Laser therapy									
Di Matteo et al,[28] 2010	Pigs	Case series	Pancreas	6	Nd:YAG laser	None	Necrosis area: 49–80 mm^2	N/A	None
diMatteo et al,[29] 2011	Humans	Case report	Hepatocellular carcinoma	1	Nd:YAG laser	None	Successful ablation at 2 mo	N/A	None
Alcohol ablation									
Aslanian et al,[31] 2005	Pigs	Case series	Pancreas	8	50% ethanol (n = 4), 98% ethanol (n = 4)	None	Necrosis, diameter: 2–8 mm (50% ethanol); 8–30 mm (98% ethanol)	N/A	98% alcohol: 4/4 pancreatitis, 1 fluid collection, 1 colonic stricture
Matthes et al,[32] 2007	Pigs	Case series	Pancreas	6	0%–100% ethanol	None	Increasing necrosis size from 40% to 100% ethanol	N/A	None
Paik et al,[38] 2016	Humans	Case series	Pancreatic neuroendocrine tumors (n = 6), pseudopapillary neoplasms (n = 2)	8	99% ethanol	None	Successful tumor ablation (75%)	N/A	1/8: acute pancreatitis - received 5 mL of alcohol
Park et al,[39] 2015	Humans	Case series	Pancreatic neuroendocrine tumor (n = 14)	11	98% ethanol	None	Successful tumor ablation (53.8% - one session; 61.5% - multiple sessions)	N/A	3/11: mild acute pancreatitis - all received >2 mL of alcohol

Abbreviations: N/A, not applicable; PFC, pancreatic fluid collection; RF, radiofrequency.

Endosonography-Guided Laser Therapy

Percutaneous laser therapy with a neodymium:yttrium aluminum garnet (Nd:YAG) laser for the ablation of neoplastic lesions was described initially for hepatocellular carcinoma and metastases to the liver via imaging guidance.[26,27] Laser-guided ablation offers the advantage of precise targeting of malignant tissue. In a porcine study, 6 swine pigs underwent successful application of EUS-guided laser ablation with no AEs.[28] In a subsequent case report by di Matteo and colleagues,[29] a patient with unresectable hepatocellular carcinoma who had failed embolization attempts underwent EUS-guided laser ablation successfully without any AEs. At 2 months after the procedure, computed tomography demonstrated successful ablation without any recurrence.

Endosonography-Guided Alcohol Ablation

Ultrasound-guided percutaneous ethanol ablation for hepatocellular malignancy was described initially in 1986.[30] Since its initial description, this procedure has been widely performed for liver masses. In a porcine study for EUS-guided alcohol ablation,[31] successful necrosis was seen in all the pigs receiving an intermediate (50%) and a high concentration (98%) of alcohol. However, pancreatitis was observed in the pigs, which received a high concentration (98%) of alcohol. In a follow-up study, increasing concentrations of alcohol from 0% to 100% were used in 6 pigs.[32] Although no pancreatitis was observed in any of the pigs, those receiving 0% and 20% did not have any tissue necrosis. The area of necrosis progressively increased with increasing concentrations of alcohol ranging from 40% to 100%.

In the first human case, hepatic metastases were ablated successfully with multiple sessions of EUS-guided injection of 98% alcohol.[33] The patient had no AEs from the procedure. Since this initial report, the procedure has been successfully performed in patients with a gastrointestinal stromal tumor,[34] insulinoma,[35] hepatocellular carcinoma,[36] and pancreatic neuroendocrine tumor.[37] Two recent series[38,39] have demonstrated successful EUS-guided alcohol ablation of small pancreatic neoplasms. Response rates from 54% to 75% were observed. A minority of patients developed recurrence, which was managed successfully with retreatment. Acute pancreatitis was observed in 10% to 30% of patients after the procedure. Interestingly, all these patients had received more than 2 mL of alcohol.

In summary, EUS-guided ethanol ablation seems to be a safe, affordable, and effective option for the treatment of small pancreatic neoplasms and hepatic masses. Multiple sessions may be required in some cases. Larger quantities (>2 mL) of high concentration (98%) alcohol seem to be associated with pancreatitis. The optimal dose and concentration of alcohol for EUS-guided injection needs to be determined.

ENDOSONOGRAPHY-GUIDED ANTITUMOR INJECTIONS

EUS-guided fine needle injection (EUS FNI) therapy offers the unique advantage of being able to deliver tumor directed therapies directly into the tumor (**Fig. 2**). Various therapies have been attempted, including immunotherapy with lymphocytic cells or dendritic cells, gene therapy with injection of mutated virus or DNA plasmid, and the injection of chemotherapeutic agents with polymers for local sustained drug delivery (**Table 3**).

Immunotherapy

The first study of EUS FNI in humans was performed by Chang and colleagues[40] in 2000. Eight patients with advanced unresectable pancreatic cancer underwent immunotherapy with injection of "cytoimplant," an allogeneic mixed lymphocytic culture. The rationale for injecting lymphocytic culture was that the lymphocyte-induced

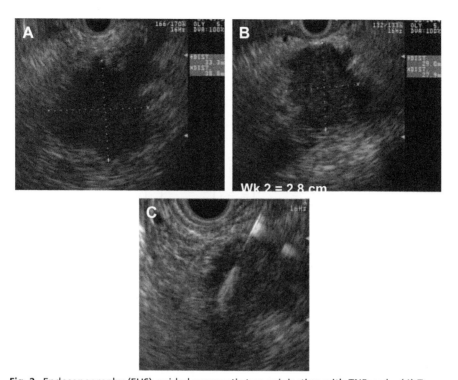

Fig. 2. Endosonography (EUS)-guided pancreatic tumor injection with TNFerade. (*A*) Tumor size is 3.9 cm at baseline (week 1) before treatment with EUS-guided gene therapy. (*B*) Tumor size has decreased to 2.8 cm after 1 week. (*C*) One month after completing treatment, the tumor size had decreased to 1.8 cm and a fine needle aspiration performed at that time was negative for malignancy. No residual tumor was found at the time of surgical resection. (*From* Chang KJ, Lee JG, Holcombe RF, et al. Endoscopic ultrasound delivery of an antitumor agent to treat a case of pancreatic cancer. Nat Clin Pract Gastroenterol Hepatol 2008;5(2):107–11; with permission.)

cytokine production could lead to activation of antitumor effector cells within tumors and result in tumor regression. Two patients had a partial tumor response and 1 had a minor response, with an overall median survival of 13.2 months. There were no procedure-related AEs. However, 7 of 8 patients developed fever, which resolved with acetaminophen. Although the response was modest in this study, it paved the way for future studies with EUS FNI therapies.

Additional pilot studies have described EUS FNI immunotherapies. In 1 study,[41] patients with advanced pancreatic cancer underwent immunotherapy with EUS FNI of dendritic cells. The authors hypothesized that, by injecting immature dendritic cells into the tumor, the cells will be exposed to tumor antigens, migrate to regional lymph nodes, present these antigens to local lymphocytes, and induce a strong tumor-directed immune response. Patients who had failed prior chemotherapy with gemcitabine were included. Stable disease or response was seen in almost one-half of the study subjects. In another similar study, patients with unresectable pancreatic cancer underwent EUS FNI with OK-432–primed dendritic cells.[42] To increase antigen exposure, all patients received gemcitabine before undergoing EUS FNI. In addition, they also received intravenous infusion of lymphokine-activated killer cells stimulated with anti-CD3 monoclonal antibody. Nearly 60% had stable disease or showed a response.

Table 3
Summary of studies describing endosonography-guided antitumor injection

Study	Humans/Animals	Design	Cancer	n	Intervention	Additional Therapy	Outcome/Comment	Survival	Adverse Events (Procedure Related, Grade ≥3)
Immunotherapy									
Chang et al,[40] 2000	Humans	Case series	Pancreatic cancer	8	Mixed lymphocytic culture (Cytoimplant)	None	Partial response (25%), minor response (12.5%)	13.2 mo (median)	Grade 3 GI toxicity (n = 3), fever responding to acetaminophen (n = 7)
Irisawa et al,[41] 2007	Humans	Case series	Pancreatic cancer	7	Immature dendritic cells	None	Stable response (28.6%); mixed response (28.6%)	9.9 mo (median)	None
Hirooka et al,[42] 2009	Humans	Case series	Pancreatic cancer	5	OK-432 primed dendritic cells	Gemcitabine, lymphocyte activated killer cells	Partial response (20%); stable disease (40%)	15.9 mo (median)	None
Gene therapy									
Hecht et al,[43] 2003	Humans	Case series	Pancreatic cancer	21	Mutated adenovirus (ONYX15)	Gemcitabine	Partial response (9.5%), minor response (9.5%); stable disease (28.6%)	7.5 mo (median)	Sepsis (n = 2), duodenal perforation (n = 2)
Citrin et al,[48] 2010	Humans	Case series	Rectal cancer	9	Mutated adenovirus (TNFerade)	Capecitabine, radiation	Rectal cancer regression grade 1 (n = 7), grade 2 (n = 2)	8/9 alive at 41.6 mo	Grade 3 hematologic toxicity (n = 2)

Chang et al,[47] 2012	Humans	Case series	Esophageal cancer	24	Mutated adenovirus (TNFerade)	Cisplatin and 5-FU, radiation	20 underwent esophagectomy, 6 had pathologic complete response	47.8 mo (median)	At a dose of 4 × 10^{11} PU, 5 of 8 patients experienced thromboembolic events
Hecht et al,[49] 2012	Humans	Case series	Pancreatic cancer	50	Mutated adenovirus (TNFerade)	5-FU, radiation	1 complete response; 7 partial or minor response; 12 stable disease	9.8 mo (median)	Cholangitis (n = 6), deep vein thrombosis (n = 6), GI bleeding (n = 6), pancreatitis (n = 2)
Herman et al,[50] 2013	Humans	Randomized controlled trial	Pancreatic cancer	304	Mutated adenovirus (TNFerade)	Cases (n = 187): TNFerade + neoadjuvant chemoradiation therapy; controls (n = 90): neoadjuvant chemoradiation therapy	Cases: Partial response (8.2%), stable disease (74.2%); Controls: Partial response (12%), stable disease (74%)	10 mo in both groups (P = .26); 6.8 mo (cases) vs 7 mo (controls; P = .51)	Grades 2-4 adverse events: 75.9% (cases) vs 65.6% (controls; P = .08)

Chemotherapy

Linghu et al,[52] 2005	Pigs	Case series	Pancreas	3	Paclitaxel (OncoGel) - 2 mL	N/A	A well-organized depot of OncoGel in pancreas tissue in all animals	N/A	None
Matthes et al,[32] 2007	Pigs	Case series	Pancreas	8	Paclitaxel (OncoGel) - 1, 2, 3, or 4 mL	N/A	On endosonography, a 2.1 ± 0.8 cm hyperechoic focus, on autopsy a 14.7 ± 5.0 mm depot was seen	N/A	None

(continued on next page)

Table 3
(continued)

Study	Humans/Animals	Design	Cancer	n	Intervention	Additional Therapy	Outcome/Comment	Survival	Adverse Events (Procedure Related, Grade ≥3)
DuVall et al,[53] 2009	Humans	Case series	Esophageal cancer	11	Paclitaxel (OncoGel)	Radiation	Partial response (18.2%); stable disease (54.5%)	N/A	Related to OncoGel (n = 5): anorexia (n = 3), nausea (n = 2), dysguesia (n = 2), esophageal pain (n = 2)
DeWitt et al,[54] 2016	Humans	Randomized, controlled trial	Esophageal cancer	137	Paclitaxel (OncoGel)	Cases: paclitaxel (OncoGel) + neoadjuvant chemoradiation therapy (n = 71); controls: neoadjuvant chemoradiation therapy (n = 65)	Pathologic complete response: cases 12.5% vs controls 26.2% (P = .046)	12-mo survival: cases, 67.8%, CI, 55.3–77.5 vs controls 68.8%, CI 55.4–78.9 (P = .41)	Grade 3 toxicity: cases 28% vs controls 17% (P = .15); grade 4 toxicity: cases 18% vs controls 15% (P = .82)
Levy et al	Humans	Case series	Pancreatic cancer	36	Gemcitabine	5-FU, radiation	Unresectable stage 3 disease: 20% were downstaged and underwent surgery	10.4 mo (median)	None

Abbreviations: 5-FU, 5-Fluorouracil; GI, gastrointestinal; N/A, not applicable.

Gene Therapy

Another novel EUS-guided treatment involves intratumoral injection of a replication deficient mutated virus. In the first such study, a mutated adenovirus (ONYX15) that replicates selectively and kills malignant cells was studied in patients with advanced pancreatic cancer.[43] Nearly one-half of patients had stable disease or showed some response. Interestingly, 2 of the 20 developed duodenal perforations. TNFerade is another replication deficient mutated adenovirus, which has been more extensively studied. Tumor necrosis factor (TNF)-α is a cytokine and has been shown to be cytotoxic to tumor cells.[44] In a prior study, systemic therapy with TNF-α for various malignancies resulted in severe toxicity, requiring discontinuation of therapy in a large proportion of study patients.[45] Thus, local delivery of TNF-α at the site of tumor is desirable. This was accomplished with the development of TNFerade virus that, when exposed to radiation or chemotherapy, expresses human TNF-α under control of the Egr-1 promoter. After an initial human study demonstrating feasibility and safety of TNFerade,[46] it has been described for various malignancies, including esophageal cancer, pancreas cancer, and rectal cancer.[47–50]

In a pilot study for locally advanced rectal cancer, EUS FNI with TNFerade in combination with neoadjuvant chemoradiation therapy was well-tolerated.[48] However, response rates were similar to prior results with neoadjuvant chemoradiation therapy. In comparison, a similar study with escalating doses of TNFerade in combination with neoadjuvant chemoradiation therapy for locally advanced esophageal cancer showed significantly greater response rates compared with historical controls.[47] However, those receiving higher doses experienced thromboembolic events requiring early termination of study. Nevertheless, the study demonstrated the safety of TNFerade at lower doses for the treatment of esophageal cancer along with an improvement in survival rates.

Two studies have evaluated the role of TNFerade for locally advanced pancreatic cancer. The first was a phase I and II study of 50 patients with locally advanced pancreatic cancer.[49] All the patients received chemotherapy (5-fluorourcil), radiation therapy, and weekly EUS FNI or percutaneous injections of TNFerade doses from 4×10^9 to 1×10^{12} PU for 5.5 weeks. The doses were well tolerated, except the 1×10^{12} PU dose, at which pancreatitis and cholangitis developed. One had a complete response, 7 had a partial or minor response, and 12 had stable disease on follow-up (see **Fig. 2**). The median survival was 9.8 months, which comparable with prior reports with chemoradiation. After this study, a large multicenter randomized controlled trial evaluated the role of TNFerade in combination with standard of care, that is, chemotherapy and radiation therapy versus standard of care alone.[50] The study did not show any difference in progression-free survival between the 2 groups. Those in the TNFerade arm experienced more grade I and II toxicities. Interestingly, on multivariate analysis, progression-free survival was inferior with EUS-guided FNI compared with percutaneous injections. This was felt to be secondary to an inability to penetrate the tumor capsule with injections during EUS and variability in endosonographer skills at the different study sites. Thus, TNFerade was safe but there was no survival benefit for locally advanced pancreatic cancer.

Although no firm conclusions can be drawn regarding the response rates given the small number of patients evaluated, these studies have demonstrated the feasibility of TNFerade as an additional therapy in the management of various gastrointestinal cancers. Unfortunately, the only randomized, controlled trial for pancreatic cancer did not show any survival benefit. The role of TNFerade in other gastrointestinal cancers needs to be further defined with additional large randomized controlled trials.

Chemotherapy

EUS-guided intratumoral injection of chemotherapeutic agents is aimed at increasing the local concentration of the drug. This procedure is appealing for the management of tumors such as pancreas cancer that have prominent desmoplastic reactions, which inhibit the ability of systemic chemotherapeutic agents to penetrate the tumor. EUS-guided FNI offers a minimally invasive method for delivery of these agents. Recently, in a study by Levy and colleagues,[51] patients with inoperable locally advanced pancreatic cancer underwent EUS-guided FNI of gemcitabine in combination with conventional therapy with 5-fluorouracil and radiation. Notably, 20% of patients with stage III unresectable cancer were downstaged and underwent R0 resection. None of the patients had any initial or delayed AEs. The study demonstrated the safety and feasibility of this form of therapy. Although the median survival did not seem to be significantly longer than historical subjects with similar stage disease, the ability to perform R0 resection in a fraction of initially inoperable cases is promising.

Over the last decade, biodegradable thermosensitive polymers have been developed that can be used for local sustained chemotherapeutic drug release in tumors. One such polymer is ReGel, which is aqueous at a high temperature (around 45°C) and is a solid gel at 37°C. In a porcine model, EUS-guided FNI of a combination of ReGel with paclitaxel (OncoGel) in the pancreas tail led to the formation of an Onco-Gel depot without any AEs.[52] In a follow-up study by the authors,[32] increasing volumes of OncoGel from 1 to 4 mL were injected in pancreas tail, which led to the formation of an OncoGel depot measuring about 1.5 cm in size, with some localized mild inflammation and sclerosis. Those that received 3 and 4 mL had high and sustained concentrations of the drug at a distance of 3 to 5 cm from the depot. Technical difficulties such as leakage of the highly viscous OncoGel were encountered during initial injections, necessitating placement of a pressure tube between the needle and the screw syringe. Accidental extrapancreatic injections in left kidney and colon were observed with 3 to 4 mL of OncoGel, without any clinical consequences.

Human studies of EUS-guided FNI with OncoGel were performed in locally advanced inoperable esophageal cancer.[53,54] In a phase II study, patients received increasing doses of Paclitaxel concentrations to achieve 0.48, 1.0, and 2.0 mg paclitaxel/cm^3 of tumor volume in the tumor and/or involved lymph nodes.[53] Most patients either had stable disease (55%) or partial response (18%) on follow-up. Systemic levels of paclitaxel were observed in all patients for 24 hours and for 3 weeks in 6 patients. Recently a large, multicenter randomized controlled trial compared a combination of EUS-guided FNI for OncoGel with neoadjuvant chemoradiation therapy versus neoadjuvant chemoradition therapy alone for locally advanced esophageal cancer.[54] The primary endpoint, namely, radiologic response by tumor volume, was not different between the 2 groups. Although the study was not powered for its secondary endpoints, the proportion of patients getting surgery, 12-month survival and AEs were not different between the 2 groups. Similar to observations with TNFerade, after promising initial studies, a subsequent randomized controlled trial failed to show any benefit in overall patient survival.

ENDOSONOGRAPHY-GUIDED CELIAC PLEXUS NEUROLYSIS

Patients with pancreatic cancer can develop abdominal pain secondary to perineural invasion by the cancer cells.[55] Treatment of this pain often requires narcotic pain medications, which can lead to opiate tolerance and side effects such as nausea, vomiting, and constipation. A nonopioid measure of controlling abdominal pain for such patients involves the injection of alcohol and a local anesthetic into the area of the celiac plexus to achieve a chemical ablation of the nerve tissue, termed CPN.

Rationale

Nociceptive stimuli from the head of the pancreas are transmitted by the splanchnic nerves to the celiac and superior mesenteric plexus, and from the body and tail of the pancreas to the celiac and splenic plexus.[55] The stimuli are then transmitted from these regions to the thalamus in the brain, where pain perception occurs. These nerve plexuses are composed of a dense network of nerves and ganglia interconnected with one another.[56] The celiac plexus is readily accessible for intervention via EUS owing to its location below and anterior to the diaphragm near the origin of celiac artery, at the level of L1 vertebra. It typically is composed of at least 2 to 5 ganglia located on either side of the origin of celiac artery, typically at the level of L1 vertebra.[56]

A percutaneous technique to block the transmission of celiac plexus impulses was described almost a century ago.[57] At present, this is performed either intraoperatively or via fluoroscopic, ultrasound, or computed tomography guidance. Because the celiac ganglia are not visualized directly via this approach, it has a higher risk of AEs owing to inadvertent injury to the diaphragm, nerve, or blood vessels. More recently, EUS-guided CPN was described by Wiersema and colleagues[58] in 1996. EUS CPN via the transgastric route offers the advantage of direct visualization of the ganglia while performing neurolysis. Patients with unresectable pancreatic cancer often have abdominal pain and are candidates for EUS CPN. For such patients, performing this procedure earlier at the time of diagnosis is recommended. In a recent randomized controlled trial, 96 patients randomized to either EUS CPN at the time of diagnosis or initial pain management with conventional medications.[59] Those with early EUS CPN had better pain scores and lower opioid requirements at 3 months compared with conventional pain management. Contraindications for performing EUS CPN include coagulopathy (International Normalized Ratio >1.6), thrombocytopenia (platelet count <50,000/μL), or use of anticoagulants or antiplatelet agents. The procedure may also not be feasible in those with a distorted anatomy secondary to a large tumor mass, bulky lymphadenopathy, or in those with an anomalous celiac artery origin.

Technique

The procedure is generally performed in the outpatient setting. After obtaining consent, the patient is placed in the left lateral decubitus position. Under continuous monitoring of respiration, oxygen saturation, blood pressure, and heart rate, the patient is typically sedated with moderate sedation or monitored anesthesia care. The linear echoendoscope is advanced into the esophagus and rotated to identify the aorta via a sagittal view (**Fig. 3**). The scope is advanced further to identify the celiac trunk arising from the aorta below the level of diaphragm. The celiac ganglion can sometimes be identified as distinct hypoechoic structures. The right ganglion is typically located 6 mm inferior to the origin of the celiac artery, whereas the left ganglion is usually located 9 mm inferior to the artery's origin.[56] At our institution, we use a standard 22-G EUS fine needle aspiration needle for the injection. However, a larger gauge needle may be used (19 G). The needle is prepared by removing the stylet and flushing with active drug (bupivacaine/alcohol). A 5-mL syringe with the active drug is attached to the hub of the needle. The EUS needle assembly is then loaded onto the biopsy channel of the scope. The needle tip is advanced across the posterior gastric wall

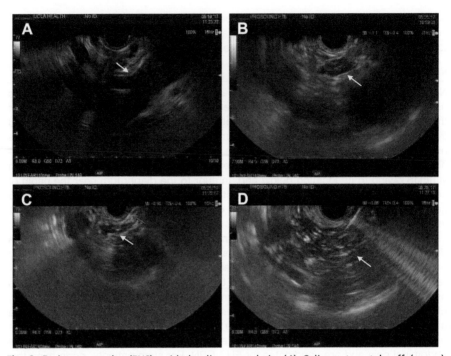

Fig. 3. Endosonography (EUS)-guided celiac neurolysis. (*A*) Celiac artery takeoff (*arrow*) from the aorta with adrenal gland seen. (*B*) A celiac ganglion is visualized (*arrow*). (*C*) EUS-guided needle injection (*red arrow*) into the celiac ganglion (*yellow arrow*). (*D*) Image after injection showing depot of injectate (*arrow*) with hyperechoic foci consistent with air.

into this space near the origin of celiac artery. Aspiration is performed to ensure that the needle is not in a vessel. At our institution, an injection of 20 mL of a 70:30 mix (by volume) of 0.25% bupivacaine and 98% alcohol is performed, although the volume and composition of the injectate varies widely. Resistance should be encountered while injecting in the space, because a lack of resistance would suggest intravascular or intraluminal injection. Bupivacaine is injected to avoid the discomfort that may occur owing to alcohol injection. After injection, an echogenic cloud typically forms at the site of injection (see **Fig. 3**).

New Techniques and Variations

Several variations to this technique have been described. Some authors have recommended a single injection centrally at the base of celiac trunk, which is referred to as a central method.[60–62] Others have recommended a bilateral technique, where the injection is performed on both sides of the celiac artery.[63,64] For bilateral injection, the scope is rotated slightly, such that the origin of celiac artery is not visualized but the aorta can be seen in sagittal view. The injection is performed in the standard fashion as described on one side of celiac trunk and repeated on the other side. Levy and colleagues[65,66] have suggested injecting preferentially into the ganglia, which can be visualized in 60% to 90% of patients. The authors recommend advancing the needle tip into the center of small ganglia (<1 cm) and injecting the agent or by advancing the needle into the deepest point of large ganglia (>1 cm) and slowly withdrawing the needle while injecting the agents. More recently, an additional injection with a 25-G needle into the superior mesenteric plexus near the origin of superior mesenteric artery has been described, termed as broad plexus neurolysis (BPN).[67] An alternate to the standard 22-G EUS fine needle aspiration needle is a needle specifically designed for CPN, the EchoTip needle by Wilson Cook Medical (Winston Salem, NC).[68] This needle does not have a stylet. It is a 20-G needle with a solid, sharp, conical tip and multiple side holes for radial delivery of the agent. However, this instrument is not available in all countries.

Adverse Events

EUS CPN is a safe procedure and AEs are infrequent. In a recent review of 661 patients undergoing CPN, AEs were reported in 21% of the patients.[69] Almost all were minor AEs: diarrhea (10%), transient hypotension (5%), exacerbation of pain (4%), and others (2%). The AEs lasted for less than 48 hours, and almost always less than 2 weeks. Diarrhea was generally mild and controlled with antidiarrheals. The hypotension was transient and responded to intravenous fluids. These AEs are felt to occur secondary to blockade of sympathetic nerves in the celiac ganglia. Major AEs are rare and were seen in 8 of 661 patients (0.2%): 4 developed ischemia to intraabdominal organs, 2 developed paraplegia, 1 had a retroperitoneal abscess, and 1 developed retroperitoneal bleeding. Two of these 8 patients died secondary to their AE (ischemia).

Effectiveness

Pain improvement has been shown in 65% to 94% of patients undergoing EUS CPN.[58,61–64,67,70–73] The high variability is likely owing to heterogeneity in studies with regard to study design, definition of pain relief, follow-up time after injection, type of procedure, and the amount of neurolytic agent injected (**Table 4**). Few studies have compared unilateral CPN with bilateral CPN. A retrospective study, which included patients with pancreatic cancer and chronic patients with pancreatitis, showed superior pain relief in those undergoing bilateral CPN.[62] Shortcomings of this study included its retrospective nature and that follow-up was performed just 1 week after CPN. However, 2 recent prospective studies have shown no difference in pain relief in those undergoing bilateral CPN versus unilateral CPN.[61,74] Although these studies were prospective with longer follow-up, they included a smaller number of patients compared with the retrospective study. Therefore, it is possible that the studies were underpowered to detect a small difference between the 2 groups.

On EUS, the celiac ganglia appeared as hypoechoic, oblong or comma-shaped structures often containing a hyperechoic focus or strand near the celiac artery.[75,76] In a large series of patients undergoing EUS, the ganglia were visualized in 81% of the patients.[65] Intuitively, it was felt that EUS-guided injection of the celiac ganglia with the neurolytic agent (CGN) would perhaps lead to a higher response rate than nontargeted injection near the celiac artery. In the initial study, 94% of patients with pancreatic cancer reported pain relief with EUS CGN.[66] Subsequently comparative studies of EUS CGN versus bilateral or central EUS CPN have consistently shown superior pain relief in those undergoing EUS CGN.[63,70]

In a further modification of the EUS CPN technique, EUS-guided BPN was described to target not only the celiac plexus, but also the superior and inferior mesenteric plexus.[67] The efficacy of EUS BPN was superior to EUS CPN for pain relief. A recent study showed that combining EUS BPN with EUS CGN provided 6 times greater pain response than either method alone.[72] Apart from BPN and CGN, other predictors of response for EUS CPN include greater pain before the procedure,[58,63]

Table 4
Summary of studies describing celiac plexus neurolysis

Reference	Study Design	n	Technique	Active Drug	Average Follow-up (wk)	Outcome	Efficacy
Wiersema et al,[58] 1996	Case series (Retrospective)	30	CPN unilateral	3 mL 0.25% bupivacaine, 10 mL 98% alcohol	10	VAS	At 12 wk: 6.6 ± 2.2–1.2 ± 1.3; 88% reduction in VAS; 28% used less opioids
Gunaratnam et al,[64] 2001	Case series (Prospective)	58	CPN bilateral	3–6 mL 0.25% bupivacaine, 10 mL 98% alcohol	24	VAS	Overall: 6.2 ± 2.4–2.1 ± 2.3; 78% reduction in VAS; 54% reduction in VAS by 2 points; no change in morphine use
Iwata et al,[60] 2011	Case series (retrospective)	32	CPN central	10 mL 0.25% bupivacaine, 20 mL 100% alcohol	1	VAS: successful if <3	68% successful
Ishiwatari et al,[71] 2015	Case series (prospective)	9	CPN central	1.4 g phenol, 12 mL of 60% glycerol	1	VAS: complete if 0 or 1, partial if 2 or 3, none if ≥ 4	Complete 44%; partial 44%; none 11%
Sahai et al,[62] 2009	Case series (retrospective-prospective)	160 (71 central, 89 bilateral); 72 pancreatic ca; 79 chronic pancreatic	CPN central vs CPN bilateral	CPB: 20 mL 0.5% bupivacaine; CPN 10 mL 0.5% bupivacaine, 20 mL 100% alcohol	1	Percent baseline pain score reduction; Positive response >50% reduction in baseline pain score	Percent baseline pain reduction 70.4% (bilateral) vs 45.9% (unilateral; $P = .0016$); positive response: 77.5% (bilateral) vs 50.7% (unilateral; $P = .0005$)

Study	Study type	N	Approach	Injectate	Follow-up (wk)	Outcome definition	Results
Le Blanc et al,[61] 2011	Randomized, parallel group study	50 (29 central, 21 bilateral)	CPN central vs CPN bilateral	20 mL 0.75% bupivacaine, 10 mL 98% alcohol	11–14	VAS: pain relief ≤4 or ≥30% baseline pain reduction; complete response: score 0 for 4 wk	Pain relief: 81% (bilateral) vs 69% (unilateral; $P = .34$); complete response: 6.9% (bilateral) vs 9.5% (unilateral)
Tellez-Avila et al,[74] 2013	Case series (retrospective)	53 (21 central, 32 bilateral)	CPN central vs CPN bilateral	Unilateral: 10 mL of 1% lidocaine, 10 mL of 98% alcohol; bilateral: 10 mL of 1% lidocaine, 20 mL of 98% alcohol	4	VAS; >50% baseline pain score reduction	VAS: central 9.5 (6–10) to 4 (0–10) vs bilateral 9 (5–10) to 3 (0–10; $P = .52$); >50% baseline pain reduction: 47.6% (central) vs 56.3% (bilateral; $P = .710$)
Levy et al	Case series (Retrospective)	17	CGN	0.25% Bupivacaine, 100% alcohol, depo-medrol (80 mg/2 mL)	2–4	Pain relief: complete, partial or none	Pain relief: partial 94%, none 6%
Ascunce et al,[63] 2011	Case series (Retrospective)	64 (24 bilateral, 40 CGN)	CPN bilateral vs CGN	10 mL 1% Lidocaine, 20 mL 98% alcohol	1	Pain relief: >2 point drop in VAS score	Pain relief: 65% (CGN) vs 25% (CPN bilateral), $P = .002$
Doi et al,[70] 2013	Randomized, controlled trial	68 (34 CPN central, 34 CGN)	CPN central vs CGN	1–2 mL 0.25%–0.5% Bupivacaine, 5–20 mL 100% alcohol	1	VAS response: positive if VAS ≤3, complete if ≤1	Positive: 73.5% (CGN) vs 45.5% (CPN central; $P = .026$); complete: CGN (50%) vs 18.2% (CPN central; $P = .01$)
Sakamoto et al,[67] 2010	Case series (prospective)	67 (34 CPN unilateral, 33 BPN)	CPN unilateral vs BPN	3 mL 1% lidocaine, 9 mL 100% alcohol	4	VAS response: good if drop ≥3, poor if drop <3	CPN: 7.8 ± 1.1–4.8 ± 2.2; BPN: 7.8 ± 1.2–3.4 ± 2.5 ($P = .05$)
Minaga et al,[72] 2016	Case series (retrospective)	112 (65 BPN, 47 BPN + CGN)	BPN ± CGN	3 mL 1% lidocaine, 9 mL 100% alcohol	4	VAS response: good if drop ≥3,	Good response: 68%; on MV analysis; BPN + CGN best predictor of response

Abbreviations: BPN, broad plexus neurolysis; CGN, celiac ganglia neurolysis; CPN, celiac plexus neurolysis; MV, multivariate; VAS, visual analog scale.

a procedure performed early in course of the pancreatic cancer,[59,77] the absence of celiac plexus invasion by cancer,[60] transient increase in pain,[66] increase in heart rate during the CPN,[78] and concomitant chemoradiation therapy.[64]

A novel approach for celiac ganglion ablation with EUS-guided irradiation with I-125 seeds was demonstrated by Wang and colleagues[14] in a porcine model. Pigs with placement of 0.8 mCi I-125 seeds had an apoptotic index (ie, proportion of apoptotic neurons) of 0.94 compared with 0 for controls on day 60 after the procedure, suggestive of successful neurolysis. In a follow-up study in humans, 23 patients underwent this procedure with pain relief in 82% of patients and reduced analgesic consumption 2 weeks after the procedure.[79] None of the patients experienced any AEs.

SUMMARY

Therapeutic EUS has the potential to play an important role in management of cancers. EUS-guided fiducial placement has a high success rate and can effectively aid in stereotactic radiotherapy. EUS-guided tumor ablation therapies can be helpful in the palliation of locally advanced tumors. Although EUS-guided antitumor injection seems to be feasible and safe in animals, initial human studies suffer from small sample size and a lack of controls groups to demonstrate efficacy and survival benefit. Unfortunately, randomized controlled trials have not shown any additional benefit from these techniques compared with conventional therapy. EUS CPN has gained popularity and is now widely performed by interventional endosonographers. The EUS CPN technique is undergoing refinement with modifications, such as EUS CGN and EUS BPN. In the future, large randomized controlled trials are needed to better determine the most appropriate indications and overall usefulness of these therapies.

REFERENCES

1. Pishvaian AC, Collins B, Gagnon G, et al. EUS-guided fiducial placement for CyberKnife radiotherapy of mediastinal and abdominal malignancies. Gastrointest Endosc 2006;64(3):412–7.

2. Ammar T, Cote GA, Creach KM, et al. Fiducial placement for stereotactic radiation by using EUS: feasibility when using a marker compatible with a standard 22-gauge needle. Gastrointest Endosc 2010;71(3):630–3.

3. Dhadham GC, Hoffe S, Harris CL, et al. Endoscopic ultrasound-guided fiducial marker placement for image-guided radiation therapy without fluoroscopy: safety and technical feasibility. Endosc Int Open 2016;4(3):E378–82.

4. Khashab MA, Kim KJ, Tryggestad EJ, et al. Comparative analysis of traditional and coiled fiducials implanted during EUS for pancreatic cancer patients receiving stereotactic body radiation therapy. Gastrointest Endosc 2012;76(5): 962–71.

5. Park WG, Yan BM, Schellenberg D, et al. EUS-guided gold fiducial insertion for image-guided radiation therapy of pancreatic cancer: 50 successful cases without fluoroscopy. Gastrointest Endosc 2010;71(3):513–8.

6. Sanders MK, Moser AJ, Khalid A, et al. EUS-guided fiducial placement for stereotactic body radiotherapy in locally advanced and recurrent pancreatic cancer. Gastrointest Endosc 2010;71(7):1178–84.

7. Law JK, Singh VK, Khashab MA, et al. Endoscopic ultrasound (EUS)-guided fiducial placement allows localization of small neuroendocrine tumors during parenchymal-sparing pancreatic surgery. Surg Endosc 2013;27(10):3921–6.

8. Okuzono T, Kanno Y, Nakahori M, et al. Preoperative endoscopic ultrasonography-guided tattooing of the pancreas with a minuscule amount of marking solution using a newly designed injector. Dig Endosc 2016;28(7):744–8.

9. DiMaio CJ, Nagula S, Goodman KA, et al. EUS-guided fiducial placement for image-guided radiation therapy in GI malignancies by using a 22-gauge needle (with videos). Gastrointest Endosc 2010;71(7):1204–10.

10. Sun S, Qingjie L, Qiyong G, et al. EUS-guided interstitial brachytherapy of the pancreas: a feasibility study. Gastrointest Endosc 2005;62(5):775–9.

11. Jin Z, Du Y, Li Z, et al. Endoscopic ultrasonography-guided interstitial implantation of iodine 125-seeds combined with chemotherapy in the treatment of unresectable pancreatic carcinoma: a prospective pilot study. Endoscopy 2008; 40(4):314–20.

12. Sun S, Ge N, Wang S, et al. Pilot trial of endoscopic ultrasound-guided interstitial chemoradiation of UICC-T4 pancreatic cancer. Endosc Ultrasound 2012;1(1): 41–7.

13. Sun S, Xu H, Xin J, et al. Endoscopic ultrasound-guided interstitial brachytherapy of unresectable pancreatic cancer: results of a pilot trial. Endoscopy 2006;38(4): 399–403.

14. Wang K, Jin Z, Du Y, et al. Evaluation of endoscopic-ultrasound-guided celiac ganglion irradiation with iodine-125 seeds: a pilot study in a porcine model. Endoscopy 2009;41(4):346–51.

15. Lah JJ, Kuo JV, Chang KJ, et al. EUS-guided brachytherapy. Gastrointest Endosc 2005;62(5):805–8.

16. Elias D, Baton O, Sideris L, et al. Necrotizing pancreatitis after radiofrequency destruction of pancreatic tumours. Eur J Surg Oncol 2004;30(1):85–7.

17. Girelli R, Frigerio I, Salvia R, et al. Feasibility and safety of radiofrequency ablation for locally advanced pancreatic cancer. Br J Surg 2010;97(2):220–5.

18. Matsui Y, Nakagawa A, Kamiyama Y, et al. Selective thermocoagulation of unresectable pancreatic cancers by using radiofrequency capacitive heating. Pancreas 2000;20(1):14–20.

19. Carrara S, Arcidiacono PG, Albarello L, et al. Endoscopic ultrasound-guided application of a new hybrid cryotherm probe in porcine pancreas: a preliminary study. Endoscopy 2008;40(4):321–6.

20. Arcidiacono PG, Carrara S, Reni M, et al. Feasibility and safety of EUS-guided cryothermal ablation in patients with locally advanced pancreatic cancer. Gastrointest Endosc 2012;76(6):1142–51.

21. Varadarajulu S, Jhala NC, Drelichman ER. EUS-guided radiofrequency ablation with a prototype electrode array system in an animal model (with video). Gastrointest Endosc 2009;70(2):372–6.

22. Pai M, Habib N, Senturk H, et al. Endoscopic ultrasound guided radiofrequency ablation, for pancreatic cystic neoplasms and neuroendocrine tumors. World J Gastrointest Surg 2015;7(4):52–9.

23. Chan HH, Nishioka NS, Mino M, et al. EUS-guided photodynamic therapy of the pancreas: a pilot study. Gastrointest Endosc 2004;59(1):95–9.

24. Yusuf TE, Matthes K, Brugge WR. EUS-guided photodynamic therapy with verteporfin for ablation of normal pancreatic tissue: a pilot study in a porcine model (with video). Gastrointest Endosc 2008;67(6):957–61.

25. Choi JH, Oh D, Lee JH, et al. Initial human experience of endoscopic ultrasound-guided photodynamic therapy with a novel photosensitizer and a flexible laser-light catheter. Endoscopy 2015;47(11):1035–8.

26. Pacella CM, Francica G, Di Lascio FM, et al. Long-term outcome of cirrhotic patients with early hepatocellular carcinoma treated with ultrasound-guided percutaneous laser ablation: a retrospective analysis. J Clin Oncol 2009;27(16):2615–21.

27. Vogl TJ, Straub R, Eichler K, et al. Colorectal carcinoma metastases in liver: laser-induced interstitial thermotherapy–local tumor control rate and survival data. Radiology 2004;230(2):450–8.

28. Di Matteo F, Martino M, Rea R, et al. EUS-guided Nd:YAG laser ablation of normal pancreatic tissue: a pilot study in a pig model. Gastrointest Endosc 2010;72(2): 358–63.

29. Di Matteo F, Grasso R, Pacella CM, et al. EUS-guided Nd:YAG laser ablation of a hepatocellular carcinoma in the caudate lobe. Gastrointest Endosc 2011;73(3):632–6.

30. Livraghi T, Festi D, Monti F, et al. US-guided percutaneous alcohol injection of small hepatic and abdominal tumors. Radiology 1986;161(2):309–12.

31. Aslanian H, Salem RR, Marginean C, et al. EUS-guided ethanol injection of normal porcine pancreas: a pilot study. Gastrointest Endosc 2005;62(5):723–7.

32. Matthes K, Mino-Kenudson M, Sahani DV, et al. Concentration-dependent ablation of pancreatic tissue by EUS-guided ethanol injection. Gastrointest Endosc 2007;65(2):272–7.

33. Barclay RL, Perez-Miranda M, Giovannini M. EUS-guided treatment of a solid hepatic metastasis. Gastrointest Endosc 2002;55(2):266–70.

34. Gunter E, Lingenfelser T, Eitelbach F, et al. EUS-guided ethanol injection for treatment of a GI stromal tumor. Gastrointest Endosc 2003;57(1):113–5.

35. Jurgensen C, Schuppan D, Neser F, et al. EUS-guided alcohol ablation of an insulinoma. Gastrointest Endosc 2006;63(7):1059–62.

36. Nakaji S, Hirata N, Iwaki K, et al. Endoscopic ultrasound (EUS)-guided ethanol injection for hepatocellular carcinoma difficult to treat with percutaneous local treatment. Endoscopy 2012;44(Suppl 2 UCTN):E380.

37. Teoh AY, Chong CC, Chan AW, et al. EUS-guided alcohol injection of pancreatic neuroendocrine tumor. Gastrointest Endosc 2015;82(1):167.

38. Paik WH, Seo DW, Dhir V, et al. Safety and efficacy of EUS-guided ethanol ablation for treating small solid pancreatic neoplasm. Medicine (Baltimore) 2016;95(4):e2538.

39. Park DH, Choi JH, Oh D, et al. Endoscopic ultrasonography-guided ethanol ablation for small pancreatic neuroendocrine tumors: results of a pilot study. Clin Endosc 2015;48(2):158–64.

40. Chang KJ, Nguyen PT, Thompson JA, et al. Phase I clinical trial of allogeneic mixed lymphocyte culture (cytoimplant) delivered by endoscopic ultrasound-guided fine-needle injection in patients with advanced pancreatic carcinoma. Cancer 2000;88(6):1325–35.

41. Irisawa A, Takagi T, Kanazawa M, et al. Endoscopic ultrasound-guided fine-needle injection of immature dendritic cells into advanced pancreatic cancer refractory to gemcitabine: a pilot study. Pancreas 2007;35(2):189–90.

42. Hirooka Y, Itoh A, Kawashima H, et al. A combination therapy of gemcitabine with immunotherapy for patients with inoperable locally advanced pancreatic cancer. Pancreas 2009;38(3):e69–74.

43. Hecht JR, Bedford R, Abbruzzese JL, et al. A phase I/II trial of intratumoral endoscopic ultrasound injection of ONYX-015 with intravenous gemcitabine in unresectable pancreatic carcinoma. Clin Cancer Res 2003;9(2):555–61.

44. Old LJ. Tumor necrosis factor (TNF). Science 1985;230(4726):630–2.

45. Hallahan DE, Vokes EE, Rubin SJ, et al. Phase I dose-escalation study of tumor necrosis factor-alpha and concomitant radiation therapy. Cancer J Sci Am 1995;1(3):204–9.

46. Senzer N, Mani S, Rosemurgy A, et al. TNFerade biologic, an adenovector with a radiation-inducible promoter, carrying the human tumor necrosis factor alpha gene: a phase I study in patients with solid tumors. J Clin Oncol 2004;22(4): 592–601.
47. Chang KJ, Reid T, Senzer N, et al. Phase I evaluation of TNFerade biologic plus chemoradiotherapy before esophagectomy for locally advanced resectable esophageal cancer. Gastrointest Endosc 2012;75(6):1139–46.e2.
48. Citrin D, Camphausen K, Wood BJ, et al. A pilot feasibility study of TNFerade biologic with capecitabine and radiation therapy followed by surgical resection for the treatment of rectal cancer. Oncology 2010;79(5–6):382–8.
49. Hecht JR, Farrell JJ, Senzer N, et al. EUS or percutaneously guided intratumoral TNFerade biologic with 5-fluorouracil and radiotherapy for first-line treatment of locally advanced pancreatic cancer: a phase I/II study. Gastrointest Endosc 2012;75(2):332–8.
50. Herman JM, Wild AT, Wang H, et al. Randomized phase III multi-institutional study of TNFerade biologic with fluorouracil and radiotherapy for locally advanced pancreatic cancer: final results. J Clin Oncol 2013;31(7):886–94.
51. Levy MJ, Alberts SR, Bamlet WR, et al. EUS-guided fine-needle injection of gemcitabine for locally advanced and metastatic pancreatic cancer. Gastrointest Endosc 2016;86(1):161–9.
52. Linghu E, Matthes K, Mino-Kenudson M, et al. Feasibility of endoscopic ultrasound-guided OncoGel (ReGel/paclitaxel) injection into the pancreas in pigs. Endoscopy 2005;37(11):1140–2.
53. DuVall GA, Tarabar D, Seidel RH, et al. Phase 2: a dose-escalation study of OncoGel (ReGel/paclitaxel), a controlled-release formulation of paclitaxel, as adjunctive local therapy to external-beam radiation in patients with inoperable esophageal cancer. Anticancer Drugs 2009;20(2):89–95.
54. DeWitt JM, Murthy SK, Ardhanari R, et al. EUS-guided paclitaxel injection as an adjunctive therapy to systemic chemotherapy and concurrent external beam radiation before surgery for localized or locoregional esophageal cancer: a multicenter prospective randomized trial. Gastrointest Endosc 2016;86(1):140–9.
55. Bapat AA, Hostetter G, Von Hoff DD, et al. Perineural invasion and associated pain in pancreatic cancer. Nat Rev Cancer 2011;11(10):695–707.
56. Ward EM, Rorie DK, Nauss LA, et al. The celiac ganglia in man: normal anatomic variations. Anesth Analg 1979;58(6):461–5.
57. Kappis M. Erfahrungen mit local anasthesie bie bauchoperationen. Vehr Dtsch Gesellsch Chir 1914;43:87–9.
58. Wiersema MJ, Wiersema LM. Endosonography-guided celiac plexus neurolysis. Gastrointest Endosc 1996;44(6):656–62.
59. Wyse JM, Carone M, Paquin SC, et al. Randomized, double-blind, controlled trial of early endoscopic ultrasound-guided celiac plexus neurolysis to prevent pain progression in patients with newly diagnosed, painful, inoperable pancreatic cancer. J Clin Oncol 2011;29(26):3541–6.
60. Iwata K, Yasuda I, Enya M, et al. Predictive factors for pain relief after endoscopic ultrasound-guided celiac plexus neurolysis. Dig Endosc 2011;23(2):140–5.
61. LeBlanc JK, Al-Haddad M, McHenry L, et al. A prospective, randomized study of EUS-guided celiac plexus neurolysis for pancreatic cancer: one injection or two? Gastrointest Endosc 2011;74(6):1300–7.
62. Sahai AV, Lemelin V, Lam E, et al. Central vs. bilateral endoscopic ultrasound-guided celiac plexus block or neurolysis: a comparative study of short-term effectiveness. Am J Gastroenterol 2009;104(2):326–9.

63. Ascunce G, Ribeiro A, Reis I, et al. EUS visualization and direct celiac ganglia neurolysis predicts better pain relief in patients with pancreatic malignancy (with video). Gastrointest Endosc 2011;73(2):267–74.
64. Gunaratnam NT, Sarma AV, Norton ID, et al. A prospective study of EUS-guided celiac plexus neurolysis for pancreatic cancer pain. Gastrointest Endosc 2001; 54(3):316–24.
65. Gleeson FC, Levy MJ, Papachristou GI, et al. Frequency of visualization of presumed celiac ganglia by endoscopic ultrasound. Endoscopy 2007;39(7):620–4.
66. Levy MJ, Topazian MD, Wiersema MJ, et al. Initial evaluation of the efficacy and safety of endoscopic ultrasound-guided direct ganglia neurolysis and block. Am J Gastroenterol 2008;103(1):98–103.
67. Sakamoto H, Kitano M, Kamata K, et al. EUS-guided broad plexus neurolysis over the superior mesenteric artery using a 25-gauge needle. Am J Gastroenterol 2010;105(12):2599–606.
68. Adler DG, Conway JD, Coffie JM, et al. EUS accessories. Gastrointest Endosc 2007;66(6):1076–81.
69. Puli SR, Reddy JB, Bechtold ML, et al. EUS-guided celiac plexus neurolysis for pain due to chronic pancreatitis or pancreatic cancer pain: a meta-analysis and systematic review. Dig Dis Sci 2009;54(11):2330–7.
70. Doi S, Yasuda I, Kawakami H, et al. Endoscopic ultrasound-guided celiac ganglia neurolysis vs. celiac plexus neurolysis: a randomized multicenter trial. Endoscopy 2013;45(5):362–9.
71. Ishiwatari H, Hayashi T, Yoshida M, et al. EUS-guided celiac plexus neurolysis by using highly viscous phenol-glycerol as a neurolytic agent (with video). Gastrointest Endosc 2015;81(2):479–83.
72. Minaga K, Kitano M, Imai H, et al. Acute spinal cord infarction after EUS-guided celiac plexus neurolysis. Gastrointest Endosc 2016;83(5):1039–40 [discussion: 1040].
73. Paik WH, Seo DW. Is endoscopic ultrasound-guided celiac ganglia neurolysis superior to celiac plexus neurolysis? Endosc Ultrasound 2013;2(3):123–4.
74. Tellez-Avila FI, Romano-Munive AF, Herrera-Esquivel Jde J, et al. Central is as effective as bilateral endoscopic ultrasound-guided celiac plexus neurolysis in patients with unresectable pancreatic cancer. Endosc Ultrasound 2013;2(3): 153–6.
75. Levy M, Rajan E, Keeney G, et al. Neural ganglia visualized by endoscopic ultrasound. Am J Gastroenterol 2006;101(8):1787–91.
76. Gerke H, Silva RG Jr, Shamoun D, et al. EUS characteristics of celiac ganglia with cytologic and histologic confirmation. Gastrointest Endosc 2006;64(1):35–9.
77. Lillemoe KD, Cameron JL, Kaufman HS, et al. Chemical splanchnicectomy in patients with unresectable pancreatic cancer. A prospective randomized trial. Ann Surg 1993;217(5):447–55 [discussion: 456–7].
78. Bang JY, Hasan MK, Sutton B, et al. Intraprocedural increase in heart rate during EUS-guided celiac plexus neurolysis: clinically relevant or just a physiologic change? Gastrointest Endosc 2016;84(5):773–9.e3.
79. Wang KX, Jin ZD, Du YQ, et al. EUS-guided celiac ganglion irradiation with iodine-125 seeds for pain control in pancreatic carcinoma: a prospective pilot study. Gastrointest Endosc 2012;76(5):945–52.
80. Goldberg SN, Mallery S, Gazelle GS, et al. EUS-guided radiofrequency ablation in the pancreas: results in a porcine model. Gastrointest Endosc 1999;50(3): 392–401.

Endoscopic Ultrasonography-Guided Techniques for Accessing and Draining the Biliary System and the Pancreatic Duct

CrossMark

Mihai Rimbaş, MD, PhD[a,b,c], Alberto Larghi, MD, PhD[c],*

KEYWORDS

- EUS-guided biliary access • EUS-guided biliary drainage
- EUS-guided pancreatic duct access • EUS-guided pancreatic duct drainage

KEY POINTS

- Endoscopic ultrasonography (EUS) access and drainage of the biliary system after failed endoscopic retrograde cholangiopancreatography (ERCP) is becoming an established alternative procedure to percutaneous intervention.
- EUS-guided pancreatic access and drainage should be considered after failed ERCP or in patients with inaccessible papilla who were diagnosed with benign main pancreatic duct strictures or disconnected pancreatic tail syndrome.
- Both EUS biliary drainage and EUS pancreatic duct drainage are technically demanding and should be performed by endoscopists adequately trained in both therapeutic EUS and ERCP and in specialized centers with interventional radiology and surgical backup.
- Because of their more favorable adverse events profile, the rendezvous procedures should be favored whenever the papilla is accessible, rather than transluminal stenting procedures.
- With the advent of dedicated accessories, the role of EUS-guided access and drainage of the biliary system and pancreatic duct is likely to increase rapidly.

Conflicts of Interest: A. Larghi is a consultant for Boston Scientific Corp; M. Rimbaş has no relevant conflicts of interest to disclose.
^a Department of Gastroenterology, Colentina Clinical Hospital, Bucharest, Romania; ^b Internal Medicine Department, Carol Davila University of Medicine, Bucharest, Romania; ^c Digestive Endoscopy Unit, Catholic University, Rome, Italy
* Corresponding author. Università Cattolica del Sacro Cuore, Largo A. Gemelli 8, Rome 00168, Italy.
E-mail address: alberto.larghi@yahoo.it

Gastrointest Endoscopy Clin N Am 27 (2017) 681–705
http://dx.doi.org/10.1016/j.giec.2017.06.006
1052-5157/17/© 2017 Elsevier Inc. All rights reserved.

INTRODUCTION: NATURE OF THE PROBLEM

Endoscopic retrograde cholangiopancreatography (ERCP) is at present the procedure of choice for achieving access and drainage of the biliary system and the pancreatic duct to treat both benign and malignant conditions. However, even in expert hands, ERCP is not technically feasible in up to 10% of patients[1–3] for various reasons, such as surgically altered anatomy, duodenal strictures or gastric outlet obstructions, tight biliary or pancreatic duct strictures, or pancreatic duct disruptions. In cases in which ERCP fails, percutaneous drainage and even surgery can be necessary for draining the biliary system, whereas surgical intervention represents the only choice to treat conditions such as pancreatic duct disruption or pancreatic duct stenosis caused by inflammation or postsurgical changes.

After Harada and colleagues[4] and Wiersema and colleagues[5] showed for the first time in 1995 and 1996 the feasibility of performing a cholangiogram or a pancreato-gram under endoscopic ultrasonography (EUS) guidance, EUS-guided biliary and pancreatic duct access and drainage have emerged as attractive, less-invasive ther-apeutic alternatives after unsuccessful ERCPs. These techniques have evolved over time and have now been reported to be technically and clinically successful in a rele-vant number of patients.

This article reviews the present status and the current evidence of interventional EUS-guided biliary and pancreatic duct access and drainage.

ENDOSCOPIC ULTRASONOGRAPHY-GUIDED BILIARY DRAINAGE

A 2011 consortium meeting involving 40 international expert advanced endoscopists intended to standardize terminology, nomenclature, and indications of EUS-guided biliary drainage (EUS-BD) concluded that, given the potential serious adverse events associated with the procedure, EUS-DB should only be performed by endoscopists trained in both EUS and ERCP, with mandatory surgical and interventional radiology backup.[6] Of interest, in a prospective 1-year cohort study at a single tertiary-care referral center with a high therapeutic endoscopy volume, including 524 native papilla ERCPs, failure occurred in only 9 cases (1.7%) of attempted ERCPs, and EUS-BD was performed in only 3 cases, being successful in all of them.[7] Therefore, in a skilled ERCP referral center, failed standard biliary cannulation is rare and EUS-BD cannot at this time replace the properly performed ERCP procedure.[8]

Indications

At present, accepted indications for EUS-BD include[9]:

- Failed conventional ERCP performed in experienced centers
- Altered anatomy by previous surgery precluding access to the papilla
- Failure to access the papilla caused by malignant involvement of the gastrointes-tinal tract
- Occluding tumor preventing access into the biliary tree
- Presence of large ascites, which represents a contraindication to percutaneous access

Techniques for Drainage

Adequate ductal dilatation is mandatory for successful stent placement, whereas rendezvous procedure can be also attempted in normal-sized bile ducts. Even for experienced endoscopists, performing at least their first 20 cases under a mentor's supervision is highly recommended.[10] Moreover, a skilled assistant is required for the long guidewire manipulation, and, because the procedure involves breaking the wall of the gastrointestinal tract, carbon dioxide (instead of air) insufflation is advised.

A therapeutic linear echoendoscope is used to achieve biliary access within a segment of the biliary tree proximal to the site of obstruction. EUS-BD can be performed with either a transgastric-transhepatic (intrahepatic) or transenteric-transcholedochal (extrahepatic) approach. Moreover, the possibility of draining the biliary tree through the gallbladder has recently been explored (**Fig. 1**).

Intrahepatic approach

For accessing the left hepatic system, the echoendoscope is positioned in the region of the cardia or the lesser curvature of the stomach, or in the jejunum in patients with prior gastrectomy, and oriented toward the left liver lobe (usually segment 3). Accessing the right liver lobe is sometimes possible from the duodenal bulb, with the transducer facing upward.

Extrahepatic approach

The common bile duct (CBD) is easily identified with the echoendoscope positioned into the duodenal bulb, or sometimes at the level of the pylorus or the gastric antrum. Depending on how the operator wants to direct the guidewire (proximally or distally), a long (with the transducer facing upward) or a short (with the transducer facing downward) scope position should be accomplished.

Gallbladder approach

Some investigators[11,12] have described gallbladder drainage to be useful for achieving biliary drainage in patients with distal biliary obstruction and patent cystic duct. In this case, before positioning the echoendoscope facing the gallbladder (either in the antrum or duodenal bulb), a careful examination of the biliary system is necessary to exclude cystic duct involvement.

Steps to Perform Endoscopic Ultrasonography-Guided Biliary Drainage

The following steps are usually done in order to complete the procedure:

- Puncture of the target duct (intrahepatic, extrahepatic) or gallbladder
- Bile aspiration and contrast injection
- Advancement and manipulation of a guidewire
- Exchange of the echoendoscope with a duodenoscope while leaving the guidewire in place (for rendezvous cases only)

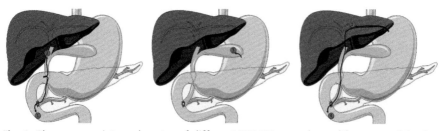

Fig. 1. The access points and routes of different EUS-BD procedures. (1) common bile duct (CBD) access from the duodenal bulb for rendezvous; (2) CBD access from the duodenal bulb for transmural stenting; (3) gallbladder drainage from the stomach when cystic duct is patent; (4) intrahepatic biliary access for rendezvous or antegrade transpapillary stenting; (5) intrahepatic biliary access for EUS-guided hepaticogastrostomy.

- Creation and dilation of a bilioenteric fistulous tract (not needed for rendezvous cases)
- Placement of a transpapillary or transmural stent (not needed for rendezvous cases)

Puncture of the duct
Puncture of the target duct is performed using a 19-gauge or a 22-gauge needle. The 19-gauge is preferred because it allows passage of larger guidewires and rapid infusion of contrast, even though its increased stiffness sometimes renders its use difficult or even impossible.

Guidewire insertion and manipulation
Once proper positioning of the tip of the needle into the biliary system is confirmed by bile aspiration and contrast injection, a hydrophilic guidewire (from 0.89 mm [0.035 inch] to 0.46 mm [0.018 inch], depending on the needle size) can be advanced into the punctured bile duct. The main benefit of using smaller-caliber (0.53 mm [0.021] or 0.46 mm [0.018 inch]) guidewires with either a 19-gauge or 22-gauge needle is their flexibility, which is helpful in maneuvering the wire though a tortuous duct and/or bypassing tight ductal strictures. Moreover, use of smaller guidewires (eg, 0.64 mm [0.025 inch] instead of .89 mm [0.035 inch]) may reduce the risk of shearing the guidewire coating, because there is more space between the guidewire and the needle tip. In contrast, these small wires often have reduced radiographic opacity, and their lack of stiffness makes maintenance of a stable position, endoscope exchange, and stent insertion more challenging. Therefore, some experts prefer to use the larger, stiffer guidewires at least for the final steps of the EUS-BD procedure.

In cases in which the guidewire can be manipulated across the ampulla into the duodenum, the procedure can be completed with either rendezvous or antegrade transpapillary stent placement (**Fig. 2**). To facilitate this process, the direction of the echoendoscope and needle should be adjusted to facilitate antegrade guidewire passage through the obstructed segment and across the papilla, with coiling of the guidewire into the small bowel. When an ideal positioning of the needle cannot be achieved, the guidewire is directed into the proximal rather than distal biliary tree. When this occurs, the guidewire may be advanced upward, where it sometimes loops, subsequently returning distally and advancing transpapillary.

Exchange of the echoendoscope (for rendezvous cases only)
If the rendezvous technique is chosen, the echoendoscope is carefully removed while leaving the guidewire in place. A duodenoscope is then passed to the papilla where a snare or biopsy forceps are used to grasp the wire, withdraw it through the accessory channel, and gain retrograde access to the bile duct to complete the procedure as a standard ERCP.

Creation of a fistulous tract (not needed for rendezvous cases)
In contrast with the EUS-guided rendezvous approach, in order to perform a direct antegrade or transluminal EUS-guided stent placement procedure, creation of a bilioenteric fistulous tract is needed. There is no best approach and the technique of choice depends on the individual endoscopist's expertise. There are 2 major ways to create the biloenteric tract: cauterization with pure-cut current with a needle knife or a small-diameter (usually 6.5-Fr) cystotome[13–15] or gradual dilation with tapered-tip catheters, cannulas, or small-diameter hydrostatic balloons.[16] Once a bilioenteric fistulous tract is created, its further dilation with 6-Fr to 9-Fr bougies or balloon

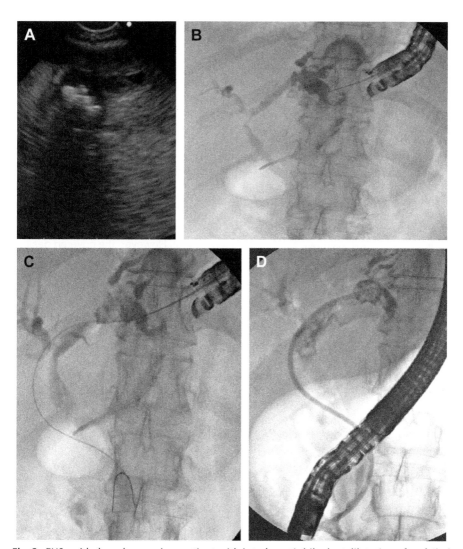

Fig. 2. EUS-guided rendezvous in a patient with intrahepatic bile duct dilatation after failed ERCP. EUS image of dilated intrahepatic left bile ducts filled with multiple stones that could not be accessed via standard ERCP (A). Fluoroscopic image of the cholangiogram after intrahepatic bile duct access with a 19-gauge needle under EUS guidance (B). Fluoroscopic image of the guidewire advanced through the papilla into the duodenum (C). After exchange of the echoendoscope with a standard duodenoscope, the procedure is continued as a standard ERCP (D).

catheters usually needs to be performed to allow passage of the proper accessories.

If a cystotome is used, the tract usually does not need to be dilated before metallic stenting. If a plastic stent is used for transmural drainage, the fistulous tract should be only minimally dilated (<4 mm) in order to prevent bile leakage. In case antegrade stenting is desired, the biliary stricture and ampulla should also be sequentially dilated under radiologic control.

Stent placement (not needed for rendezvous cases)

Once proper dilatation is reached, placement of a transpapillary or a transmural stent can be accomplished. Options for EUS-BD include plastic and partially covered or fully covered self-expandable metal stents (FC-SEMSs). The main disadvantage of plastic stents is the high risk of bile leakage into the peritoneal space, which may cause bile peritonitis. In contrast, because of expandability, an FC-SEMS automatically seals the gap between the stent and the fistula, thus preventing bile leakage from occurring.[17] Considering also the propensity of the plastic stents to become clogged much more easily than the metallic stents, the latter are being used more and more often for EUS-guided biliary drainage, either transluminally or as antegrade stenting.[18,19] The design of the metal stents must be covered at least in the transluminal region (eg, Wallstent, Boston Scientific; Bonastent, Sewoon Medical Co Ltd; Niti-S Biliary, Taewoong Medical), with a diameter of 8 or 10 mm in order to adequately seal the newly created bilioenteric tract and provide good drainage.

For EUS-guided hepaticogastrostomy, long tubular standard biliary self-expandable metal stents have so far been used (**Fig. 3**). However, the covered design of the intrahepatic portion of the stent can close the intrahepatic biliary radicals, with reported focal cholangitis or liver abscess formation.[10] For this reason, a novel generation of stents half uncovered in the extrahepatic portion have been developed and are now available for this indication (the GIOBOR stent, Taewoong Company).[20,21]

For EUS-guided choledochoduodenostomy, tubular fully covered standard biliary metal stents with a length of more than 4 cm have been used so far in order to prevent stent inward migration; however, with these stents reintervention is sometimes difficult and the distal portion of the stent may cause duodenal trauma and even perforation.[22,23] Lumen-apposing fully covered self-expandable metal stents that were initially developed for drainage of pancreatic fluid collections are now available and can be used for this indication. Their advantage is that, by sealing the 2 hollow organs together, they reduce the risk of bile leakage. Moreover, with the advent of the novel cautery-enhanced delivery system (Hot AXIOS device, Boston Scientific), the EUS-BD procedure can now be performed as 1 step (**Fig. 4**), without the need for prior needle puncture or guidewire insertion, and even without the need for fluoroscopy use.[24] However, care must be taken, because it cannot be used in a nondilated bile duct, and a distance of 10 mm or less between the two apposed structures is needed in order to prevent pressure necrosis.

Outcomes

Most of the available studies are retrospective and have grouped together the outcomes of individual procedural approaches. Results of all the relevant published studies with at least 30 patients enrolled are shown in **Table 1**. The mean combined technical and clinical success rates in these 27 studies are 91% and 86%, respectively.

In a recently published systematic review that included 42 studies and 1192 patients, the cumulative technical success rate (TSR), and functional success rate (FSR) were 94.5% and 92.5%, respectively, for all EUS-guided techniques.[51] For EUS rendezvous, the TSR and FSR were 89.7% and 100%, respectively. Moreover, the FSR of studies using plastic stents versus those using metal stents was not statistically different (98.2% vs 94.5%, respectively).

There are still many controversies, which reflects the lack of properly designed studies. In the same systematic review of the literature[51] a suboptimal FSR for benign disease (only 82.3%) of EUS-BD has been found, which made the investigators conclude that malignant diseases represent a better indication for this technique.

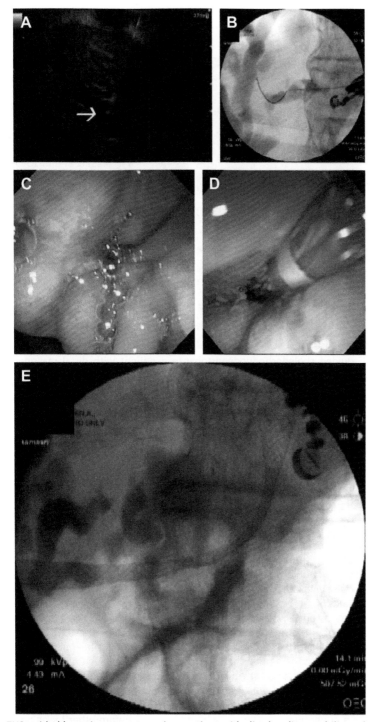

Fig. 3. EUS-guided hepaticogastrostomy in a patient with distal malignant biliary obstruction and failed ERCP. EUS-guided puncture of the dilated intrahepatic left biliary ducts (*A*), followed by contrast injection and guidewire advancement (*B*). The tract is then gradually dilated with bougies (*C*) and then a metal stent is inserted under both endoscopic (*D*) and radiologic control (*E*). *The arrow* points at the dilated intrahepatic left biliary ducts, as stated in explanation for frame (*A*). (*Courtesy of* Uwe Will, MD, Department of Gastroenterology, Municipal Hospital, Gera, Germany.)

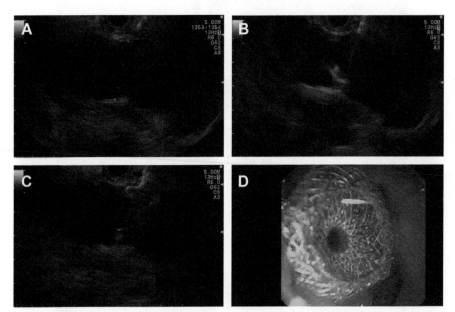

Fig. 4. EUS-guided choledochoduodenostomy in a patient with distal malignant biliary obstruction and failed ERCP. Direct EUS-guided access of a dilated bile duct (*A*) with an electrocautery-enhanced device (*B*), followed by stent deployment under EUS control only (*C*). The endoscopic control at the end of the procedure shows the lumen-apposing metal stent with its proximal flange opened in the duodenal bulb and good drainage of bile (*D*).

This low success rate has also been shown in a recent review[52] and may just be related to the difficulty in directing the guidewire toward the papilla in normal cases in which the CBD is not dilated and stenting is not an option.

Wang and colleagues[51] also compared the outcome of transgastric versus transduodenal procedures and found no differences in terms of technical success and clinical success. Similar results have also been found in other recent studies.[43,52,53] Based on these results, an algorithm for EUS-BD has recently been proposed, which is mainly based on the accessibility or not of the papilla. If the papilla is accessible, EUS rendezvous should be attempted first, whereas in cases of inaccessible papilla one of the other available approaches should be used based on the endoscopist's preference (**Fig. 5**).

One small study on 12 patients has evaluated the possibility of drainage of the biliary system by draining the gallbladder. TSR and FSR of 100% and 91.7% respectively were found,[11] making this technique potentially useful for patients in whom ERCP has failed and who have a patent cystic duct.

In the situation of patients with surgically altered anatomy, the TSR and FSR are reported to be 89.2% and 91.1%, respectively, for EUS-BD.[54] These figures are higher than those reported for enteroscopy-assisted ERCP (69.4% and 61.7%, respectively).[55] As a consequence, EUS-BD should be used before other techniques in this clinical scenario.

Importantly, if EUS-BD fails after penetrating the biliary system at least with a needle, immediate drainage by an alternative technique must be performed, to avoid the risk of fistula formation and spillage of bile from the biliary system into the peritoneum.

Table 1
Outcome of endoscopic ultrasonography-guided biliary drainage evaluated in relevant studies with more than 30 patients

Study	Design	No. of Patients	Technical Success (%)	Clinical Success (%)	Complications (%)
Maranki et al,[25] 2009	RS	49	84	73	16
Park et al,[26] 2011	PS	57	97	89	20
Shah et al,[27] 2012	RS	66	85	85	9
Iwashita et al,[28] 2012	RS	40	73	NR	13
Dhir et al,[29] 2012	RS	58	98	NR	3
Villa et al,[30] 2012	RS	106	69	NR	23
Park et al,[31] 2013	PS	45	91	87	11
Dhir et al,[32] 2013	RS	35	97	NR	23
Khashab et al,[33] 2013	RS	35	94	91	9
Gupta et al,[34] 2014	RS	240	87	NR	35
Dhir et al,[35] 2014	RS	68	96	NR	21
Kawakubo et al,[36] 2014	RS	64	95	NR	19
Dhir et al,[37] 2015	RS	104	93	92	9
Poincloux et al,[38] 2015	RS	101	98	92	12
Sportes et al,[39] 2015	RS	31	100	81	16
Sharaiha et al,[40] 2016	RS	47	92	62	>13
Kunda et al,[41] 2016	RS	57	98	95	7
Khashab et al,[42] 2016	PS	96	96	90	11
Khashab et al,[43] 2016	RS	121	93	83	17
Khashab et al,[44] 2016	RS	49	98	88	20
Tyberg et al,[45] 2016	PS	52	96	77	10
Cho et al,[46] 2017	PS	54	100	94	17
Nakai et al,[21] 2016	RS	33	100	100	9
Nakai et al,[47] 2017	RS	56	95	NR	21
Khumbhari et al,[48] 2016	RS	87	93	82	NR
Torres-Ruiz et al,[49] 2016	RS	35	81	73	>11
Lee et al,[50] 2016	RCT	34	94	82	9
Total		1820	91	86	17

Abbreviations: NR, not reported; PS, prospective study; RCT, randomized controlled trial; RS, retrospective study.

Adverse Events

Rates of adverse events seem to be even more variable among the different studies, with an average complication rate in the 27 reported studies of 17% (range, 3%–35%) (see **Table 1**). In the recent systematic review involving 42 studies and 1192 patients,[51] the adverse event rate of EUS-BD was 23.3%. Among the most common adverse events that are associated with EUS-BD are bleeding (either during the procedure or afterward), bile leakage into the peritoneum, stent migration, cholangitis, and abdominal pain (**Table 2**). Most of these adverse events are either self-limited or could be managed conservatively. However, in a study on 101 procedures at a single center, 6 procedure-related deaths were reported, 5 of them occurring among the first 50 patients,[38] thus indicating the importance of training and the need for a learning curve to become highly proficient.

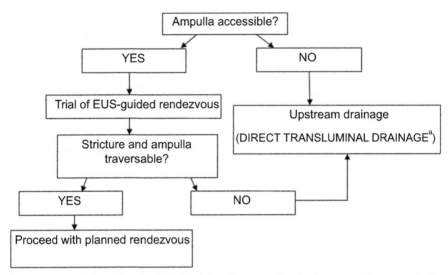

Fig. 5. Proposed algorithm for EUS-BD. [a] For direct transluminal access, either the extrahepatic or intrahepatic approach can be tried; if the first choice is unsuccessful, convert to the other approach, if feasible. (*From* Khashab MA, Valeshabad AK, Modayil R, et al. EUS-guided biliary drainage by using a standardized approach for malignant biliary obstruction: rendezvous versus direct transluminal techniques (with videos). Gastrointest Endosc 2013;78:736; with permission.)

In one study, the use of nonaxial cautery and plastic stent placement seemed to be independently associated with occurrence of adverse events.[43] Similarly, in the large systematic review, the rate of adverse events associated with the use of metal stents was 17.5%, which is significantly lower than that of plastic stents (31.0%) ($P = .013$).[51] In the same meta-analysis, no differences were found in terms of complication rates between the transgastric and the transduodenal approaches.[51] Similar results have also been found in a recent study by Artifon and colleagues,[53] and in another one by Khashab and colleagues,[43] but not in a recent review by Dhir and colleagues.[52] In the Dhir and colleagues[52] review, considering only studies with more than 50 enrolled patients, complications were encountered significantly more frequently for the transgastric approach than for the transduodenal approach (18.9% vs 10.3%). Properly designed multicenter prospective studies are needed to clarify which approach should be used.

Another recent meta-analysis reported a reduced rate of adverse events of EUS rendezvous compared with EUS-guided transmural drainage (11% vs 21%, respectively).[57] The theoretic advantage of the rendezvous approach is the ability to avoid the potential risk of bile leakage related to the fistula formation, an advantage that is lost with the antegrade approach. Dhir and colleagues[29] performed a retrospective nonrandomized study in a highly selective cohort of patients in whom they compared safety and efficacy of EUS rendezvous bile duct drainage versus precut papillotomy after failed ERCP. The rate of technical success was significantly higher in the EUS-BD group than in the precut papillotomy group (98.3% vs 90.3%; $P = .03$). The only failure in the EUS group occurred in a patient with a pancreatic head tumor and was caused by the inability to pass the guidewire across the biliary stricture. The high success rate reported in the EUS group might partly be explained by the use of a 260-cm guidewire instead of the commonly used 450-cm guidewire to have a

Table 2
Side effects related to the procedure encountered during or after endoscopic
ultrasonography-guided biliary drainage, as reported in a recent systematic review

	Reported Frequency (%)	Comments
Common Adverse Events		
Bleeding	4.03	
Bile leakage	4.03	
Pneumoperitoneum	3.02	Usually small; not a complication per se
Stent migration	2.68	The covered biliary metal stents are theoretically more prone to migration than the uncovered ones[56]
Cholangitis	2.43	Possibly triggered by the duodenobiliary reflux after fistula tract formation
Abdominal pain	1.51	
Peritonitis	1.26	
Rare Adverse Events		
Stent occlusion	1.09	
Biloma	0.59	
Pancreatitis	0.50	Associated with the rendezvous technique
Perforation	0.50	
Death	0.50	
Fever	0.34	
Sepsis	0.34	
Bacteremia	0.17	
Transient ileus	0.08	
Sheared guidewire	0.08	Not a complication per se
Retrogastric collection	0.08	
Arteriobiliary fistula	0.08	

From Wang K, Zhu J, Xing L, et al. Assessment of efficacy and safety of EUS-guided biliary drainage: a systematic review. Gastrointest Endosc 2016;83:1222; with permission.

better ability to steer and by the use of a small biopsy forceps to anchor the guidewire in the stomach during endoscope exchange to prevent its incidental slippage. Occurrence of complications was similar in the two groups (6.9% in the precut group vs 3.4% in the EUS group; $P = .27$), but the severe ones (ie, severe pancreatitis and bleeding) were only observed in the precut group.

One of the studies with the lowest technical success and the highest complication rate is the study by Villa and colleagues,[30] considering 19 centers, most of which included very few patients. These data emphasize the existence and the importance of the learning curve on the technical and complication rates for EUS-BD.

At present, efforts are being made to develop dedicated accessories capable of simplifying the procedure and decreasing the rate of adverse events.[58,59] In a recent study[46] enrolling 54 consecutive patients, including 21 EUS-guided hepaticogastrostomies and 33 EUS-guided choledochoduodenostomies, the use of a novel hybrid half-covered metallic stent (to prevent bile leakage in the distal portion) with double anchoring flaps (median and distal) (Standard Sci-Tech Inc) resulted in no events of stent migration (either distal or proximal) during follow-up. Similarly, a lumen-apposing self-expandable metal stent designed for choledochoduodenostomy (Hot AXIOS, Boston Scientific Corp) coupled with an electrocautery-enhanced delivery system allows an easy creation of a more stable biliary anastomosis.[60] A retrospective study involving 57 patients in whom the stent was used for choledochoduodenostomy both with and without the electrocautery-enhanced device resulted in a procedure-related complication rate of 7%, with no mortality, and a reintervention rate of 9.3%, mainly for sump syndrome.[41] In addition, a tubular stent 8 or 10 cm long that is 50% uncovered (intrabiliary part, in order to prevent migration) and 50% covered (transmural and intragastric portion, in order to prevent bile leakage) (the GIOBOR stent, Taewoong Company) has been tested in a study of 22 patients, in all of whom no bile leakage has been observed after the procedure.[20]

Comparison with Percutaneous Drainage, Endoscopic Retrograde Cholangiopancreatography or Surgery

In a recent meta-analysis including 9 studies with 483 patients comparing EUS-BD with percutaneous transhepatic biliary drainage (PTBD), no difference in technical success between the two procedures was reported,[61] but EUS-BD was associated with better clinical success (odds ratio [OR], 0.45), fewer postprocedure adverse events (OR, 0.23), and much lower rates of reintervention (OR, 0.13). EUS-BD seems to be more cost-effective than PTBD.

Recently, there is increasing evidence that EUS-BD can be as good as ERCP to achieve palliation of distal malignant biliary obstruction. An international multicenter retrospective study involving 208 patients compared ERCP with EUS for this indication.[37] In the EUS study group, 68 patients (65.4%) underwent choledochoduodenostomy and the remaining 36 hepaticogastrostomy. Duodenal stenosis was present in 6.7% of the ERCP group versus 62.5% of the EUS group ($P = .0001$). Comparing ERCP and EUS, similar TSRs (94.23% vs 93.26%) and adverse events (8.65% and 8.65%) were found. The rate of composite success (technical success with >50% reduction in bilirubin concentration within 2 weeks) was significantly superior for the EUS group compared with the ERCP group, in particular in patients with standard access (93.93% vs 79.58%; $P = .0001$). This finding can have a major clinical impact, making possible early administration of chemotherapy when drainage is performed under EUS compared with standard ERCP. In a similar retrospective study from Japan, 26 patients underwent EUS-guided choledochoduodenostomy and 56 underwent standard ERCP.[62] Clinical success rates were comparable between the two groups, with a significantly shorter duration of the procedure and a significantly lower rate of pancreatitis in patients who underwent choledochoduodenostomy compared with standard ERCP. Moreover, the need for reintervention at 1 year was similar in the two groups. All these results prompted the investigators to conclude that EUS-guided choledochoduodenostomy should be considered as the first-line treatment of patients with malignant distal biliary obstruction.

Compared with surgery, in a small prospective study enrolling 32 patients, technical and clinical success, as well as patient survival, were similar in patients who underwent surgical biliary bypass and EUS-guided choledochoduodenostomy drainage after failed ERCP,[63] but at a cost of increased morbidity in the surgical arm.

Endoscopic Ultrasonography-Guided Biliary Drainage as a Primary Treatment of Distal Common Bile Duct Obstruction

The only study performed in naive patients who did not undergo previous ERCP is a prospective Japanese study in which EUS-guided choledochoduodenostomy with direct metallic stent placement was performed using a prototype forward-viewing echoendoscope.[22] In 94% of the cases, the procedure was technically and clinically successful, with 2 cases (11%) of focal peritonitis resolved with conservative treatment. During follow-up (median, 187 days; range, 29–607 days), only 3 metallic stent occlusion events occurred in 2 patients, with successful stent cleaning in all 3 cases.

ENDOSCOPIC ULTRASONOGRAPHY-GUIDED PANCREATIC DUCT ACCESS AND DRAINAGE

From its first description,[4] EUS-guided access and drainage of the main pancreatic duct slowly became accepted as a therapeutic option in certain clinical circumstances, mainly when ductal hypertension is thought to be associated with pain, or when there is a leak of pancreatic juice from ductal injury.[64,65]

Indications

Accepted indications for EUS-guided pancreatic duct drainage (EUS-PDD) include[3,65]:

- Symptomatic obstruction of the main pancreatic duct after failed ERCP and cancer are excluded
- Symptomatic ductal stones after failed extracorporeal shock wave lithotripsy
- Symptomatic obstruction of the main pancreatic duct in patients with inaccessible papilla in the presence of postsurgical anatomy (gastrectomy, Roux-en-Y anastomosis, post-Whipple procedure)
- Disconnected pancreatic tail syndrome

Techniques for Drainage

EUS-guided pancreatic drainage can be performed with either an anterograde or a retrograde pancreatic ductal approach, and also with the rendezvous procedure (**Fig. 6**). With the anterograde approach, the stent insertion or rendezvous procedure occurs in the direction of the ampulla, whereas retrograde stenting is performed with insertion in the caudal direction. Although some clinicians prefer accessing the main pancreatic duct (MPD) from the stomach, including in patients with surgically altered

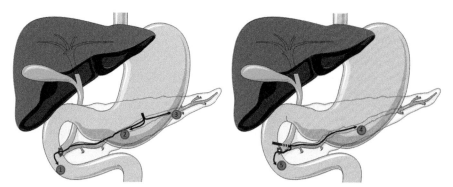

Fig. 6. The access points and routes of different EUS-PDD procedures. Transgastric approach: (1) transgastric trans-stenotic transpapillary pancreatic duct access for rendezvous or antegrade stenting; (2) transgastric pancreatic duct access for antegrade stenting; (3) transgastric pancreatic duct access for retrograde stenting. Transduodenal approach: (4) transduodenal pancreatic duct access for retrograde stenting; (5) transduodenal trans-stenotic transpapillary pancreatic duct access for rendezvous or antegrade stenting.

anatomy, others use the retrograde approach because the long scope position in the duodenal bulb allows better stability and facilitates the ability to push the stent. Placement of a stent in a transpancreatic fashion, with one end in the gastric lumen and the other through the pancreatic duct in the small bowel, has also been described.[66]

Steps to Perform Endoscopic Ultrasonography-Guided Pancreatic Duct Drainage

The procedural steps are similar to those of the biliary drainage. However, EUS-PDD is definitively more demanding and challenging than EUS-BD. The stability of the EUS scope in the stomach is low and does not allow the application of forces that act on the instrument or the accessories that are being used. Perhaps the most important factor in determining the success of the procedure is the careful planning of the puncture site and direction.[67]

Needle puncture

The choice of the puncturing site should favor a place with a short distance between the EUS transducer and the MPD. The degree of ductal dilatation and the presence of chronic pancreatitis changes of the pancreatic parenchyma should be carefully considered.[68] The 19-gauge needle that is generally preferred for accessing a larger duct can be stiff and not able to traverse extensive fibrotic parenchyma. In difficult cases, such as those with a nondilated pancreatic duct or a very hard pancreas, the puncture can be facilitated in a couple of ways.[67,68] First, a puncture deeper than the level of the MPD should be done followed by withdrawal of the needle until it reaches the duct. Second, complete removal of the stylet should be done to increase needle flexibility and maneuverability. Moreover, in certain occasions, using a smaller (22-gauge) needle to obtain the initial access to the duct can increase the rate of procedural success.

If antegrade stenting is planned, the MPD is ideally accessed at the body-tail region to be able to direct the guidewire toward the head of the pancreas, whereas for retrograde stenting the MPD is optimally accessed at the head with the guidewire directed toward the tail region. Thus, a longer length of the stent is positioned in the MPD.[65,67,69] In this regard it is ideal to get the long axis of the needle as parallel as possible with the direction of the MPD, which offers a larger area to target and facilitates insertion of the guidewire, of the dilation devices, and of the stent (**Fig. 7**).[70]

Once inside the MPD, pancreatogram is performed under fluoroscopic control, usually after aspiration of pancreatic juice.[71] The quantity of injected contrast should be limited in order to avoid a significant increase in ductal pressure with a consequent increased risk of postprocedural pancreatitis.[72]

Guidewire insertion and manipulation

The guidewire size should be chosen considering especially its stiffness and capability to traverse tight strictures. Rendezvous procedures often require the use of a hydrophilic guidewire (eg, 0.64-mm [0.025-inch] or 0.89-mm [0.035-inch] Visiglide, Olympus Corp; Glidewire, Jagwire, Boston Scientific; 0.81-mm [0.032-inch] Radifocus, Terumo). Thinner guidewires (0.53 mm [0.021 inch] or 0.46 mm [0.018 inch) that can work with a 22-gauge needle are useful for passing tortuous and/or tight strictures, but are poorly visible fluoroscopically, kink easily, and lack stiffness, therefore should be exchanged with the larger and stiffer wires once passed through the stricture.[68] The guidewire should be advanced as far as possible into the bowel for rendezvous and into the MPD for stenting.

Exchange of the echoendoscope with a duodenoscope (for rendezvous cases only)

When the guidewire is advanced from the stomach or the duodenum through the papilla into the duodenum a rendezvous procedure can be done (**Fig. 8**). The

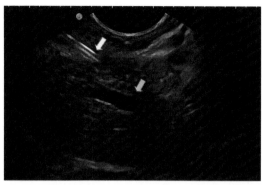

Fig. 7. Correct position to perform EUS-guided puncture of the pancreatic duct. The needle (*white arrow*) needs to be parallel to the long axis of the Wirsung duct (*yellow arrow*) for a successful EUS-PDD procedure. (*Courtesy of* Uwe Will, MD, Department of Gastroenterology, Municipal Hospital, Gera, Germany.)

echoendoscope is removed leaving the guidewire in place and a duodenoscope is passed alongside the guidewire to the papilla where the wire is grasped and withdrawn through the working channel, thus gaining retrograde access to the pancreatic duct. The procedure is then continued as a standard ERCP.

Creation and dilation of the pancreatic-enteric fistulous tract (not needed for rendezvous cases)

Creation and dilation of the newly formed fistulous tract is needed before stenting, to the size of the MPD and of the stent. Given the often hardened pancreatic parenchyma, it is difficult to dilate the tract using dilation catheters (eg, 5-Fr to 8.5-Fr Soehendra dilation catheters, Cook Medical; Proforma cannula, Conmed Endoscopic Technologies) or balloons (eg, Titan Biliary Dilation Balloon, Cook Medical; Hurricane Biliary Dilation Balloon, Boston Scientific) alone, even if in a step-up fashion. Some investigators report that initial dilation with the needle sheath can aid the subsequent passages.[72] Others favor the initial advancement of an over-the-wire diathermy catheter or needle knife (eg, 6.5-F Endoflex, Voerde; Microknife, Boston Scientific; Will's ring knife, MTW Endoskopie) with a short burst of pure-cut current for tract dissection and fistula creation, followed by dilation with a 4-mm balloon or catheter for easier stent placement,[73–76] whereas others avoid their use because of the fear of cautery-related adverse events, and therefore serially exchange multiple devices over the guidewire.[68] Regardless of personal choice in deciding which equipment to use, continuous EUS and fluoroscopic imaging are useful at this stage to maintain a stable scope position.[67]

Placement of a transpapillary or transmural stent (not needed for rendezvous cases)

Once proper dilatation is reached, placement of a transpapillary or transmural stent can be accomplished under continuous fluoroscopy with endoscopic control.

Standard plastic stents are suitable for this indication, preferably with the feature of being pulled back to avoid stent positioning into the abdominal cavity (eg, Flexim; Boston Scientific Corp, Marlborough, MA; Trough-Pass Gadelius Tokyo, Japan). Moreover, a dedicated stent for EUS-PDD has been developed by Itoi and colleagues,[77] and fully covered SEMSs and lumen-apposing fully covered SEMSs have been reported to be effective after overcoming the fear of blocking side-branch ducts **(Fig. 9)**.[71,78]

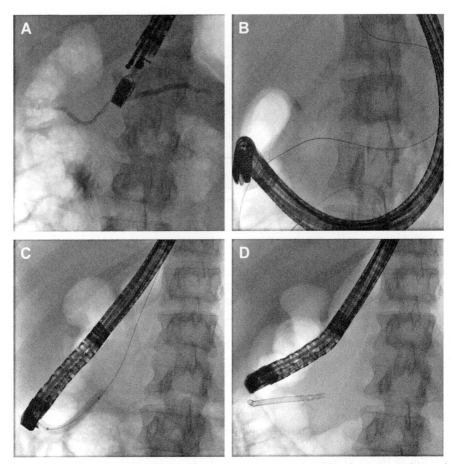

Fig. 8. EUS-guided pancreatic duct rendezvous in a patient with a dilated pancreatic duct and chronic abdominal pain. EUS-guided puncture of a dilated Wirsung duct in the region of the pancreatic isthmus, followed after contrast injection (*A*) by guidewire insertion through the papilla (*B*) and a rendezvous procedure by exchange with a duodenoscope and performance of balloon dilation of the pancreatic duct stricture (*C*) and pancreatic stent insertion (*D*). (*Courtesy of* Uwe Will, MD, Department of Gastroenterology, Municipal Hospital, Gera, Germany.)

Outcomes

Most published studies are retrospective and, in most of the cases, a transgastric approach has been used. Results of all relevant published studies with at least 10 patients enrolled are shown in **Table 3**. The mean combined technical and clinical success rates in these 12 studies are 79% and 78%, respectively.

Two recent studies have reported the largest series published to date. In one multicenter study (4 centers over a 10-year period), Tyberg and colleagues[66] performed EUS-PDD in 80 patients, including 6 with malignancy. In 35 patients (41%) an anastomotic stricture was present. Technical success was achieved in 89% of patients. All stents were 5-Fr to 10-Fr double-pigtail plastic stents. Clinical success was achieved in 81% of patients. Note that the method of approach (anterograde/retrograde) trended toward being a predictor of complete symptom resolution (95% in patients

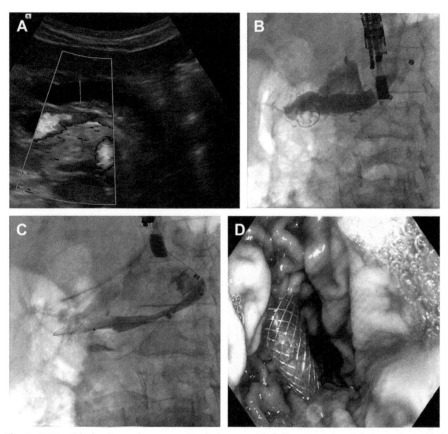

Fig. 9. EUS-guided antegrade pancreatic drainage with fully covered metal stent placement in a patient with pancreatic duct stenosis and multiple failed ERCPs. EUS visualization of a dilated Wirsung duct from the gastric body (*A*) followed by contrast injection and guidewire advancement (*B*). After cautery dilation of the tract, a fully covered metal stent is then deployed across the stricture under radiologic (*C*) and endoscopic control (*D*). (*Courtesy of* Uwe Will, MD, Department of Gastroenterology, Municipal Hospital, Gera, Germany.)

with a retrograde stent placement vs 76% of patients with anterograde stent placement; $P = .067$), but not of technical success ($P = .23$).

In the second article, Will and colleagues[71] described a single-center experience over a 12-year period. They treated 94 symptomatic patients with enlarged pancreatic ducts in whom active cancer was excluded. In all 94 patients, puncture of the pancreatic duct was achieved and pancreatography done, and this showed no need for further intervention in 10 of them. Moreover, in 1 subject, Histoacryl injection into the tail segment of the pancreatic duct was performed. In the remaining 83 patients, successful placement of drainage at the first attempt was achieved in only 47 (56.6%) of them. Of the 26 patients undergoing transluminal (retrograde) drainage, plastic stents were used in 11 and metal stents in 12, whereas the remaining 3 of these patients received placement of a enteropancreaticogastric drain (antegrade internal drainage) using a double-pigtail plastic stent. In the remaining 21 patients, transpapillary drainage with a rendezvous procedure could be achieved, plastic stents being placed in almost all cases (n = 19), with only 2 covered self-expanding metal stents

Table 3
Outcome of endoscopic ultrasonography-guided pancreatic duct drainage evaluated in relevant studies with more than 10 patients

Study	Design	No. of Patients	Technical Success (%)	Clinical Success (%)	Complications (%)
Tessier et al,[73] 2007	RS	36	92	69	14
Kahaleh et al,[75] 2007	PS	12	83	NR	17
Will et al,[79] 2007	PS	12	67	NR	17
Barkay et al,[80] 2010	RS	21	48	NR	10
Ergun et al,[81] 2011	RS	20	90	72	10
Shah et al,[27] 2012	RS	22	86	NR	18
Villa et al,[30] 2012	RS	19	58	NR	26
Kurihara et al,[82] 2013	RS	14	93	93	7
Fujii et al,[83] 2013	RS	45	73	60	6
Will et al,[71] 2015	RS	83	63	82	22
Tyberg et al,[66] 2017	PS	80	89	81	20
Chen et al,[84] 2017	RS	40	92.5	87.5	35
Total		404	79	78	18

placed. Three of the 36 patients who were not initially successfully drained showed distinct clinical improvement after guidewire manipulation in the pancreatic duct only, whereas another 12 showed clinical improvement after additional cystotome and/or balloon manipulation at the transenteric access site. The median follow-up of the 26 patients who underwent successful transgastric/transduodenal EUS-PDD was 9.5 months (range, 1–82 months). Reinterventions were required for pain (n = 3), stent dislocation (n = 3), stent occlusion (n = 2), and technical problems (n = 9). These results indicate that endoscopic treatment should be repeated if necessary, stent revisions being recommended 2 to 3 months after the index procedure.[3] If stent dysfunction occurs, it should be exchanged if the MPD remains dilated or the patient is symptomatic.[71,73] Serial dilations and repeated stent exchanges are often required for fistula maturation until stents can be removed.

In patients with post-Whipple anatomy, a recent international multicenter retrospective study in 7 tertiary centers comparing EUS-PDD and enteroscopy-assisted ERCP (e-ERP) in 66 patients[84] showed technical success in 92.5% in the EUS-PDD group compared with 20% in the e-ERP group (OR, 49.3; P<.001). Similarly, clinical success (per patient) was more frequently attained in the EUS-PDD group compared with the e-ERP group (87.5% vs 23.1%; OR, 23.3; P<.001).

Based on their experience presented earlier, Will and colleagues[71] proposed a treatment algorithm (**Fig. 10**). The first step is the evaluation of accessibility of the papilla. If the papilla is endoscopically accessible, an EUS rendezvous procedure should be attempted first. When the papilla cannot be reached, the decision of which approach to use should be guided by patient anatomy. If the pancreas is in situ and the patient underwent previous Roux-en-Y reconstruction, Billroth II gastric resection or gastroenterostomy, EUS-guided pancreaticogastrostomy, or EUS-guided pancreaticoduodenostomy should be performed. In patients with previous Whipple procedure or pancreaticojejunostomy with suspected anastomotic stenosis, antegrade internal drainage should be the approach of choice. In addition, in patients with a pancreatic duct stricture that cannot be traversed with the guidewire or in patients with a disconnected duct, an EUS-guided pancreaticogastrostomy should be done.

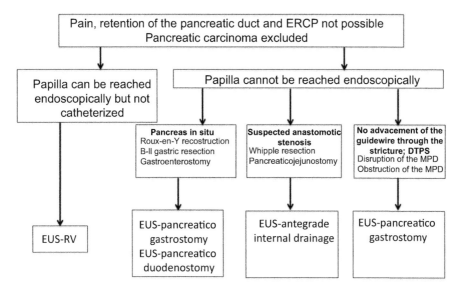

Fig. 10. Proposed algorithm for EUS-guided pancreatic duct drainage. DTPS, disconnected pancreatic tail syndrome. (*From* Will U, Reichel A, Fueldner F, et al. Endoscopic ultrasonography-guided drainage for patients with symptomatic obstruction and enlargement of the pancreatic duct. World J Gastroenterol 2015; 21:13146; with permission.)

Adverse Events

In a recent review of the literature by Fujii-Lau and colleagues[65] the overall pooled adverse events rate from small retrospective series was 18% (n = 42) in a total of 222 patients (with or without surgically altered anatomy) and included abdominal pain in 40%, bleeding in 10%, pancreatitis in 7%, pancreatic abscess formation in 5%, perforation in 5%, shaving of the guidewire coating in 5%, pneumoperitoneum in 2%, postprocedural fever in 2%, and perigastric or peripancreatic fluid collections (with or without aneurysm formation) in 6%. Also in our search, including 12 relevant studies, the complication rate of EUS-PDD was 18% (see **Table 3**).

In one recent study on 80 patients in whom plastic stents have been used,[66] immediate adverse events occurred in 20% of patients (n = 16) after EUS-PDD, with major complications including 6 cases of post-ERCP pancreatitis after rendezvous, 4 pancreatic fluid collections, 1 MPD leak, and 1 perforation. Most importantly, 6 of the 16 complications occurred in patients in whom technical success was not achieved (post-ERCP pancreatitis in 5 cases, and pancreatic fluid collection in 1 case). Delayed (>24 hours postprocedurally) complications occurred in 9 patients (11%).

Adverse events occurred in 24 out 111 (21.6%) interventions in the second largest recent study and included major and intermediate complications such as perforation (1 case), abscess formation (4 cases), bleeding (7 cases), moderately severe pancreatitis (6 cases), pressure ulcer formation (1 case), perigastric fluid (2 cases), and bronchopulmonary aspiration (1 case).[71]

CONTROVERSIES AND FUTURE DIRECTIONS

All the available evidence on EUS-BD and EUS-PDD indicates that these are technically challenging procedures that need to be performed by expert endoscopists and in a setting with multidisciplinary support in case of the occurrence of complications. Consensus on the best approach to be used based on the clinical scenario is still unclear and a better definition of such parameters is needed in order to be able to compare outcomes from different studies.

An unsettled issue is the requirements for training, because of the technical difficulty of the procedures and the potential for serious adverse events. Most experts agree that training should include not only interventional EUS techniques but also ERCP. Moreover, the number of procedures to be performed in order to become proficient in EUS-BD and EUS-PPD drainage needs to be better clarified.

Most likely the number of EUS-PDD cases will remain limited because of the low number of indications, whereas EUS-BD will probably grow in parallel with the development of dedicated accessories. In this regard, despite some reports favorably comparing EUS-BD with standard ERCP, it seems premature to perform EUS-BD before ERCP and well-designed comparative studies with clear end points are needed before this change can take place. The potential of EUS-BD is huge, but it needs to be associated with the development of dedicated accessories and standardization of techniques, and should be evidence driven to bring EUS-BD to another level.

SUMMARY

- EUS access and drainage of the biliary system after failed ERCP is becoming an established alternative procedure to percutaneous intervention
- EUS-guided pancreatic access and drainage should be considered after failed ERCP or in patients with inaccessible papilla who were diagnosed with benign MPD strictures or disconnected pancreatic tail syndrome
- Both EUS-BD and EUS-PDD are technically demanding and should be performed by endoscopists adequately trained in both therapeutic EUS and ERCP and in specialized centers with interventional radiology and surgical backup
- Because of their more favorable adverse events profile, the rendezvous procedures should be favored whenever the papilla is accessible rather than transluminal stenting procedures
- With the advent of dedicated accessories, the role of EUS-guided access and drainage of the biliary system and pancreatic duct is likely to increase rapidly.

REFERENCES

1. Ekelenkamp VE, de Man RA, Ter Borg F, et al. Prospective evaluation of ERCP performance: results of a nationwide quality registry. Endoscopy 2015;47:503–7.
2. Williams EJ, Ogollah R, Thomas P, et al. What predicts failed cannulation and therapy at ERCP? Results of a large-scale multicenter analysis. Endoscopy 2012;44:674–83.
3. Widmer J, Sharaiha RZ, Kahaleh M. Endoscopic ultrasonography–guided drainage of the pancreatic duct. Gastrointest Endosc Clin N Am 2013;23:847–61.
4. Harada N, Kouzu T, Arima M, et al. Endoscopic ultrasound-guided pancreatography: a case report. Endoscopy 1995;27:612–5.
5. Wiersema MJ, Sandusky D, Carr R, et al. Endosonography-guided cholangiopancreatography. Gastrointest Endosc 1996;43:102–6.
6. Kahaleh M, Artifon EL, Perez-Miranda M, et al. Endoscopic ultrasonography guided biliary drainage: summary of consortium meeting, May 7th, 2011, Chicago. World J Gastroenterol 2013;19:1372–9.
7. Holt BA, Hawes R, Hasan M, et al. Biliary drainage: role of EUS guidance. Gastrointest Endosc 2016;83:160–5.

8. Tonozuka R, Itoi T, Tsuchiya T, et al. EUS-guided biliary drainage is infrequently used even in high-volume centers of interventional EUS. Gastrointest Endosc 2016;84:206–7.
9. Kedia P, Gaidhane M, Kahaleh M. Endoscopic guided biliary drainage: how can we achieve efficient biliary drainage? Clin Endosc 2013;46:543–51.
10. Hara K, Yamao K, Mizuno N, et al. Endoscopic ultrasonography-guided biliary drainage: who, when, which, and how? World J Gastroenterol 2016;22:1297–303.
11. Imai H, Kitano M, Omoto S, et al. EUS-guided gallbladder drainage for rescue treatment of malignant distal biliary obstruction after unsuccessful ERCP. Gastrointest Endosc 2016;84:147–51.
12. Itoi T, Binmoeller K, Itokawa F, et al. Endoscopic ultrasonography-guided cholecystogastrostomy using a lumen-apposing metal stent as an alternative to extrahepatic bile duct drainage in pancreatic cancer with duodenal invasion. Dig Endosc 2013;25:137–41.
13. Varadarajulu S, Hawes RH. EUS-guided biliary drainage: taxing and not ready. Gastrointest Endosc 2013;78:742–3.
14. Park DH, Song TJ, Eum J, et al. EUS-guided hepaticogastrostomy with a fully covered metal stent as the biliary diversion technique for an occluded biliary metal stent after a failed ERCP (with videos). Gastrointest Endosc 2010;71:413–9.
15. Artifon EL, Takada J, Okawa L, et al. EUS-guided choledochoduodenostomy for biliary drainage in unresectable pancreatic cancer: a case series. JOP 2010;11:597–600.
16. Prachayakul V, Aswakul P. A novel technique for endoscopic ultrasound-guided biliary drainage. World J Gastroenterol 2013;19:4758–63.
17. Artifon ELA, Ferreira FC, Sakai P. EUS guided biliary drainage. Korean J Radiol 2012;13:S74–82.
18. Artifon EL, Safatle-Ribeiro AV, Ferreira FC, et al. EUS-guided antegrade transhepatic placement of a self-expandable metal stent in hepaticojejunal anastomosis. J Oncol Pract 2011;12:610–3.
19. Nguyen-Tang T, Binmoeller KF, Sanchez-Yague A, et al. Endoscopic ultrasound (EUS)-guided transhepatic anterograde self-expandable metal stent (SEMS) placement across malignant biliary obstruction. Endoscopy 2010;42:232–6.
20. Giovannini M, Pesenti C, Bories E, et al. EUS guided hepatico-gastrostomy using a new design partially covered stent (GIOBOR Stent). Gastrointest Endosc 2012;75:AB441.
21. Nakai Y, Isayama H, Yamamoto N, et al. Safety and effectiveness of a long, partially covered metal stent for endoscopic ultrasound-guided hepaticogastrostomy in patients with malignant biliary obstruction. Endoscopy 2016;48:1125–8.
22. Hara K, Yamao K, Hijioka S, et al. Prospective clinical study of endoscopic ultrasound-guided choledochoduodenostomy with direct metallic stent placement using a forward-viewing echoendoscope. Endoscopy 2013;45:392–6.
23. Rimbaş M, Kunda R, Larghi A. Endoscopic ultrasound-guided choledochoduodenostomy as a primary treatment for malignant distal biliary obstruction: is it time for a randomized controlled study? Endoscopy 2016;48:686.
24. Attili F, Rimbaş M, Galasso D, et al. Fluoroless endoscopic ultrasound-guided biliary drainage after failed ERCP with a novel lumen-apposing metal stent mounted on a cautery-tipped delivery system. Endoscopy 2015;47(Suppl 1):E619–20.
25. Maranki J, Hernandez AJ, Arslan B, et al. Interventional endoscopic ultrasound-guided cholangiography: long-term experience of an emerging alternative to percutaneous transhepatic cholangiography. Endoscopy 2009;41:532–8.

26. Park DH, Jang JW, Lee SS, et al. EUS-guided biliary drainage with transluminal stenting after failed ERCP: predictors of adverse events and long-term results. Gastrointest Endosc 2011;74:1276–84.

27. Shah JN, Marson F, Weilert F, et al. Single-operator, single-session EUS-guided anterograde cholangiopancreatography in failed ERCP or inaccessible papilla. Gastrointest Endosc 2012;75:56–64.

28. Iwashita T, Lee JG, Shinoura S, et al. Endoscopic ultrasound-guided rendezvous for biliary access after failed cannulation. Endoscopy 2012;44:60–5.

29. Dhir V, Bhandari S, Bapat M, et al. Comparison of EUS-guided rendezvous and precut papillotomy techniques for biliary access (with videos). Gastrointest Endosc 2012;75:354–9.

30. Villa JJ, Pérez-Miranda M, Vazquez-Sequeiros E, et al. Initial experience with EUS-guided cholangiopancreatography for biliary and pancreatic duct drainage: a Spanish national survey. Gastrointest Endosc 2012;76:1133–41.

31. Park DH, Jeong SU, Lee BU, et al. Prospective evaluation of a treatment algorithm with enhanced guidewire manipulation protocol for EUS-guided biliary drainage after failed ERCP (with video). Gastrointest Endosc 2013;78:91–101.

32. Dhir V, Bhandari S, Bapat M, et al. Comparison of transhepatic and extrahepatic routes for EUS-guided rendezvous procedure for distal CBD obstruction. United European Gastroenterol J 2013;1:103–8.

33. Khashab MA, Valeshabad AK, Modayil R, et al. EUS-guided biliary drainage by using a standardized approach for malignant biliary obstruction: rendezvous versus direct transluminal techniques (with videos). Gastrointest Endosc 2013; 78:734–41.

34. Gupta K, Perez-Miranda M, Kahaleh M, et al. Endoscopic ultrasound-assisted bile duct access and drainage: multicenter, long-term analysis of approach, outcomes, and complications of a technique in evolution. J Clin Gastroenterol 2014; 48:80–7.

35. Dhir V, Artifon EL, Gupta K, et al. Multicenter study on endoscopic ultrasound-guided expandable biliary metal stent placement: choice of access route, direction of stent insertion, and drainage route. Dig Endosc 2014;26:430–5.

36. Kawakubo K, Isayama H, Kato H, et al. Multicenter retrospective study of endoscopic ultrasound-guided biliary drainage for malignant biliary obstruction in Japan. J Hepatobiliary Pancreat Sci 2014;21:328–34.

37. Dhir V, Itoi T, Khashab MA, et al. Multicenter comparative evaluation of endoscopic placement of expandable metal stents for malignant distal common bile duct obstruction by ERCP or EUS-guided approach. Gastrointest Endosc 2015; 81:913–23.

38. Poincloux L, Rouquette O, Buc E, et al. Endoscopic ultrasound-guided biliary drainage after failed ERCP: cumulative experience of 101 procedures at a single center. Endoscopy 2015;47:794–801.

39. Sportes AMC, Grabar S, Leblanc S, et al. Comparative trial of EUS-guided hepatico-gastrostomy and percutaneous transhepatic biliary drainage for malignant obstructive jaundice after failed ERCP. Gastrointest Endosc 2016;83:AB522–3.

40. Sharaiha RZ, Kumta NA, Desai AP, et al. Endoscopic ultrasound-guided biliary drainage versus percutaneous transhepatic biliary drainage: predictors of successful outcome in patients who fail endoscopic retrograde cholangiopancreatography. Surg Endosc 2016;30:5500–5.

41. Kunda R, Perez-Miranda M, Will U, et al. EUS-guided choledochoduodenostomy for malignant distal biliary obstruction using a lumen apposing fully covered metal stent after failed ERCP. Surg Endosc 2016;30:5002–8.

42. Khashab MA, Van der Merwe S, Kunda R, et al. Prospective international multi-center study on endoscopic ultrasound-guided biliary drainage for patients with malignant distal biliary obstruction after failed endoscopic retrograde cholangiopancreatography. Endosc Int Open 2016;4:E487–96.
43. Khashab MA, Messallam AA, Penas I, et al. International multicenter comparative trial of transluminal EUS-guided biliary drainage via hepatogastrostomy vs choledochoduodenostomy approaches. Endosc Int Open 2016;4:E175–81.
44. Khashab MA, El Zein MH, Sharzehi K, et al. EUS-guided biliary drainage or enteroscopy-assisted ERCP in patients with surgical anatomy and biliary obstruction: an international comparative study. Endosc Int Open 2016;4:E1322–7.
45. Tyberg A, Desai AP, Kumta NA, et al. EUS-guided biliary drainage after failed ERCP: a novel algorithm individualized based on patient anatomy. Gatrointest Endosc 2016;84:941–6.
46. Cho DH, Lee SS, Oh D, et al. Long term outcomes of a newly developed hybrid metal stent for EUS-guided biliary drainage (with videos). Gastrointest Endosc 2017;85(5):1067–75.
47. Nakai Y, Isayama H, Yamamoto N, et al. Indications for endoscopic ultrasonography (EUS)-guided biliary intervention: does EUS always come after failed endoscopic retrograde cholangiopancreatography? Dig Endosc 2017;29(2):218–25.
48. Khumbhari V, Peñas I, Tieu AH, et al. Interventional EUS using a flexible 19-gauge needle: an international multicenter experience in 162 patients. Dig Dis Sci 2016; 61:3552–9.
49. Torres-Ruiz MF, Alonso-Larraga JO, Del Monte JS, et al. Biliary drainage in malignant obstruction: a comparative study between EUS-guided vs percutaneous drainage in patients with failed ERCP. Gastrointest Endosc 2016;83:AB356.
50. Lee TH, Choi JH, Park DH, et al. Similar efficacies of endoscopic ultrasound-guided transmural and percutaneous drainage for malignant distal biliary obstruction. Clin Gastroenterol Hepatol 2016;14:1011–9.e3.
51. Wang K, Zhu J, Xing L, et al. Assessment of efficacy and safety of EUS-guided biliary drainage: a systematic review. Gastrointest Endosc 2016;83:1218–27.
52. Dhir V, Isayama H, Itoi T, et al. EUS-guided biliary and pancreatic duct interventions. Dig Endosc 2017;29(4):472–85.
53. Artifon EL, Marson FP, Gaidhane M, et al. Hepaticogastrostomy or choledochoduodenostomy for distal malignant biliary obstruction after failed ERCP: Is there any difference? Gastrointest Endosc 2015;81:950–9.
54. Siripun A, Sripongpun P, Ovartlarnporn B. Endoscopic ultrasound-guided biliary intervention in patients with surgically altered anatomy. World J Gastrointest Endosc 2015;7:283–9.
55. Inamdar S, Slattery E, Sejpal DV, et al. Systematic review and meta-analysis of single-balloon enteroscopy-assisted ERCP in patients with surgically altered GI anatomy. Gastrointest Endosc 2015;82:9–19.
56. Lee JH, Krishna SG, Singh A, et al. Comparison of the utility of covered metal stents versus uncovered metal stents in the management of malignant biliary strictures in 749 patients. Gastrointest Endosc 2013;78:312–24.
57. Alvarez-Sanchez MV, Jenssen C, Faiss S, et al. Interventional endoscopic ultrasonography: an overview of safety and complications. Surg Endosc 2014;28: 712–34.
58. Umeda J, Itoi T, Tsuchiya T, et al. A newly designed plastic stent for EUS-guided hepaticogastrostomy: a prospective preliminary feasibility study (with videos). Gastrointest Endosc 2015;82:390–6.e2.

59. Park DH, Lee TH, Paik WH, et al. Feasibility and safety of a novel dedicated device for one-step EUS-guided biliary drainage: a randomized trial. J Gastroenterol Hepatol 2015;30:1461–6.

60. Rimbaş M, Attili F, Larghi A. Single-session EUS-guided FNA and biliary drainage with use of a biflanged lumen apposing stent on an electrocautery enhanced delivery system: one-stop shop for unresectable pancreatic mass with duodenal obstruction. Gastrointest Endosc 2015;82:405.

61. Sharaiha RZ, Khan MA, Kamal F, et al. Efficacy and safety of EUS-guided biliary drainage in comparison with percutaneous biliary drainage when ERCP fails: a systematic review and meta-analysis. Gastrointest Endosc 2017;85(5):904–14.

62. Kawakubo K, Kawakami H, Kuwatani M, et al. Endoscopic ultrasound-guided choledochoduodenostomy vs. transpapillary stenting for distal biliary obstruction. Endoscopy 2016;48:164–9.

63. Artifon EL, Loureiro JF, Baron TH, et al. Surgery or EUS-guided choledochoduodenostomy for malignant distal biliary obstruction after ERCP failure. Endosc Ultrasound 2015;4:235–43.

64. Fabbri C, Luigiano C, Lisotti A, et al. Endoscopic ultrasound-guided treatments: are we getting evidence based–a systematic review. World J Gastroenterol 2014; 20:8424–48.

65. Fujii-Lau LL, Levy MJ. Endoscopic ultrasound-guided pancreatic duct drainage. J Hepatobiliary Pancreat Sci 2015;22:51–7.

66. Tyberg A, Sharaiha RZ, Kedia P, et al. EUS-guided pancreatic drainage for pancreatic strictures after failed ERCP: a multicenter international collaborative study. Gastrointest Endosc 2017;85:164–9.

67. Itoi T, Yasuda I, Kurihara T, et al. Technique of endoscopic ultrasonography-guided pancreatic duct intervention (with videos). J Hepatobiliary Pancreat Sci 2014;21:E4–9.

68. Chapman CG, Waxman I, Siddiqui UD. Endoscopic ultrasound (EUS)-guided pancreatic duct drainage: the basics of when and how to perform EUS-guided pancreatic duct interventions. Clin Endosc 2016;49:161–7.

69. Oh D, Park do H, Cho MK, et al. Feasibility and safety of a fully covered self-expandable metal stent with antimigration properties for EUS-guided pancreatic duct drainage: early and midterm outcomes (with video). Gastrointest Endosc 2016;83:366–73.e2.

70. Gines A, Varadarajulu S, Napoleon B. EUS 2008 Working Group document: evaluation of EUS-guided pancreatic-duct drainage (with video). Gastrointest Endosc 2009;69:S43–8.

71. Will U, Reichel A, Fueldner F, et al. Endoscopic ultrasonography-guided drainage for patients with symptomatic obstruction and enlargement of the pancreatic duct. World J Gastroenterol 2015;21:13140–51.

72. Levy MJ. EUS-guided drainage of biliary and pancreatic ductal systems. In: Hawes RH, Fockens P, Varadarajulu S, editors. Endosonography: expert consult. 2nd edition. Philadelphia: Elsevier Saunders; 2010. p. 264–74.

73. Tessier G, Bories E, Arvanitakis M, et al. EUS-guided pancreatogastrostomy and pancreatobulbostomy for the treatment of pain in patients with pancreatic ductal dilatation inaccessible for transpapillary endoscopic therapy. Gastrointest Endosc 2007;65:233–41.

74. Francois E, Kahaleh M, Giovannini M, et al. EUS-guided pancreaticogastrostomy. Gastrointest Endosc 2002;56:128–33.

75. Kahaleh M, Hernandez AJ, Tokar J, et al. EUS-guided pancreaticogastrostomy: analysis of its efficacy to drain inaccessible pancreatic ducts. Gastrointest Endosc 2007;65:224–30.
76. Varadarajulu S, Trevino JM. Review of EUS-guided pancreatic duct drainage (with video). Gastrointest Endosc 2009;69:S200–2.
77. Itoi T, Sofuni A, Tsuchiya T, et al. Initial valuation of a new plastic pancreatic duct stent for endoscopic ultrasonography-guided placement. Endoscopy 2015;47: 462–5.
78. Ogura T, Onda S, Takagi W, et al. Placement of a 6 mm, fully covered metal stent for main pancreatic head duct stricture due to chronic pancreatitis: a pilot study (with video). Therap Adv Gastroenterol 2016;9:722–8.
79. Will U, Fueldner F, Thieme A, et al. Transgastric pancreatography and EUS-guided drainage of the pancreatic duct. J Hepatobiliary Pancreat Surg 2007; 14:377–82.
80. Barkay O, Sheman S, McHenry L, et al. Therapeutic EUS-assisted endoscopic retrograde pancreatography after failed pancreatic duct cannulation at ERCP. Gastrointest Endosc 2010;7:1166–73.
81. Ergun M, Aouattah T, Gillain C, et al. Endoscopic ultrasound-guided transluminal drainage of pancreatic duct obstruction: long-term outcome. Endoscopy 2011; 43:518–25.
82. Kurihara T, Itoi T, Sofuni A, et al. Endoscopic ultrasonography-guided pancreatic duct drainage after failed endoscopic retrograde cholangiopancreatography in patients with malignant and benign pancreatic duct obstructions. Dig Endosc 2013;25:109–16.
83. Fujii LL, Topazian MD, Abu Dayyeh BK, et al. EUS-guided pancreatic duct intervention: outcomes of a single tertiary-care referral center experience. Gastrointest Endosc 2013;78:854–64.e1.
84. Chen YI, Levy MJ, Moreels TG, et al. An international multicenter study comparing EUS-guided pancreatic duct drainage with enteroscopy-assisted endoscopic retrograde pancreatography after Whipple surgery. Gastrointest Endosc 2017;85:170–7.

Endoscopic Ultrasound–Guided Gastrojejunostomy

Sunil Amin, MD, MPH, Amrita Sethi, MD*

KEYWORDS

- Endoscopic ultrasonography • Gastrojejunostomy • Anastomosis
- Gastric outlet obstruction • Lumen-apposing metal stent

KEY POINTS

- EUS-guided gastrojejunostomy is an emerging modality for the treatment of gastric outlet obstruction.
- Provided patients are chosen carefully and anatomy is favorable, clinical success rates are 90% in the hands of an expert endoscopist.
- A one-step procedure using a cautery-tipped lumen-apposing metal stent (LAMS) results in higher technical success and shorter procedure times by obviating multiple long wire exchanges.
- Although early retrospective data compare favorably with enteral stenting and surgical gastrojejunostomy, prospective studies are needed before recommending EUS-GJ as the standard of care for benign or malignant gastric outlet obstruction.

 Video content accompanies this article at http://www.giendo.theclinics.com.

INTRODUCTION: NATURE OF THE PROBLEM

Gastric outlet obstruction (GOO) is a common complication of advanced upper gastrointestinal and pancreatic malignancies. Surgical gastrojejunostomy is currently the standard of care for palliative treatment; however, limitations include prolonged recovery times delaying chemotherapy, delayed gastric emptying/gastroparesis, and the costs associated with operating room time. Enteral stenting is a less durable option for patients with a life expectancy less than 2 months, but, beyond this time-frame, such complications as stent migration or stent occlusion are common.[1] More recently, endoscopic ultrasound (EUS)-guided gastrojejunostomy or gastroenterostomy (EUS-GJ, EUS-GE) with placement of a biflanged lumen-apposing metal stent

Disclosure Statement: Dr A. Sethi serves as a paid consultant for Boston Scientific Corp and Olympus America.
Division of Digestive and Liver Diseases, Department of Medicine, Columbia University Medical Center, 161 Fort Washington Avenue, 852A, New York, NY 10032, USA
* Corresponding author.
E-mail address: as3614@cumc.columbia.edu

Gastrointest Endoscopy Clin N Am 27 (2017) 707–713
http://dx.doi.org/10.1016/j.giec.2017.06.009
1052-5157/17/© 2017 Elsevier Inc. All rights reserved.

(LAMS) has emerged as a third option that may provide long-term luminal patency without the surgical limitations described previously. Provided candidates are chosen appropriately, early data suggest good outcomes with acceptable complication rates. This article discusses the indications, techniques, complications, postoperative care, and early outcomes for this emerging procedure.

INDICATIONS/CONTRAINDICATIONS

Several requirements must be met before consideration of an EUS-GJ (**Table 1**). First, a target area of duodenal or jejunal lumen must be located by EUS within 2 cm of the gastric wall. Any distance longer than 2 cm may result in incomplete apposition of the lumens by the metal stent. Second, one must be cognizant of the possibility of malignant invasion into the wall of the stomach. Direct puncture through tumor may result in an increased risk of complications, such as bleeding and incomplete apposition. Third, because a dilating balloon is often passed distally through the duodenum to locate an appropriate area of jejunum to target for distal site of anastomosis, severe outlet obstruction resulting in the inability to advance a wire to the jejunum may render the procedure not feasible. Fourth, the endoscopist must be able to maintain access to the free floating jejunum after initial EUS-guided puncture. Multiple exchanges over the wire make this component more challenging, and thus the one-step cautery-assisted stent deployment method is preferred (discussed later). Ascites also hinder attempts at maintaining access to the jejunum. Fifth, an appropriate lumen-apposing stent must be available with the ability to hold the two lumens together and maintain patency. A standard covered metal stent may not be appropriate. Finally, care must be taken to ensure that no downstream luminal obstruction exists distal to the jejunum puncture site. In this setting, which may occur in the setting of peritoneal carcinomatosis or extensive lymphadenopathy, the procedure does not provide symptomatic relief.

TECHNIQUE/PROCEDURE

To date, four primary techniques have been described to create a EUS-GJ: (1) water immersion,[2] (2) water-inflated balloon technique,[3,4] (3) endoscopic ultronsonographically guided double-balloon-occluded GJ bypass (EPASS),[5] and (4) the free-hand technique.[4,6] Although slightly different with regards to method of locating the jejunal loop before EUS-guided transgastric puncture, all four methods require a therapeutic linear echoendoscope and use a biflanged LAMS to ultimately create the GJ. Before

Table 1 Indications and contraindications for EUS-GJ	
Indications	**Contraindications**
Malignant obstruction in the gastric antrum or first, second, or third parts of duodenum	Malignant obstruction downstream of jejunal puncture site
	Target puncture site >2 cm from gastric wall
	Malignant invasion through wall of stomach (relative)
	Ascites (relative)
	Inability to pass wire through obstruction (unless using free-hand technique)

starting the procedure, regardless of technique, the patient is given intravenous anti-biotics, intubated, and placed in a supine position. Intravenous glucagon may be used intermittently to decrease small bowel peristalsis.

To perform the water-immersion technique, a large amount of water is infused either through the working channel of the linear echoendoscope or after direct puncture with a 22-gauge needle into the proximal small bowel.[2,5] This infusion distends the jejunal lumen and facilitates endosonographic localization of a suitable transgastric puncture site. Either a one-step or two-step procedure is then performed to create the GJ. In the one-step procedure, a cautery-tipped 10.8F catheter of a 15-mm LAMS (AXIOS-EC, Boston Scientific, Natick, MA) is then used to simultaneously puncture the water-distended jejunal loop and perform stent deployment. Using the less preferable two-step procedure, a 19-gauge needle (as opposed to the cautery-tipped stent cath-eter) is used to puncture the water-distended jejunal loop and a 0.035-inch wire is advanced distally. The 19-gauge needle is then exchanged under endosonographic guidance, leaving the wire in place, for a 6-mm dilating balloon. The gastrojejunal tract is then flash-dilated to allow for passage of the 10.8F LAMS delivery catheter, which is subsequently passed over the wire transgastrically into the jejunum. More aggressive dilation is discouraged because this may result in peritoneal leakage during the long-wire exchange.[5,7] The LAMS is then deployed with one flange in the jejunum and one flange in the stomach. Finally, the lumen of the LAMS is dilated to 15 mm using a 12 to 13.5 to 15 mm through-the-scope balloon dilator.

The water-inflated balloon technique is similar to the water-filling technique; how-ever, a biliary retrieval or dilating balloon catheter is passed into the jejunum over a wire that has been preplaced under fluoroscopic guidance, and inflated (with contrast or water) as a means of localizing a jejunal loop instead of a bolus of water. Once the inflated balloon is localized endosonographically, transgastric puncture is performed with the goal of bursting the balloon.[3] This initial puncture can be done directly with the 10.8F cautery-tipped LAMS catheter (hot) or with a 19-gauge needle and subse-quent guidewire placement and dilation before introduction of the stent catheter (non-cautery enhanced version) (Video 1).Variations on the use of an assisted device to fill and subsequently localize a jejunal loop have also been described with a nasobiliary drain and ultraslim endoscope passed through the stricture.[4]

To perform the EPASS procedure, a proprietary double-balloon enteric tube (Create Medic Co, Ltd, Yokohama, Japan) is passed over a 0.089-inch guidewire or through an overtube into the jejunum beyond the ligament of Treitz.[5] The two balloons are then inflated and saline/contrast is used to fill and distend the lumen between the balloons allowing for easy transgastric endosonographic localization. The subsequent puncture and stent deployment is then done using the one- or two-step method described previously.

Finally, the free-hand technique is more natural orifice transluminal endoscopic surgery based. To accomplish this technique, a transgastric puncture into the peri-toneum is first performed with a 19-gauge needle under EUS guidance. A guidewire is placed through the needle into the peritoneum, and the linear echoendoscope is exchanged for a double-channel gastroscope over the wire. An incision on the gastric wall is then made with a needle knife (inserted through the second channel) and the gastrostomy is dilated to 15 mm. The gastroscope is then passed into the peritoneum where a jejunal loop is located and incised with the needle knife, followed by subsequent advancement and coiling of the guidewire in the jejunum. The distal flange of the LAMS is then deployed in the jejunum, the gastroscope is pulled back in the stomach, and the proximal flange deployed in the stomach, thus creating the GJ.[6]

COMPLICATIONS AND MANAGEMENT

To date, there have been no procedural-related deaths associated with EUS-GJ. Nevertheless, several complications, such as postprocedural pain, stent maldeployment, perforation leading to peritonitis, and bleeding, have been reported. In their series of 26 patients, Tyberg and colleagues[4] report adverse events of peritonitis, bleeding, and surgery in three patients (11.5%). Although not noted to be device or procedure related, there was one death caused by peritonitis noted in this series 1 day postprocedure in which the stent was removed and the defect was endoscopically closed. This patient had ascites and peritoneal carcinomatosis, raising the consideration of the need for careful patient selection. In a series of 10 patients by Khashab and colleagues,[3] no patients suffered from procedure-related adverse events. However, only 3 of the 10 patients had malignant GOO, whereas the other seven had benign obstruction. Among 20 patients with malignant GOO who underwent EUS-GJ using the EPASS technique, Itoi and colleagues[5] report two (10%) adverse events. Both were cases of stent deployment that were immediately noticed and treated with stent removal and conservative management. The authors noted, however, that in the setting of poor overall prognosis and progressive cancer with concomitant acute cholangitis, stent maldeployment may be a fatal event, similar to the series discussed previously.

PERIPROCEDURAL CARE

There is no consensus on the optimal periprocedural management of patients undergoing EUS-GJ. However, most proceduralists would agree that outpatients should be kept on noting by mouth or given a clear liquid diet for several days before the procedure to minimize gastric residue. Postprocedurally, patients should be admitted to the hospital ward for observation, maintained on broad-spectrum antibiotics for at least 7 days, and kept nothing by mouth for 24 to 48 hours. Thereafter, pending clinical course, clear liquids are introduced and the diet advanced as tolerated up to a soft diet. It is important that patients be instructed to follow traditional dietary recommendations after enteral stent placement, including drinking liquids during and after each meal, cutting food into small pieces and chewing thoroughly, sitting upright during meals and for 1 to 2 hours afterward, and avoiding fresh fruits and vegetables.

OUTCOMES

Initial outcomes of EUS-GJ have been promising, regardless of technique, and for a variety of different indications. The largest series to date has been a prospective, multicenter, international collaboration compiled by Tyberg and colleagues,[4] in which 26 patients with GOO (malignant, 17; benign, 9) were treated with EUS-GJ creation using a LAMS. Technical success, defined as successful creation of the EUS-GJ, was achieved in 92% of patients, whereas clinical success, defined as the ability of a patient to tolerate an oral diet, was achieved in 85% of patients. Adverse events, such as bleeding, peritonitis, and surgery, occurred in three patients (11.5%). Limitations of this study are the lack of consistency with regards to the method of GJ creation (balloon assisted, directed GJ, and water distention all used) and the type of stent used (AXIOS-EC used in only 35%).

Itoi and colleagues[5] report a second large series of 20 patients with malignant GOO treated with EUS-GJ. The authors use a special double-balloon enteric tube to perform an EPASS procedure (described previously). The double-balloon enteric tube allows water to fill between the two balloons thereby distending the lumen and creating a window for EUS-guided transgastric access. Technical success was 90% and all 18 patients reported an increase in their GOO scoring system score postprocedure. Both the mean (0.6 ± 0.75 vs 2.94 ± 0.23; $P<.001$) and median (0 vs 3; $P<.001$) post-GOO scoring system score scores were significantly higher than the pre-GOO scores. Furthermore, no stent migration or occlusion was noted in any of the 18 technically successful cases after a median of 100 days follow-up. There are two important considerations with regards to this study. First, all cases were performed using the electrocautery-tipped stent delivery system (AXIOS-EC). Second, when the authors abandoned the use of an over-the-wire method to advance the LAMS into the jejunal lumen in favor of free-style catheter advancement, technical success increased from 82% to 100%. In the opinion of the authors, pushing the guidewire causes the jejunum to move away from the stomach, potentially resulting in maldeployment of the LAMS.

The third largest series of EUS-GJ is a retrospective series from two tertiary care centers published by Khashab and colleagues[3] in 2015. Seven patients with benign obstruction and three patients with malignant GOO were treated with EUS-GJ using the direct EUS-GE or balloon-assisted EUS-GE technique. Technical success was achieved in 90% of patients and clinical success was achieved in 100% of patients. Mean procedural time was 96 minutes (range, 45–152 minutes) and mean length of hospital stay was 2.2 days. There were no procedural-related adverse events in this study.

With regards to smaller studies and alternative indications, Barthet and coworkers[6] used a natural orifice transluminal endoscopic surgery approach EUS-GJ to treat three patients with GOO. After obtaining EUS-guided access to the peritoneum through the gastric wall, a needle knife was used to incise a loop of jejunum through which a cold AXIOS stent was deployed transgastrically. Technical and clinical success was achieved in all three patients, with minimal complications. Shah and colleagues[8] describe a case of afferent loop syndrome successfully treated with the creation of a EUS-GJ. The authors report that this procedure was feasible because of a fixed position of the afferent limb. Finally, although not EUS-guided, Ryou and colleagues[9] describe the creation of endoscopic anastomoses using magnets for lumen compression and subsequent necrosis.

To date, there are two studies available comparing EUS-GE with other modalities, such as enteral stenting or surgical GJ (SGJ) to treat malignant GOO. In their retrospective series of 82 patients, Chen and colleagues[10] compared 30 patients who underwent EUS-GE with 52 patients who underwent enteral stenting at four centers between 2008 and 2015. Although there was no difference in technical or clinical success between the two modalities (86.7% EUS-GE vs 94.2% enteral stenting [$P = .2$] and 83.3% EUS-GE versus 67.3% enteral stenting [$P = .12$]), symptom recurrence and need for reintervention was significantly lower among the EUS-GE group (4.0% vs 28.6%; $P = .015$). On multivariable analysis controlling for covariates, enteral stenting was associated with a 12.8-fold greater odds of reintervention than EUS-GE (odds ratio, 12.8; $P = .027$).

In a nonrandomized, multicenter, international retrospective comparative study, EUS-GE and SGJ for malignant GOO were compared in 30 patients and 60 patients, respectively.[11] Three methods of EUS-GE were performed including balloon-assisted EUS-GE, EPASS, and direct puncture technique. Although the EUS-GE group was derived from three centers, all the surgical patients were from one center. LAMS were used in all EUS-GE procedures. Although the technical success rate was significantly higher in the SGJ group (100% vs 87%; odds ratio, 3.4; $P = .009$), there was no significant difference in the clinic success rate between the two groups. Multivariate analysis revealed that the only predictor of clinical success was the absence of peritoneal carcinomatosis. There was a nonsignificant lower rate of adverse events in the EUS-GE group, and these included clinically relevant stent misdeployment (n = 3) and abdominal pain (n = 2). There were similar rates of GOO recurrence, time to reintervention, and mean Length of Hospital Stay.

CURRENT CONTROVERSIES/FUTURE CONSIDERATIONS

Given the technical and clinical success achieved by several groups using a variety of different techniques (>90%), there is no current consensus on the optimal method for performing EUS-GJ. Of the techniques discussed previously, Itoi and colleagues propose the superiority of their double-balloon occluded method (EPASS) over the water-filling technique or the water-inflated balloon technique. The primary argument against the water-filling technique is that rapid infusion of water may lead to electrolyte complications, such as hyponatremia, cardiovascular compromise from fluid overload, or misguided EUS puncture into a distended colon. In terms of the water-inflated balloon technique, although initial EUS puncture may be easy, manually apposing the lumen of the jejunum to the stomach under EUS guidance is difficult and may result in inability to deploy the LAMS. Although a balloon snare apparatus has been described to aid in this purpose by allowing tension to be applied to both ends of the guidewire to prevent the small bowel from moving away from the gastric wall, the use of a cautery-tipped LAMS essentially minimizes this problem (Video 2).[12] One-step EPASS does seem to be time-saving, however, with a mean procedure time of only 25.5 minutes.[5]

Although early data for EUS-GJ are promising, the procedure cannot yet be endorsed as the standard of care for GOO. Going forward, prospective studies are needed to clarify several issues. First, EUS-GE must be compared in a prospective fashion with enteral stenting and SGJ. If the early data hold true and EUS-GJ results in similar rates of technical and clinical success without more adverse events, the optimal method of performing EUS-GE must then be determined. There are little long-term data on stent patency, migration rates, and long-term outcomes beyond several months and there is a need to determine how these outcomes change with regards to cause of GOO (ie, benign or malignant disease).

SUMMARY

GOO is a common complication of upper gastrointestinal and pancreatic malignancies, for which multiple treatment modalities exist. EUS-GJ is emerging as a new option that may provide a more durable solution than enteral stenting with shorter recovery time and less cost than SGJ. Nevertheless, patients must be chosen carefully and favorable anatomy is required to achieve clinical success. Several techniques for performing EUS-GJ have been described with favorable outcomes including the direct-EUS, balloon-assisted, and free-hand methods, although no one technique has yet emerged as superior. Most experts agree, however, that a one-step procedure with a cautery-tipped LAMS (which obviates multiple long-wire exchanges) results in higher rates of technical success and shorter procedure times. In terms of outcomes, early retrospective data suggest that EUS-GJ is comparable with regards to clinical efficacy (90% clinical success rate) and adverse events to enteral stenting and SGJ. Nevertheless, prospective studies comparing these different modalities of treatment for GOO and the various techniques of performing EUS-GJ are warranted before recommending this new and innovative procedure as standard of care.

SUPPLEMENTARY DATA

Supplementary data related to this article can be found online at http://dx.doi.org/10.1016/j.giec.2017.06.009.

REFERENCES

1. Jeurnink SM, Steyerberg EW, van Hooft JE, et al. Surgical gastrojejunostomy or endoscopic stent placement for the palliation of malignant gastric outlet obstruction (SUSTENT study): a multicenter randomized trial. Gastrointest Endosc 2010; 71(3):490–9.
2. Binmoeller KF, Shah JN. Endoscopic ultrasound-guided gastroenterostomy using novel tools designed for transluminal therapy: a porcine study. Endoscopy 2012; 44(5):499–503.
3. Khashab MA, Kumbhari V, Grimm IS, et al. EUS-guided gastroenterostomy: the first U.S. clinical experience (with video). Gastrointest Endosc 2015;82(5):932–8.
4. Tyberg A, Perez-Miranda M, Sanchez-Ocaña R, et al. Endoscopic ultrasound-guided gastrojejunostomy with a lumen-apposing metal stent: a multicenter, international experience. Endosc Int Open 2016;4(3):E276–81.
5. Itoi T, Ishii K, Ikeuchi N, et al. Prospective evaluation of endoscopic ultrasonography-guided double-balloon-occluded gastrojejunostomy bypass (EPASS) for malignant gastric outlet obstruction. Gut 2016;65(2):193–5.
6. Barthet M, Binmoeller KF, Vanbiervliet G, et al. Natural orifice transluminal endoscopic surgery gastroenterostomy with a biflanged lumen-apposing stent: first clinical experience (with videos). Gastrointest Endosc 2015;81(1):215–8.
7. Itoi T, Baron TH, Mouen K, et al. Technical review of EUS-guided gastroenterostomy in 2017. Dig Endosc 2017;29(4):495–502.
8. Shah A, Khanna L, Sethi A. Treatment of afferent limb syndrome: novel approach with endoscopic ultrasound-guided creation of a gastrojejunostomy fistula and placement of lumen-apposing stent. Endoscopy 2015;47(Suppl 1 UCTN): E309–10.
9. Ryou M, Agoston AT, Thompson CC. Endoscopic intestinal bypass creation by using self-assembling magnets in a porcine model. Gastrointest Endosc 2016; 83(4):821–5.
10. Chen Y-I, Itoi T, Baron TH, et al. EUS-guided gastroenterostomy is comparable to enteral stenting with fewer re-interventions in malignant gastric outlet obstruction. Surg Endosc 2017;31(7):2946–52.
11. Khashab MA, Bukhari M, Baron TH, et al. International multicenter comparative trial of endoscopic ultrasonography-guided gastroenterostomy versus surgical gastrojejunostomy for the treatment of malignant gastric outlet obstruction. Endosc Int Open 2017;5(4):E275.
12. Ngamruengphong S, Kumbhari V, Tieu AH, et al. A novel "balloon/snare apparatus" technique to facilitate easy creation of fistula tract during EUS-guided gastroenterostomy. Gastrointest Endosc 2016;84(3):527.

Endoscopic Ultrasonography–guided Drainage of Pancreatic Collections, Including the Role of Necrosectomy

Ryan Law, DO[a], Todd H. Baron, MD[b],*

KEYWORDS

- Acute pancreatitis • Pancreatic necrosis/therapy • Endoscopic therapy
- Minimally invasive • Pancreatitis/adverse events • Drainage/methods
- Therapeutic irrigation

KEY POINTS

- Pancreatic ductal injury often leads to development of pancreatic fluid collections with or without solid necrotic debris.
- Endoscopic intervention is considered the current standard of care for management of symptomatic pancreatic fluid collections.
- Cross-sectional imaging is paramount before any endoscopic intervention to determine the cavity size, location of potential access sites, and relevant adjacent anatomic structures.
- Direct endoscopic necrosectomy can be performed using various techniques but remains a time-intensive procedure.
- The most common adverse events associated with endoscopic management of pancreatic collections are bleeding and perforation.

INTRODUCTION

Injury to the pancreas may occur as a result of varying insults; however, regardless of the cause, resultant parenchymal inflammation occurs, often leading to disruption of the main pancreatic duct and/or secondary branches. Following ductal

Disclosure: R. Law has no conflicts of interest/disclosures; T.H. Baron and W.L. Gore receive support from Boston Scientific, Olympus, and Cook Endoscopy.
[a] Division of Gastroenterology, University of Michigan, 3912 Taubman Center, 1500 East Medical Center Drive, SPC 5362, Ann Arbor, MI 48109-5362, USA; [b] Division of Gastroenterology and Hepatology, The University of North Carolina at Chapel Hill, 130 Mason Farm Road, CB 7080, Chapel Hill, NC 27599-0001, USA
* Corresponding author.
E-mail address: todd_baron@med.unc.edu

injury, leakage of pancreatic contents promotes formation of fluid-filled pancreatic or peripancreatic collections with or without the presence of solid debris. A minority of patients (approximately 5%–10%) develop evidence of glandular necrosis, often in combination with necrosis of adjacent structures.[1] Clinically severe acute pancreatitis evolves over several weeks, culminating in walled-off necrosis (WON) in many cases (**Fig. 1**).[1,2] The aim of endoscopic therapy in this setting is to provide drainage of liquid contents and mechanical removal of necrotic tissue, if necessary. Endoscopic intervention remains the current standard of care for patients with WON following acute pancreatitis. Minimally invasive approaches, including flexible endoscopic and percutaneous therapy, either alone or in combination, are commonly used by most major medical centers.[3] This article focuses on the indications, techniques, and outcomes of endoscopic therapy and management of pancreatic fluid collections (PFCs).

Indications and Timing of Intervention

Cross-sectional imaging should be performed before initiation of endoscopic intervention to assess the properties of the collection (ie, size, shape, wall thickness, contents), discern adjacent relevant vascularity, and ascertain the relationship between the cavity and true gastrointestinal lumen. Thorough review of cross-sectional imaging is crucial. The computed tomography (CT) and MRI appearance of PFCs can vary widely. Compared with CT, MRI reliably delineates liquid and solid components. On CT, nondependent air seen within a cavity indicates the presence of solid debris but does not represent infection with gas-forming microorganisms, as is often cited. Most commonly, such nondependent air enters through a fistulous connection from the gastrointestinal lumen. As described later, this fistulous tract can be used for transmural entry into the cavity, either for egress of liquefied contents or to enable endoscopic debridement. Coronal CT/MRI images can be useful, often complementing the standard axial images (see **Fig. 1**). Although liquefactive necrosis is generally evident, pancreatic necrosis can appear as nonenhancement of the pancreatic parenchyma and surrounding structures or may be more indistinct, resembling a pseudocyst. This uncertainty often compels therapeutic endoscopists to pursue standard

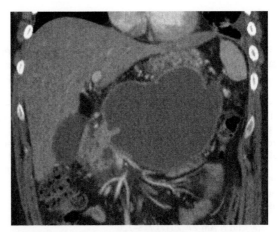

Fig. 1. Coronal computed tomography image of WON. The collection is compressing the stomach, and the patient had clinical gastric outlet obstruction.

pseudocyst drainage methods, which are insufficient at freeing adherent necrotic tissue, and may potentiate serious infection. Understanding the burden of necrosis, the presence or absence of extension into the paracolic gutters, and interactions between multiple cavities, if present, guides the index procedure and streamlines subsequent interventions.

When WON is readily apparent on cross-sectional imaging, consideration can be given to determining the bacteriologic status of the collection, because overt signs/symptoms of infection (eg, leukocytosis, fever) may not be evident. Endoscopic ultrasonography (EUS)–guided drainage or percutaneous fine-needle aspiration (FNA) to sample the contents of the collection are available but are infrequently performed in clinical practice because the decision to intervene is most commonly based on clinical criteria. In addition, EUS-FNA is not sterile and can cause infection of sterile necrosis. When objective findings of infected necrosis are present, urgent intervention is mandatory using either endoscopic (ie, drainage with or without necrosectomy) or percutaneous techniques.

The indications and timing for drainage of sterile fluid or pancreatic necrosis remain controversial. Commonly, peripancreatic collections remain immature and not amenable to endoscopic drainage until at least 4 weeks after the onset of pancreatitis. This interval allows organization of the internal contents of the collection and development of an external rind. Overall, endoscopic intervention should be deferred for as long as possible in patients who remain clinical stable. Common indications for drainage of sterile contents include (1) evidence of gastric outlet obstruction (clinical or radiologic), (2) evidence of biliary obstruction, (3) persistent abdominal discomfort, or (4) failure to thrive (fatigue, anorexia, weight loss). The radiologic appearance (ie, size, shape, location) of a necrotic collection on cross-sectional imaging may be incongruent with the patient's clinical status, and is an insufficient indication for intervention by itself. Historically, a size cutoff of greater than 6 cm was considered an indication for intervention; however, many patients with collections larger than 6 cm may remain asymptomatic with low risk for rupture, bleeding, or infection.

EUS can be used as an adjunct to cross-sectional image before intervention. EUS allows assessment of the presence or absence of significant solid debris that may alter the management strategy. In addition, if there is doubt as to whether the collection represents a true pseudocyst/WON or other noninflammatory cystic lesion, EUS can provide a definitive diagnosis using ultrasonographic features. EUS findings of WON manifest as hyperechoic areas within the collection, which can appear as free-floating debris (**Fig. 2**) or areas of adherent solid material. This solid material can range from a small percentage to nearly the entire collection with a minimal liquid component. If the diagnosis remains in question, aspiration and analysis of cystic contents, biopsy of the cavity wall, and even probe-based confocal endomicroscopy passed through an FNA needle can also be performed. After verification that the lesion is a PFC, and it is decided to proceed with endoscopic drainage, EUS can guide transmural drainage, as discussed later.

Procedural Technique

Before any intervention, the International Normalized Ratio and platelet count should be assessed and corrected, if necessary. Broad-spectrum antibiotics should be initiated if patients are not already receiving them. Recommended broad-spectrum agents include intravenous penicillins (ie, piperacillin/tazobactam), quinolones (ie, levofloxacin), and carbapenems (ie, meropenem). Antibiotic treatment should

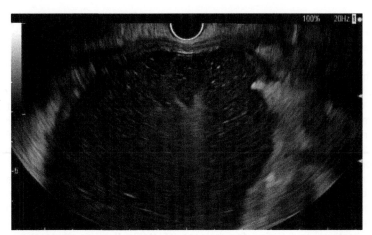

Fig. 2. Echoendoscopic view of WON from patient shown in **Fig. 1**. Note the presence of scattered debris within the cavity.

subsequently be modified when microbiologic data from intraprocedural cultures are obtained. In general, the authors perform all procedures, pseudocyst drainage, and direct endoscopic necrosectomy (DEN), with anesthesia support given high patient acuity, potential length of the procedure, and increased risk for adverse events compared with other endoscopic procedures.

Endoscopic management of PFCs is predicated on evacuation of liquid and/or solid debris from the cavity. An initial transmural puncture, either transgastric or transduodenal, facilitates access to the collection and drains liquid contents. Collections located within or adjacent to the pancreatic body or tail are drained transgastrically, whereas transduodenal access is best for collections located near the pancreatic head and genu. For PFCs composed predominately of liquefied material, transpapillary drainage may be a viable option either alone or in conjunction with transmural drainage.

Several methods to obtain transmural access have been described. When extrinsic compression leads to endoscopically evident luminal protrusion, non–EUS-guided punctures aided by fluoroscopic guidance can be successfully performed (>95%) with low adverse event rates (<5%) when performed by experienced endoscopists.[4] However, most endoscopists concur that EUS-guided access is superior and should be used whenever available. EUS guidance allows precision targeting of the cavity while mitigating the risk of inadvertent injury to adjacent vasculature or intraabdominal structures. In addition, EUS permits real-time assessment of the extent, volume, and density of material within the collection.[5] Transmural access can be gained using a variety of endoscopic devices, including electrocautery-based instruments such as needle knives and specialized cystenterostomy devices (Cystotome, Cook Endoscopy, Winston-Salem, NC), and noncautery tools such as EUS-FNA needles. A recently introduced, lumen-apposing metal stent equipped with an electrocautery-enhanced delivery system (described later) has simplified the management of PFCs. On entrance into the cavity there is often visible extravasation of liquefied contents into the lumen. Aspiration of cyst fluid through an FNA needle, and/or the injection of radiopaque contrast in the cavity under fluoroscopy, can also be used to confirm access.

Following drainage of liquefied contents, FNA or other aspiration needles are advantageous because they permit guidewire passage through the needle core into the cavity (ie, Seldinger technique). A specialized 19-gauge FNA needle (EchoTip Ultra

HD ultrasonography access needle, Cook Endoscopy) designed specifically for EUS-guided drainage procedures may be helpful. A generous length of guidewire is then passed into the collection before tract dilation using a biliary dilating balloon. If the guidewire is lost inadvertently, easily reaccessing the cavity may be problematic, despite prior tract dilation. Blind attempts at passage of the guidewire into the cavity may increase the risk for adverse events. Some endoscopists elect to place 1 (or more) double-pigtail plastic stents during the index procedure with a plan for necrosectomy during subsequent procedures, if necessary. For drainage of purely liquid collections (pancreatic pseudocysts), the authors balloon dilate the tract to 8 to 10 mm followed by placement of 2 10-Fr double-pigtail stents (length of 3–5 cm) to mitigate concerns for stent migration into or out of the cavity. Double-pigtail stents also prevent trauma from impaction into the lumen or cavity wall. The authors recommend placing an endoscopically visible, indelible mark at the midpoint of the stent before placement, if markers are not present on the stent. This technique guards against inadvertent deployment of the entire plastic stent within the collection. Small-bore (10 mm), fully covered, biliary self-expandable metal stents (SEMS) can also be placed for management of collections that are predominately liquid. An SEMS with a diameter of 10 mm only requires a 4-mm balloon dilation (to allow passage of the delivery system). An alternative option to plastic stents or smaller bore SEMS is placement of a large-caliber (16–23mm midbody diameter) SEMS across the dilated lumen wall.[6–10] Use of large-diameter, covered esophageal SEMS facilitates DEN procedures, at the index procedure and/or in subsequent procedures, and circumvents balloon dilation of the tract before each debridement.[7] The shortest available SEMS lengths are 6 to 7 cm, often resulting in excess stent length protruding into gastrointestinal lumen or the necrotic cavity, and possibly leading to impaction as the cavity collapses. Stents can be trimmed using argon plasma coagulation, although minimal disruption of the SEMS interstices is paramount. A double-pigtail plastic stent can also be placed within the deployed SEMS to serve as a buffer between the stent flange and the lumen/cavity wall, and to inhibit necrotic debris from occluding the SEMS.

The recent development of lumen-apposing stents (LAMS) (AXIOS; Boston Scientific, Marlborough, MA) provides solutions to many of the limitations of previous drainage techniques (**Figs. 3** and **4**). These stents are currently available with midbody

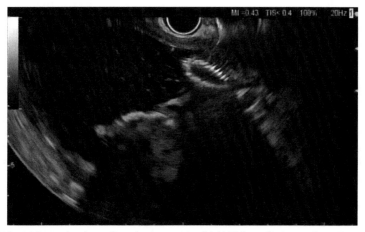

Fig. 3. Echoendoscopic view after deployment of LAMS from same patient. Note a large piece of dense solid debris (hyperechoic) within the cavity.

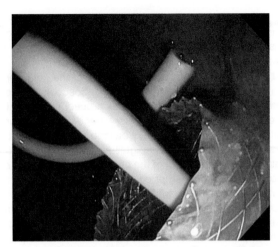

Fig. 4. Endoscopic view of deployed LAMS with 15-mm diameter from same patient as seen from the stomach. An indwelling 10-Fr plastic double-pigtail stent is seen within the LAMS.

luminal diameters of 10 and 15 mm and corresponding external flange diameters of 21 and 24 mm, respectively, with total stent length between the flanges of 1 cm. The short length of these LAMS is ideal for DEN. In addition, the 15-mm version affords apposition of the gastric wall and cavity wall while allowing repeated endoscope passage during debridement procedures.[11,12] A 20-mm iteration of the device is US Food and Drug Administration approved and expected to be commercially available soon. There are 2 types of AXIOS stent delivery systems. The initial iteration requires a placement approach similar to plastic stent or standard SEMS placement (ie, 1-puncture, 2-guidewire placement; 3-tract dilation, 4-stent deployment), whereas the newer version includes an electrocautery-enhanced tip allowing for puncture and tract dilation in 1 step, followed by stent deployment, with or without the use of a guidewire. Many endoscopists place 1 double-pigtail plastic stent within the LAMS (see **Fig. 4**) to maintain stent patency, prevent stent impaction, facilitate removal if a buried stent occurs, and leave room for plastic pigtail stents to treat disconnected ducts as the cavity resolves.

Various techniques can be used for removal of solid debris from necrotic collections. A 7-Fr nasocystic irrigation tube can be placed into the cavity, adjacent to transmural stents, to permit intermittent irrigation with escape of disrupted necrosis through 1 or more transmural exit sites.[13,14] Up to 200 mL of normal saline (with or without 3% hydrogen peroxide) is vigorously infused through the tube every 2 to 4 hours initially to lavage debris from the cavity. Nasocystic irrigation tubes are rarely used in current clinical practice, mostly because of patient intolerance.[15] Dual-modality therapy is a variation of the nasocystic drainage technique that uses the combination of endoscopic and percutaneous therapy, in lieu of a transnasal tube.[16] This technique combines percutaneous drain placement, used as the irrigation conduit, and endoscopic transmural drainage, for egress of debrided necrotic tissue. As mentioned earlier, spontaneous fistulous tracts can provide egress for liquefied debris and allow access for debridement of necrosis, in select cases.[17] If possible, the tract should be balloon dilated to a diameter greater than or equal to 15 mm to allow egress of the remaining liquid and facilitate DEN.

The objective of each DEN procedure should be to remove all possible necrosis. DEN is a labor-intensive intervention that is performed by passing an endoscope transmurally into the collection. Both diagnostic and therapeutic endoscopes can be used, each with intrinsic benefits and limitations. Diagnostic endoscopes have better flexibility but a smaller working channel compared with therapeutic endoscopes. Depending on the manufacturer, each can offer a high-flow water jet that is used to fragment and irrigate necrotic debris. As previously alluded to, the use of hydrogen peroxide lavage may aid in liquefying necrotic tissue during DEN, although evidence from comparative trials is lacking.[18] Mechanical debridement can be accomplished with various endoscopic accessories (eg, stone retrieval baskets, polypectomy snares, polyp retrieval nets, grasping forceps). Regardless of the device, once the necrotic tissue is freed, it is extracted from the cavity and deposited in the lumen. Larger pieces may be cut into smaller pieces using a polypectomy snare with or without electrocautery, then cleared from the collection to avoid unnecessary transmural passage into and out of the cavity. The consistency of necrotic tissue is variable from one patient to another, ranging from solid debris that is densely adherent to tissue that is loosely attached and easy to remove. Some endoscopists opt to perform DEN immediately after the initial transmural puncture, whereas others advocate debridement starting with the subsequent procedure; however, no data exist to advocate one approach rather than the other.

Assuming clinical stability and absence of intraprocedural adverse events, patients may resume (or initiate) oral intake on the day of the procedure. The authors routinely continue peroral antibiotics for several weeks, often until the cavity completely resolves as determined by cross-sectional imaging. Repeat interventions are almost universally necessary for WON when plastic stents are used, compared with large-diameter SEMS, and include stent removal, followed by debridement, then stent replacement. Future procedures can be scheduled if incomplete debridement is recognized,[19] or performed as determined by clinical status and/or cross-sectional imaging findings. The overall clinical picture, in conjunction with logistical issues (eg, inpatient/outpatient status, distance from treatment center) often determine the procedure frequency. Patients requiring ongoing hospitalization often require frequent procedures (every 1–2 days), whereas stable outpatients can generally tolerate 1 to 2 weeks between DEN. In patients with persistent collections despite several interventions, endoscopic retrograde cholangiopancreatography should be considered to assess for an ongoing pancreatic duct disruption. Adjunctive transpapillary stenting of the pancreatic duct can be considered; however, stenting only minimizes leakage of additional pancreatic fluid into the cavity, and is insufficient to use as a drainage route for pancreatic debris. As the cavity resolves, external drains should be removed before removal of internal drains. Internal drains are then endoscopically removed after complete resolution of the collection. This approach is intended to prevent formation of gastrocutaneous/enterocutaneous fistulae.

In our current practice the authors place large-diameter LAMS with an internal 10-Fr double-pigtail plastic stent. This approach is intended to prevent impaction of the necrotic material within the LAMS lumen and allows continued egress of liquid material. The double-pigtail stent also protects the gastric wall and cavity wall as the collection recedes and minimizes the risk of a buried LAMS. An additional advantage of LAMS is the short overall length (~1 cm) and lack of exposed edges that are involuted at full expansion. LAMS also promote a certain degree of procedural efficiency and safety because dilation of the tract is unnecessary before each session. The authors ask patients to discontinue any acid-suppressive medications to promote acid-induced debridement. We reserve DEN for patients who fail to improve or clinically deteriorate. Studies are being performed that suggest that the need for DEN following LAMS placement is based on percentage of necrosis within the WON cavity.

Outcomes

Outcome data following endoscopic intervention of pancreatic pseudocysts is challenging to interpret. For example, there is notable heterogeneity across patient populations and interventions within series. Frequently, studies have included patients receiving both transpapillary and/or transmural drainage. Overall, successful drainage of liquefied collections is achieved in ~90% of patients with acceptable adverse event (5%–10%) and recurrence (5%–20%) rates.[20–22]

Many case series have shown the efficacy of DEN[15,23–26] when plastic stents were used as the primary drainage strategy. Patients with WON have substantial variation in: (1) collection size/shape, (2) overall burden of necrosis, (3) extensions of necrosis into the paracolic gutters, (3) medical comorbidities, and (4) time from onset of necrotizing pancreatitis to intervention. Given this patient heterogeneity and varying definitions of success/failure, comparison of outcomes between reported series remains challenging. In available literature, the 2 most widely used definitions of successful outcomes are complete nonsurgical resolution (including percutaneous drainage) and resolution caused by flexible endoscopy alone.[15]

Data from 2 systematic reviews suggest that complete resolution of pancreatic necrosis can be obtained in 81% of patients using endoscopy alone with a mean number of 4 procedures necessary for resolution.[27,28] The adverse event rates from these studies were 21% and 36%. Furthermore, 2 large retrospective studies have shown resolution in approximately 90% of patients with a lower rate of adverse events (~14%).[15,24]

Limited outcome data in patients treated with transmural placement of esophageal SEMS or LAMS to facilitate DEN have begun to emerge. A recent retrospective study from 2 US medical centers found that resolution could be achieved in 88% of patients using an esophageal SEMS for transmural access.[10] A mean of 5 DEN procedures were required for complete endoscopic resolution, with adverse events occurring in 6% of patients. A similar study from Attam and colleagues[29] revealed similar findings (90% resolution, median 3 procedures). Outcomes following LAMS placement for DEN have also been reported with high rates of success (technical >95%; clinical >80%) and acceptable risk of serious adverse events (<7%).[30,31]

As described, both double-pigtail plastic stents and SEMS/LAMS can be used to establish and maintain tract patency in patients requiring repeated DEN. Clinical judgment should be used to determine the optimal strategy on a case-by-case basis, because both techniques have high clinical resolution rates (>80%).

ALTERNATIVE TREATMENT STRATEGIES

Patients with WON are best managed by a multidisciplinary approach in tertiary care medical centers. Alternative options to endoscopic intervention include (1) nutritional support with parenteral or enteral supplementation, (2) percutaneous drainage, and (3) surgical drainage. A multicenter, randomized controlled trial (Transluminal ENdoscopic versus Surgical necrOsectomy in patients with infected pancreatic Necrosis [TENSION] trial) designed to compare outcomes between a endoscopic step-up approach (transmural drainage plus or minus DEN) and a surgical step-up approach (percutaneous drainage plus or minus surgical necrosectomy) is ongoing.[32]

Percutaneous DEN has previously been described. This technique requires placement of a large-caliber, fully covered SEMS (20–25 mm in diameter) or flexible overtube to perform debridement of WON.[33,34] The SEMS remains in place between interventions with an overlying ostomy appliance to prevent soiling. The stent can then be removed when the cavity resolves. Video-assisted retroperitoneal debridement is a similar technique performed by gastrointestinal surgeons using rigid endoscopes through percutaneous tracts to access and treat WON in areas inaccessible from the gastrointestinal lumen.[35] This method is most commonly used when treating necrosis that extends into the paracolic gutters. Paracolic gutter extensions can be challenging to manage, especially when the WON extends into the pelvis, and are often unresolved with endoscopic therapy alone.

STRATEGIES ASSOCIATED WITH ENDOSCOPIC INTERVENTION OF PANCREATIC COLLECTIONS

The authors recommend that surgical and interventional radiology support be available during DEN procedures. Life-threatening adverse events can occur when performing endoscopic intervention for WON, either intraprocedurally or postprocedurally. Recent data show a mortality of 6% for patients undergoing DEN.[28] The most serious adverse events of necrosectomy include perforation and bleeding.

Bleeding can occur at any time during the intervention (ie, transmural puncture, dilation, necrosectomy) but most frequently occurs at the puncture site. Supportive measures are generally adequate because bleeding is usually self-limited and resolves by the completion of the procedure. Endoscopic hemostasis, surgical intervention, or angiographic embolization may be required in rare instances. Minor recalcitrant bleeding during the procedure can be managed by endoscopic injection of dilute (1:10,000) epinephrine, balloon tamponade, endoscopic clips (either through the scope [TTS] or over the scope), or electrocautery. Severe bleeding occurring at the transmural entry site can be managed by placement of a large-diameter, fully covered esophageal SEMS.[36,37] Intracavitary bleeding during debridement occurs but is typically self-limited.

Perforation may occur at the transmural access site or within the cavity wall, and can rarely result in tension pneumoperitoneum, a life-threatening emergency requiring needle decompression.[38] Perforations at the entry site occur because of separation of the lumen wall and the cavity wall. This condition can occur during creation of the tract or during DEN. Management options for this scenario include TTS endoclips or placement of a large-caliber SEMS,[37] similar to management of bleeding described earlier. Egress of gastric contents must be avoided/limited to minimize the risk of peritonitis. The gastric wall of the body and antrum is extremely forgiving and often closes rapidly without clinical consequence. Many patients can be managed with conservative measures (ie, nil per os status, nasogastric suction, antibiotics) alone. Management of transduodenal perforations is a subject of debate. Some endoscopists think that transduodenal perforation may also be managed conservatively, because the perforation occurs into the retroperitoneum. Large perforations through the cavity wall generate more concern, and often require surgical or percutaneous intervention.

Sufficient removal of fluid and solid debris is essential during DEN, because infectious adverse events can occur from inadequate drainage. As mentioned previously, patients should be maintained on antibiotics during the management of WON. Patients showing signs/symptoms of infection (ie, leukocytosis, fever/chills, culture positivity) should have their antibiotic coverage broadened. Patients may require concomitant placement of 1 or more percutaneous drainage catheters to achieve source control. This requirement most commonly occurs in patients with WON expanding into the paracolic gutters.[13]

Less common adverse events include air embolism and stent migration. Fatal air embolism has been described following DEN.[39] Because of this concern, nearly all medical centers managing WON have shifted from air to CO_2 for insufflation during endoscopic intervention. Stent migration (double-pigtail plastic stents or SEMS) may occur during or after endoscopic placement. Stents can migrate into the collection or out of the collection, both with significant clinical implications. Endoscopic retrieval of migrated stents into the cavity is feasible, assuming that migration is identified promptly. Delayed recognition of migration either into the cavity or into the stomach may lead to premature closure of the transmural puncture site, requiring a new puncture to remove inwardly migrated SEMS.

REFERENCES

1. Banks PA, Bollen TL, Dervenis C, et al. Classification of acute pancreatitis–2012: revision of the Atlanta classification and definitions by international consensus. Gut 2013;62:102–11.
2. Bakker OJ, van Santvoort H, Besselink MG, et al. Extrapancreatic necrosis without pancreatic parenchymal necrosis: a separate entity in necrotising pancreatitis? Gut 2013;62:1475–80.
3. van Santvoort HC, Besselink MG, Bakker OJ, et al. A step-up approach or open necrosectomy for necrotizing pancreatitis. N Engl J Med 2010;362:1491–502.
4. Chahal P, Papachristou GI, Baron TH. Endoscopic transmural entry into pancreatic fluid collections using a dedicated aspiration needle without endoscopic ultrasound guidance: success and complication rates. Surg Endosc 2007;21: 1726–32.
5. Jurgensen C, Arlt A, Neser F, et al. Endoscopic ultrasound criteria to predict the need for intervention in pancreatic necrosis. BMC Gastroenterol 2012;12:48.
6. Antillon MR, Bechtold ML, Bartalos CR, et al. Transgastric endoscopic necrosectomy with temporary metallic esophageal stent placement for the treatment of infected pancreatic necrosis (with video). Gastrointest Endosc 2009;69:178–80.
7. Belle S, Collet P, Post S, et al. Temporary cystogastrostomy with self-expanding metallic stents for pancreatic necrosis. Endoscopy 2010;42:493–5.
8. Itoi T, Nageshwar Reddy D, Yasuda I. New fully-covered self-expandable metal stent for endoscopic ultrasonography-guided intervention in infectious walled-off pancreatic necrosis (with video). J Hepatobiliary Pancreat Sci 2013;20:403–6.
9. Krishnan A, Ramakrishnan R. EUS-guided endoscopic necrosectomy and temporary cystogastrostomy for infected pancreatic necrosis with self-expanding metallic stents. Surg Laparosc Endosc Percutan Tech 2012;22:e319–21.
10. Sarkaria S, Sethi A, Rondon C, et al. Pancreatic necrosectomy using covered esophageal stents: a novel approach. J Clin Gastroenterol 2014;48:145–52.
11. Shah RJ, Shah JN, Waxman I, et al. Safety and efficacy of endoscopic ultrasound-guided drainage of pancreatic fluid collections with lumen-apposing covered self-expanding metal stents. Clin Gastroenterol Hepatol 2015;13: 747–52.
12. Siddiqui AA, Adler DG, Nieto J, et al. EUS-guided drainage of peripancreatic fluid collections and necrosis by using a novel lumen-apposing stent: a large retrospective, multicenter U.S. experience (with videos). Gastrointest Endosc 2016; 83:699–707.
13. Papachristou GI, Takahashi N, Chahal P, et al. Peroral endoscopic drainage/ debridement of walled-off pancreatic necrosis. Ann Surg 2007;245:943–51.
14. Varadarajulu S, Phadnis MA, Christein JD, et al. Multiple transluminal gateway technique for EUS-guided drainage of symptomatic walled-off pancreatic necrosis. Gastrointest Endosc 2011;74:74–80.

15. Gardner TB, Chahal P, Papachristou GI, et al. A comparison of direct endoscopic necrosectomy with transmural endoscopic drainage for the treatment of walled-off pancreatic necrosis. Gastrointest Endosc 2009;69:1085–94.

16. Ross A, Gluck M, Irani S, et al. Combined endoscopic and percutaneous drainage of organized pancreatic necrosis. Gastrointest Endosc 2010;71:79–84.

17. Kang SG, Park do H, Kwon TH, et al. Transduodenal endoscopic necrosectomy via pancreaticoduodenal fistula for infected peripancreatic necrosis with left pararenal space extension (with videos). Gastrointest Endosc 2008;67:380–3.

18. Abdelhafez M, Elnegouly M, Hasab Allah MS, et al. Transluminal retroperitoneal endoscopic necrosectomy with the use of hydrogen peroxide and without external irrigation: a novel approach for the treatment of walled-off pancreatic necrosis. Surg Endosc 2013;27:3911–20.

19. Coelho D, Ardengh JC, Eulalio JM, et al. Management of infected and sterile pancreatic necrosis by programmed endoscopic necrosectomy. Dig Dis 2008; 26:364–9.

20. Johnson MD, Walsh RM, Henderson JM, et al. Surgical versus nonsurgical management of pancreatic pseudocysts. J Clin Gastroenterol 2009;43:586–90.

21. Varadarajulu S, Wilcox CM, Latif S, et al. Management of pancreatic fluid collections: a changing of the guard from surgery to endoscopy. Am Surg 2011;77:1650–5.

22. Varadarajulu S, Christein JD, Tamhane A, et al. Prospective randomized trial comparing EUS and EGD for transmural drainage of pancreatic pseudocysts (with videos). Gastrointest Endosc 2008;68:1102–11.

23. Charnley RM, Lochan R, Gray H, et al. Endoscopic necrosectomy as primary therapy in the management of infected pancreatic necrosis. Endoscopy 2006; 38:925–8.

24. Gardner TB, Coelho-Prabhu N, Gordon SR, et al. Direct endoscopic necrosectomy for the treatment of walled-off pancreatic necrosis: results from a multicenter U.S. series. Gastrointest Endosc 2011;73:718–26.

25. Seewald S, Groth S, Omar S, et al. Aggressive endoscopic therapy for pancreatic necrosis and pancreatic abscess: a new safe and effective treatment algorithm (videos). Gastrointest Endosc 2005;62:92–100.

26. Voermans RP, Veldkamp MC, Rauws EA, et al. Endoscopic transmural debridement of symptomatic organized pancreatic necrosis (with videos). Gastrointest Endosc 2007;66:909–16.

27. Puli SR, Graumlich JF, Pamulaparthy SR, et al. Endoscopic transmural necrosectomy for walled-off pancreatic necrosis: a systematic review and meta-analysis. Can J Gastroenterol Hepatol 2014;28:50–3.

28. van Brunschot S, Fockens P, Bakker OJ, et al. Endoscopic transluminal necrosectomy in necrotising pancreatitis: a systematic review. Surg Endosc 2014;28(5): 1425–38.

29. Attam R, Trikudanathan G, Arain M, et al. Endoscopic transluminal drainage and necrosectomy by using a novel, through-the-scope, fully covered, large-bore esophageal metal stent: preliminary experience in 10 patients. Gastrointest Endosc 2014;80:312–8.

30. Walter D, Will U, Sanchez-Yague A, et al. A novel lumen-apposing metal stent for endoscopic ultrasound-guided drainage of pancreatic fluid collections: a prospective cohort study. Endoscopy 2015;47:63–7.

31. Rinninella E, Kunda R, Dollhopf M, et al. EUS-guided drainage of pancreatic fluid collections using a novel lumen-apposing metal stent on an electrocautery-enhanced delivery system: a large retrospective study (with video). Gastrointest Endosc 2015;82:1039–46.

32. van Brunschot S, van Grinsven J, Voermans RP, et al. Transluminal endoscopic step-up approach versus minimally invasive surgical step-up approach in patients with infected necrotising pancreatitis (TENSION trial): design and rationale of a randomised controlled multicenter trial [ISRCTN09186711]. BMC Gastroenterol 2013;13:161.
33. Yamamoto N, Isayama H, Takahara N, et al. Percutaneous direct-endoscopic necrosectomy for walled-off pancreatic necrosis. Endoscopy 2013;45(Suppl 2 UCTN):E44–5.
34. Navarrete C, Castillo C, Caracci M, et al. Wide percutaneous access to pancreatic necrosis with self-expandable stent: new application (with video). Gastrointest Endosc 2011;73:609–10.
35. Horvath K, Freeny P, Escallon J, et al. Safety and efficacy of video-assisted retroperitoneal debridement for infected pancreatic collections: a multicenter, prospective, single-arm phase 2 study. Arch Surg 2010;145:817–25.
36. Akbar A, Reddy DN, Baron TH. Placement of fully covered self-expandable metal stents to control entry-related bleeding during transmural drainage of pancreatic fluid collections (with video). Gastrointest Endosc 2012;76:1060–3.
37. Iwashita T, Lee JG, Nakai Y, et al. Successful management of arterial bleeding complicating endoscopic ultrasound-guided cystogastrostomy using a covered metallic stent. Endoscopy 2012;44(Suppl 2 UCTN):E370–1.
38. Baron TH, Wong Kee Song LM, Zielinski MD, et al. A comprehensive approach to the management of acute endoscopic perforations (with videos). Gastrointest Endosc 2012;76:838–59.
39. Seifert H, Biermer M, Schmitt W, et al. Transluminal endoscopic necrosectomy after acute pancreatitis: a multicentre study with long-term follow-up (the GEPARD Study). Gut 2009;58:1260–6.

Endoscopic Ultrasound-Guided Drainage of Pelvic Fluid Collections

SriHari Mahadev, MD, MS, David S. Lee, MD*

KEYWORDS

- Endoscopic ultrasonography • Drainage • Pelvic abscess
- Therapeutic endoscopic ultrasound • Intra-abdominal abscess
- Transrectal drainage

KEY POINTS

- Pelvic collections can result from surgical complications, or from diseases involving the reproductive organs or alimentary tract.
- Endoscopic ultrasound (EUS) provides an effective, low-risk alternative to surgical and percutaneous methods for drainage of pelvic collections.
- Successful treatment involves a multidisciplinary approach with proper surgical backup and careful patient selection.
- Because of its many advantages and low risk for adverse events, EUS drainage has been increasingly the preferred first line option for these collections.
- Options for drainage include either stent/drain placement or aspiration and lavage depending on the etiology, maturity, and size of the cyst.

INTRODUCTION

Fluid collections in the pelvis occur following surgery, or as a result of perforation of pelvic viscera due to medical conditions involving the alimentary tract (eg, diverticulitis, appendicitis, or inflammatory bowel disease), or reproductive tracts (prostate, gynecologic organs).[1] Drainage of pelvic collections is essential for source control of infection, and can be achieved via 1 of 3 approaches: surgical, percutaneous, and transluminal. Advances in endosonography equipment and techniques have allowed the endoscopist to safely and reliably access structures adjacent to the gastrointestinal tract under direct visualization.[2] More recently, the advent of lumen-apposing stents with integrated dilation and deployment systems have further simplified the

Disclosure Statement: No disclosures to declare.
Division of Digestive and Liver Diseases, Department of Medicine, Columbia University Medical Center, 630 West 168th Street, P&S 3-401, New York, NY 10032, USA
* Corresponding author.
E-mail address: dsl2155@cumc.columbia.edu

technique of endosonographic drainage. As such, endoscopic ultrasound (EUS)-guided transluminal drainage in the pelvis is increasingly viewed as the first-line, least-invasive approach. EUS offers certain advantages over competing approaches, in particular decreased pain at the puncture site, and the ability to dilate and achieve a widely patent tract for rapid drainage. This article summarizes appropriate patient selection, safety considerations, technique, and the available evidence on outcomes of EUS-guided abscess drainage in the pelvis.

INDICATIONS AND PREPROCEDURE CONSIDERATIONS

Careful preassessment and anatomic evaluation are essential for safe and effective EUS-guided drainage in the pelvis. Dedicated imaging via contrast-enhanced computed tomography (CT) of the abdomen and pelvis or MRI should be undertaken to delineate the relationships between the collection, surrounding structures, and the rectosigmoid lumen. Although transvaginal ultrasound-guided drainage is an option in female patients and may afford easier access to anterior pelvic collections, it is outside the scope of practice of most gastrointestinal endoscopists. Hence this article will focus on the transrectal approach.

Imaging characteristics of the pelvic collection should be taken into consideration, including location, size, loculation, maturity, etiology, mucosal disruption, and ascites. These will be discussed in detail in the following sections.

Location

The collection should be in a space that can be brought to within 2 cm of the ultrasound transducer. Extraperitoneal collections adjacent to the rectum are ideally suited for EUS-guided drainage. In both sexes, the pararectal and presacral spaces are easily accessed. Anterior to the rectum, the rectouterine space in females and the rectovesical space in males are also suitable. Collections that are anterior to the uterus in women and anterior to the bladder in men are best accessed via alternative routes. Abscesses that are superior to the peritoneal reflection, often sequelae of sigmoid diverticulitis, can be drained through the sigmoid colon; however, this poses greater technical challenges, and limited data are available on outcomes; as such, the role of EUS for these collections remains uncertain, and may require a forward-viewing EUS scope that is not readily available to many endosonographers. Perineal collections that are located inferior to the dentate line are best drained via the percutaneous (transgluteal) approach.

Size

The EUS technique is best suited to collections larger than 4 cm. Smaller collections may be drained endoscopically, but can often resolve with antibiotics alone.

Loculation

Multiple loculations reduce the likelihood of successful drainage, as does high-density debris.

Maturity

A well-circumscribed rim around the collection is necessary to support the creation of a fistula with stents and minimize the risk of free wall perforation. Aspiration alone, without leaving a stent, may be considered for immature collections if urgent drainage is indicated in the setting of clinical instability (**Fig. 1**).

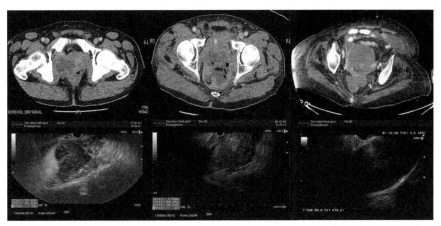

Fig. 1. (*Left*): Lytic bone lesion (A) with a pelvic collection (B) caused by multiple myeloma and osteomyelitis successfully drained with aspiration and lavage with corresponding EUS image below. (*Middle*): A multiloculated fluid collection with EUS imaging below showing a solid mass. Pathology consistent with prostate cancer. (*Right*): Pelvic abscess due to a gynecologic procedure with mature wall.

Etiology

The organ from which the collection arises is not always evident radiologically; however, attention should be paid to etiology and differential diagnosis of the collection before draining it. The most common cause of a pelvic collection is an anastamotic leak following colorectal surgery, and most abscesses arise from perforation of the gastrointestinal tract. The technique is, however, also applicable to other etiologies of pelvic collection, and successful EUS-guided drainage of collections arising from the prostate, uterus, tubo-ovarian organs, and bone/periosteum has been reported. There is some evidence that success rates for drainage of diverticular abscesses are lower than for other etiologies.[3]

Mucosal Disruption

Inflammation or ulceration in the vicinity of the access site should prompt consideration for drainage via an alternative route. Active inflammatory bowel disease involving the rectum or perianal region may predispose patients to local complications if transrectal drainage is attempted. Although EUS-guided pelvic drainage has been successfully reported in patients with Crohn disease, there are insufficient data to evaluate its safety in this patient population, and the technique should be employed with caution. Abscesses and collections that appear to invade or involve the bowel wall should raise concerns, as they may indicate a malignant etiology, and may increase the risk of free wall perforation if drainage is attempted.

Ascites

The presence of intervening ascites is a contraindication to transluminal drainage.

PATIENT PREPARATION

Septic patients should be stabilized with fluids and antibiotics prior to attempting drainage. Antibiotics should be administered prior to the procedure and for several days thereafter. The specific antibiotic agent should be tailored to the suspected etiology and local antibiotic resistance patterns.

Coagulation parameters should be checked prior to the procedure and coagulopathy reversed, as per society guidelines for high-risk endoscopic procedures.

Bowel preparation, either with oral lavage solutions or enemas, is essential to allow for optimal endosonographic visualization, and to minimize the risk of soiling in the event of a perforation. The availability of surgical backup in the event of a perforation is recommended, and it is essential to work within a multidisciplinary team with colorectal surgery, interventional radiology, and, as applicable, urology and gynecology.

Patients should empty the bladder, or a urinary catheter should be placed prior to the procedure, to minimize the risk of inadvertent bladder puncture. The balloon of a Foley catheter can be easily visualized endosonographically and can help to distinguish the bladder from the collection of interest. Puncture with a 19-gauge needle has not been reported to result in injury to the bladder unless the tract is dilated.

Adequate procedural sedation, administered either by an anesthesia specialist or by the endoscopist, is essential. Although EUS-guided pelvic drainage is similar to flexible sigmoidoscopy, sedation is more important, as manipulating a therapeutic echoendoscope adjacent to an infected pelvic collection may cause significant discomfort. Moreover, patient movement after puncture can cause dislodgement and loss of access to the collection, with attendant risk for perforation and adverse outcomes.

Appropriate surgical backup is essential. Management of patients with pelvic collections should involve input from colorectal, urologic, or gynecologic surgeons as appropriate. Surgical colleagues should be aware of the decision to proceed with endoscopic drainage, and ideally be in-house to manage emergent complications, should they arise.

The procedure is typically performed with the patient in the left lateral decubitus position, as with flexible sigmoidoscopy.

EQUIPMENT

EUS-guided pelvic drainage requires the use of a therapeutic echoendoscope with a working channel of at least 3 mm caliber in order to permit the passage of a 19-gauge fine-needle aspiration (FNA) needle. Currently available therapeutic curvilinear-array echoendoscopes include the Olympus GF-UCT140/160/180 range (Olympus Corporation, Tokyo, Japan) with a 3.7 mm channel, and the Pentax EG 38UT (Pentax Medical, Tokyo, Japan) with a 3.8 mm channel, both of which afford the passage of a 10 F stent. The Pentax FG 38UX (Pentax Medical, Tokyo, Japan) has a smaller 3.2 mm channel that will permit only an 8.5 F stent. There is limited experience with the use of recently developed forward-viewing echoendoscopes; however, it appears they may offer advantages in obtaining optimal positioning and maintaining visualization during the procedure.[4] The Olympus XGIF-UCT160J-AL5 has a 3.7 mm working channel and has been reported to have been used successfully for pelvic abscess drainage in 1 series.[5] CO_2 insufflation is preferred over air to minimize the risk of cardiopulmonary distress from tension pneumoperitoneum and/or compartment syndrome.[6]

Accessories required for pelvic abscess drainage vary by intended drainage technique and will be addressed.

TECHNIQUE

With the development of drainage devices with integrated deployment systems, several alternative techniques for EUS-guided pelvic abscess drainage have emerged. The traditional wire-guided technique is described here.

Needle Aspiration and Wire-Guided Access

Inspection
Following ultrasound visualization of the collection, the endoscopist should maneuver the endoscope into a stable position and apply color Doppler to exclude the presence of intervening vasculature. Consideration should be given to distinguishing the collection from the urinary bladder.

Puncture
In the traditional wire-guided technique, access is gained to the collection using a 19-gauge FNA needle and confirmed with injection of contrast on fluoroscopy (**Fig. 2**). The needle stylet is then removed and the abscess contents aspirated and sent for cytology, Gram stain, and culture. Thick purulent debris may limit fluid return. If no fluid is obtained, then the cavity should be irrigated with 10 to 20 mL of normal saline followed by repeat aspiration. For small collections, or circumstances in which creation of a fistula is undesirable, aspiration and lavage alone may be sufficient to achieve source control and stabilization of sepsis, at least temporarily.

Wire access
For more definitive drainage, a 0.035 mm guidewire is passed into and coiled at least twice within the collection. Initial access to the tract over the wire may then be performed with a 5 F endoscopic retrograde cholangio-pancreatography (ERCP) catheter or a needle knife followed by passage of an 8 to 10 mm biliary or through-the-scope (TTS) dilation balloon. Electrocautery-assisted advancement of a 10 F cystotome over the wire under EUS control is an alternative to balloon dilation.[7]

Stenting
The tract may then be maintained using one or more double-pigtail plastic stents (typically 7–10 F outer diameter, 4–5 cm long). A 10 F, 80 cm single-pigtail transrectal

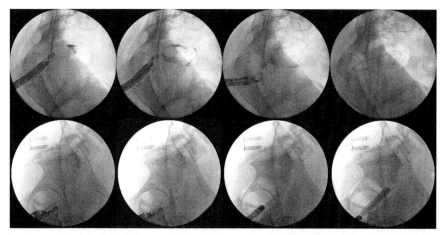

Fig. 2. (*Top images from left to right*) EUS FNA of the abscess cavity with contrast injection. Wire is then advanced into the cavity. After initial needle knife cautery of the tract, dilation of the tract is performed with a TTS dilation balloon. A 10 F double-pigtail catheter is then deployed over the wire. (*Bottom images from left to right*) EUS access to the cyst cavity is obtained with Hot Axios cautery. The inner flange is then deployed with gentle retraction. The stent is then fully deployed. Dilation of the lumen of the stent was performed to increase drainage.

drainage catheter can also be deployed, especially for collections with thick or loculated contents that may benefit from frequent irrigation with 50 mL of sterile normal saline every 4 to 6 hours.

Integrated Systems

Integrated puncture, dilation, and stent deployment systems have emerged to streamline the process of EUS drainage. The Giovannini Needle-Wire Oasis system (Cook Medical, Bloomington, Indiana) comprises 3 devices: a needle-wire, a 5.5 F dilator catheter, and an 8.5 F stent. The system allows for 1-step puncture, dilation, and stenting, and has been successfully reported for pelvic abscess drainage.[8]

Lumen-Apposing Stents

More recently, short fully-covered metal stents with accentuated, dumbbell-shaped flanges have emerged. These lumen-apposing metal stents (LAMS) exert radial forces that dilate the tract at the same time as the flanges apply compressive force to appose the cavity and lumen walls together, limiting the risk of migration. LAMS have been rapidly adopted for drainage of pancreatic fluid collections, where they have been shown to be easy to use, safe, and effective.[9] In the United States, the Axios stent (Boston Scientific, Natick, Massachusetts) is currently available, and comes in 2 sizes: 10 mm and 15 mm luminal diameters, with 21 mm and 24 mm flange diameters respectively, and a common saddle length of 10 mm. The Axios is deployed through a 10.8 F TTS catheter under EUS guidance. The initial iteration of the device required wire-guided access to the collection. In the latest iteration, the Axios may be deployed via direct electrocautery-assisted puncture of the cavity, obviating the need for wire guidance altogether, reducing the overall procedure time. LAMS have streamlined the process of stent placement; however, due to their short length, they are not suitable for collections that are located much greater than 1 cm away from the transducer.

TECHNICAL CONSIDERATIONS
Aspiration Alone?

There are circumstances in which leaving a stent or physical drain in the pelvic collection may not be desirable. Some examples include

- If the source of the collection is unclear, and a there is concern regarding formation of a fistulous tract, such as a recto-urethral fistula arising from a prostatic collection
- If coagulopathy or clinical instability limits tract dilation
- If there is a concern regarding a malignant etiology
- If the collection is too small to accommodate a stent
- If the collection is more than 20 mm away from the colorectal lumen

If drainage is still needed for source control or for identification of the causative organism, aspiration alone or irrigation and aspiration with a 19-gauge needle can be performed and may temporize the patient until a more definitive intervention can be arranged. For small collections, aspiration can permit resolution of the collection with antibiotics targeted to culture data, with 4 of 4 patients who underwent aspiration in 1 series experiencing complete resolution.[10] There are no available trials comparing aspiration alone with drain/stent placement; however, within the urology literature, transrectal ultrasound-guided needle aspiration has been reported to have high rates of success.[11,12]

Is Fluoroscopy Necessary?

Fluoroscopy is needed for wire-tip control, where a wire is used to guide access to the collection. As such, it is obligatory when dilation and stent placement over a wire is anticipated. For aspiration alone, and for cautery-assisted LAMS, fluoroscopy may be considered optional, as these can be performed under ultrasound guidance alone. The authors would suggest, however, that fluoroscopy should be used whenever available, as it permits routine intraprocedural assessment for complications—in particular perforation resulting in pneumoperitoneum—which may not otherwise be readily clinically apparent, especially with the use of CO_2 insufflation.

Transcolonic Versus Transrectal Drainage?

Drainage of collections is feasible through the rectum if the collection is located in the inferior pelvis. Collections that are located at or above the pelvic rim may be inaccessible from the rectum and require the endoscope to be maneuvered more proximally into the sigmoid colon in order the achieve a drainage window. Several challenges arise in conducting transcolonic drainage. First, the sigmoid colon is highly mobile, and achieving a stable position from which to safely access the collection is more difficult than from the rectum. Second, currently available therapeutic curvilinear echoendoscopes have relatively oblique camera visualization and limited tip deflection that make navigating the tortuous sigmoid colon difficult. Third, the sharp angulation of the sigmoid turns may make it difficult to puncture the collection directly en face rather than tangentially, potentially increasing the risk of perforation. There are few data comparing outcomes from transcolonic and transrectal drainage. In the 1 retrospective cohort study that has addressed the issue, a trend toward lower treatment success (70% vs 96%) was seen with transcolonic drainage; however, the difference was not statistically significant, and neither group experienced procedural complications.[3] The study was limited by small sample size, including only 11 transcolonic cases, which limited the ability to detect a difference. There are 2 other reports in the literature of perforations in patients who underwent transcolonic drainage of diverticular and Crohn abscesses, suggesting that there may be a higher risk of complications with transcolonic drainage that may not be conclusively demonstrated in the absence of large series with numerous adverse events.[10,13] Some of the potential challenges of transcolonic drainage may be overcome with the use of forward-viewing therapeutic echoendoscopes as they become more readily available.

POSTPROCEDURE CARE

Recommendations for postprocedure care are based largely on expert opinion rather than evidence. Patients who have successfully undergone transrectal drainage can be resumed on regular oral or enteral feeds; however, they should be maintained on a bowel regimen to reduce the risk of fecal impaction adjacent to rectal prostheses. Follow-up CT should be obtained at 36 to 48 hours to ensure that the collection is responding with a decrease in size. External drainage catheters are typically discontinued in the inpatient setting once symptomatic improvement is achieved and CT response is confirmed, because of their inconvenience. Plastic stents may stay in place after discharge and can be retrieved at follow-up outpatient sigmoidoscopy in 2 to 4 weeks following complete abscess resolution, although spontaneous migration and expulsion are not uncommon. Prompt removal of LAMS is of greater urgency than for plastic stents, as late complications including stent burial, migration, and severe bleeding have been reported with prolonged LAMS placement, beginning 3 weeks after transgastric placement for drainage of pancreatic necrosis.[14,15]

Table 1
Summary of case series on endoscopic ultrasound-guided drainage of pelvic abscesses

Author, Year	Origin	# Cases	Abscess Etiology	Mean Maximum Diameter	Technique	Technical Success (%)	Treatment Success (%)	Complications
Manvar,[a] 2017	United States	11	5 postoperative 6 other	70 mm	4 LAMS 7 cautery-assisted LAMS	100	100	None
Poincloux,[10] 2017	France	37	31 postoperative 6 other	60 mm[b]	29 double pigtail stents 4 aspiration 4 LAMS	100	87	1 perforation 1 rectal pain
Ratone,[17] 2016	France	7	5 postoperative 2 other	71 mm	Double-pigtail stents	100	n/a	None
Puri,[16] 2014	India	30	15 postoperative 5 diverticular 4 prostatic 6 other	49 mm	17 double-pigtail stents 5 aspiration 5 aspiration, dilation	100	93	None
Hadithi,[7] 2014	Holland	8	4 diverticular 2 postoperative 2 other	73 mm	Double-pigtail stents	100	100	None
Luigiano,[18] 2013	Italy	2	1 postoperative 1 diverticular	—	FCSEMS	100	100	None
Ramesh et al,[3] 2013	USA	38	25 postoperative 5 diverticular 8 other	68 mm	Double-pigtail stents	100	86	None

Study	Country	N	Collection type	Size	Technique			Complications
Ulla-Rocha,[8] 2012	Spain	3	Postoperative	47 mm	NWOA	100	100	None
Puri,[19] 2010	India	14	9 post-op, 3 diverticular	73 mm	9 double-pigtail stents, 3 aspiration, 2 aspiration, dilation	100	93	None
Piraka,[13] 2009	USA	3	1 postoperative, 1 diverticular, 1 Crohn	65 mm	2 double-pigtail stents, 1 aspiration alone	100	100	1 perforation
Varadarajulu,[20] 2009	United States	25	17 postoperative, 3 diverticular, 5 other	69 mm	25 double-pigtail stents, 10 double-pigtail stents + transrectal catheter	100	96	None
Trevino,[21] 2008	United States	4	2 postoperative, 2 other	93 mm	Double-pigtail stents + transrectal catheter	100	100	None
Varadarajulu,[22] 2007	United States	4	4 postoperative	72 mm	Transrectal catheter	100	100	None
Giovannini et al,[23] 2003	France	12	11 postoperative, 1 other	49 mm	9 straight plastic stents, 3 aspiration	100	89	None

Abbreviations: FCSEMS, fully-covered self-expanding metal stent; NWOA, needle-wire oasis system, Cook Corporation.
[a] Unpublished data, to be presented at DDW 2017 courtesy of Dr. Sammy Ho and Dr. Amar Manvar.
[b] Median.

OUTCOMES

Despite over a decade of cumulative experience worldwide with EUS-guided drainage of pelvic collections, there have been no large multicenter cohort studies published evaluating the technique. **Table 1** provides a detailed summary of the literature to date on outcomes of EUS-guided drainage of pelvic collections. Based on the limited available evidence, the technique appears to be safe and effective, with near-perfect rates of technical success (albeit in carefully selected cohorts), and favorable clinical outcomes, with treatment success as defined by the authors of the original studies ranging from 86% to 100%.

The highest-quality data available come from a prospective cohort study performed by Ramesh and colleagues,[3] who enrolled 38 consecutive patients who underwent lower EUS-guided drainage of abdominopelvic collections over a 7-year period at 1 center. Most collections were either postsurgical (66%) or diverticular (13%) in etiology. The procedural technique in all cases involved puncture with a 19-gauge FNA needle, followed by aspiration, and access to the collection with a 0.035 inch wire. Dilation was then performed over the wire using a 4.5 F ERCP catheter, followed by a 6 to 8 mm biliary balloon. Following dilation, 1 or 2 7 F, 4 cm double pigtail plastic stents were placed. In addition, for large (>8 cm) collections, a 10 F drainage catheter was placed and flushed every 4 hours with 200 mL of normal saline until clear aspirate was returned, at which point the catheter was removed. The study explicitly compared outcomes of transcolonic (11 cases) and transrectal (27 cases) drainage, finding no difference in rates of technical success (100% for each). There was a trend toward lower treatment success in the transcolonic group (70% vs 96%, $P = .053$), and higher rate of surgical intervention (27% vs 4%, $P = .06$) due to failure of EUS-guided drainage to resolve the collections. No serious complications were noted in either group.

The second-largest series from Poincloux and colleagues,[10] retrospectively reviewed 37 patients who underwent EUS-guided pelvic abscess drainage at 2 centers in France. Most (84%) collections were postsurgical in etiology, with the remainder attributed to sigmoid diverticulitis, Crohn disease, and other medical disease. The authors used a variety of techniques. For 4 patients with collections greater than 20 mm from the lumen, aspiration alone was performed. Most patients were stented via puncture of the cavity with a 10 F electrocautery-assisted cystotome, followed by contents aspiration, 0.035 inch guidewire insertion, and deployment of 1 or more double pigtail plastic transmural stents. In place of the plastic stents, a 10 × 30 mm LAMS was deployed in 4 cases. Some patients underwent 19-gauge needle puncture, wire access, and tract dilation via a needle-knife catheter and over-the-wire balloons, followed by plastic stent placement. The authors reported that stent insertion was technically successful in all 33 patients (100%) in whom stent placement was attempted. Stents were retained for a mean duration of 1.7 months. A second EUS-guided drainage procedure was required in 5 patients because of stent migration or inadequate response; all of these patients had a successful clinical outcome. Long-term clinical success was reported in 32 of 37 patients (87%) over the follow-up period, which averaged 64 months. Complications reported in this series included 2 minor (stent migration, rectal discomfort) and 1 major (perforation) event. The perforation was discovered on day 1 following transcolonic LAMS placement for a diverticular abscess, and required surgery.

Puri and colleagues[16] reported the results of 30 patients with pelvic abscess, of postsurgical (45%), diverticular (15%) and prostatic (12%) etiologies. Of note, 3 patients were excluded from analysis because of unfavorable abscess characteristics, including organized debris in 2 cases, and distance greater than 20 mm from the transducer in 1 case. The authors reported technically successful drainage in 93% of patients analyzed. However, 2 patients with diverticular abscess who underwent aspiration alone (7%) went on to surgery, and 5 patients (17%) required repeat EUS intervention. No serious adverse events were reported.

In their review of the available evidence, including recent unpublished data, the current authors found a total of 198 cases reported (see **Table 1**). Most studies were small and did not have well-defined or prespecified outcome criteria. The use of LAMS for pelvic abscess drainage is clearly a new and emerging area for which there are few data, with only 15 cases. LAMS also provide a larger lumen that may give an option to debris-filled collections and provide access for endoscopic debridement similar to necrosectomy in pancreatic necrosis. There is certainly a need for higher-quality, systematic prospective studies to evaluate this technique.

COMPLICATIONS

EUS-guided drainage of pelvic collections appears to be safe. Aside from 2 perforations noted by Poicloux and colleagues and Piraka and colleagues, significant complications have not been reported in the almost 200 cases summarized in **Table 1**. Spontaneous migration and expulsion of plastic stents are frequent, and the authors feel it should not be classified as a complication. One series by Hadithi and colleagues[7] reported dislodgement in 6 of 8 patients (75%) who underwent drainage, in part because of placement of small-caliber 7 F stents. All 6 patients who experienced spontaneous stent migration, however, had a favorable clinical outcome. It is likely that involution of the collection is partly responsible for plastic stent expulsion; hence, it does not appear to interfere with the success of the procedure. Serious late complications from LAMS have been reported with their use in drainage of pancreatic collections, and careful attention needs to be paid to prompt removal of these stents.

SUMMARY

EUS-guided drainage has been established as a safe and effective alternative to more invasive percutaneous and surgical approaches for management of pelvic collections, and should be considered first-line in suitable cases. The technique offers advantages including the straightforward nature of the procedure, decreased patient discomfort, rapid resolution due to large-caliber drains, and few reported complications. Although it is appropriate to a variety of clinical scenarios, there are limitations to the technique. In particular, collections that are greater than 20 mm from the EUS transducer may be difficult to access; there may be intervening structures, and transcolonic drainage may present special challenges. It is anticipated that the applications for the procedure will widen with widespread access to forward-viewing therapeutic echoendoscopes.

ACKNOWLEDGMENTS

The authors would like to thank Dr. Sammy Ho and Dr. Amar Manvar for their assistance with accessing unpublished data.

REFERENCES

1. Varadarajulu S, Lee YT, EUS 2008 Working Group. EUS 2008 Working Group document: evaluation of EUS-guided drainage of pelvic-fluid collections (with video). Gastrointest Endosc 2009;69:S32–6.

2. Sarkaria S, Lee HS, Gaidhane M, et al. Advances in endoscopic ultrasound-guided biliary drainage: a comprehensive review. Gut Liver 2013;7:129–36.

3. Ramesh J, Bang JY, Trevino J, et al. Comparison of outcomes between endoscopic ultrasound-guided transcolonic and transrectal drainage of abdominopelvic abscesses. J Gastroenterol Hepatol 2013;28:620–5.

4. Iwashita T, Nakai Y, Lee JG, et al. Newly-developed, forward-viewing echoendoscope: a comparative pilot study to the standard echoendoscope in the imaging of abdominal organs and feasibility of endoscopic ultrasound-guided interventions. J Gastroenterol Hepatol 2012;27:362–7.

5. Trevino JM, Varadarajulu S. Initial experience with the prototype forward-viewing echoendoscope for therapeutic interventions other than pancreatic pseudocyst drainage (with videos). Gastrointest Endosc 2009;69:361–5.

6. Lo S, Fugii-Lau LI, Enestvedt BK, et al. The use of carbon dioxide in gastrointestinal endoscopy. Gastrointest Endosc 2016;83(5):857–65.

7. Hadithi M, Bruno MJ. Endoscopic ultrasound-guided drainage of pelvic abscess: a case series of 8 patients. World J Gastrointest Endosc 2014;6:373–8.

8. Ulla-Rocha JL, Vilar-Cao Z, Sardina-Ferreiro R. EUS-guided drainage and stent placement for postoperative intra-abdominal and pelvic fluid collections in oncological surgery. Therap Adv Gastroenterol 2012;5:95–102.

9. Sharaiha RZ, Tyberg A, Khashab MA, et al. Endoscopic therapy with lumen-apposing metal stents is safe and effective for patients with pancreatic walled-off necrosis. Clin Gastroenterol Hepatol 2016;14:1797–803.

10. Poincloux L, Caillol F, Allimant C, et al. Long-term outcome of endoscopic ultrasound-guided pelvic abscess drainage: a two-center series. Endoscopy 2017;49(5):484–90.

11. Tiwari P, Pal DK, Tripathi A, et al. Prostatic abscess: diagnosis and management in the modern antibiotic era. Saudi J Kidney Dis Transpl 2011;22:298–301.

12. Fabiani A, Filosa A, Maurelli V, et al. Diagnostic and therapeutic utility of transrectal ultrasound in urological office prostatic abscess management: a short report from a single urologic center. Arch Ital Urol Androl 2014;86:344–8.

13. Piraka C, Shah RJ, Fukami N, et al. EUS-guided transesophageal, transgastric, and transcolonic drainage of intra-abdominal fluid collections and abscesses. Gastrointest Endosc 2009;70:786–92.

14. Bang JY, Hasan M, Navaneethan U, et al. Lumen-apposing metal stents (LAMS) for pancreatic fluid collection (PFC) drainage: may not be business as usual. Gut 2016. [Epub ahead of print].

15. Stecher SS, Simon P, Friesecke S, et al. Delayed severe bleeding complications after treatment of pancreatic fluid collections with lumen-apposing metal stents. Gut 2017. [Epub ahead of print].

16. Puri R, Choudhary NS, Kotecha H, et al. Endoscopic ultrasound-guided pelvic and prostatic abscess drainage: experience in 30 patients. Indian J Gastroenterol 2014;33:410–3.

17. Ratone JP, Bertrand J, Godat S, et al. Transrectal drainage of pelvic collections: Experience of a single center. Endosc Ultrasound 2016;5:108–10.

18. Luigiano C, Togliani T, Cennamo V, et al. Transrectal endoscopic ultrasound-guided drainage of pelvic abscess with placement of a fully covered self-expandable metal stent. Endoscopy 2013;45(Suppl 2 UCTN):E245–6.

19. Puri R, Eloubeidi MA, Sud R, et al. Endoscopic ultrasound-guided drainage of pelvic abscess without fluoroscopy guidance. J Gastroenterol Hepatol 2010;25:1416–9.

20. Varadarajulu S, Drelichman ER. Effectiveness of EUS in drainage of pelvic abscesses in 25 consecutive patients (with video). Gastrointest Endosc 2009;70: 1121–7.
21. Trevino JM, Drelichman ER, Varadarajulu S. Modified technique for EUS-guided drainage of pelvic abscess (with video). Gastrointest Endosc 2008;68:1215–9.
22. Varadarajulu S, Drelichman ER. EUS-guided drainage of pelvic abscess (with video). Gastrointest Endosc 2007;66:372–6.
23. Giovannini M, Bories E, Moutardier V, et al. Drainage of deep pelvic abscesses using therapeutic echo endoscopy. Endoscopy 2003;35:511–4.

Endoscopic Ultrasonography–Guided Hemostasis Techniques

Everson Luiz de Almeida Artifon, MD, PhD[a],*,
Fernando Pavinato Marson, MD, PhD[a], Muhammad Ali Khan, MD[b]

KEYWORDS

- EUS-guided hemostasis • Gastrointestinal bleeding • Endoscopic hemostasis
- EUS-guided vascular access

KEY POINTS

- Endoscopic ultrasonography (EUS) provides an easy access route to important vessels in the abdomen and mediastinum.
- Sclerosants, cyanoacrylate, and coils can be delivered through standard fine-needle aspiration needles.
- Compared with endoscopy-only approaches, the luminal contents like blood and clots do not impair echographic visualization of fundal gastric varices.
- EUS-guided hemostasis may play an important role in patients with refractory gastrointestinal bleeding.

INTRODUCTION

Endoscopic ultrasonography (EUS) was initially introduced as a diagnostic modality in early 1980s,[1] but with the advent of the curved linear array echoendoscope it has transformed into a therapeutic modality capable of a multitude of EUS-guided interventions. In the last few years, EUS-guided vascular access and injection emerged as a new possibility to achieve hemostasis. This novel technique was first reported by Levy and colleagues[2] in 2008 in 5 patients with refractory nonvariceal upper gastrointestinal (GI) bleeding that included a GI stromal tumor (GIST), Dieulafoy lesion, and a duodenal ulcer. EUS assessment can detect bleeding vessels located in the wall of the GI tract that cannot be identified or successfully treated endoscopically. EUS provides real-time high-quality sonographic images of both the GI wall and major arterial and

Disclosure: The authors have nothing to disclose.
[a] Department of Surgery, University of São Paulo, Rua Dr. Ovídio Pires de Campos, 255 - Cerqueira César, São Paulo, São Paulo 05403-000, Brazil; [b] Department of Gastroenterology and Hepatology, University of Tennessee Health Science Center, 956 Court Avenue, Suite H 314, Memphis, TN 38163, USA
* Corresponding author.
E-mail address: eartifon@hotmail.com

venous vessels like the splenoportal confluence, splenic artery, and hepatic artery that can be punctured and obliterated. Smaller branches can be identified and traced to their feeding vessels using EUS. This technique may allow a rescue EUS-guided therapy by means of fine-needle injection of sclerosants or coils, similar to the procedures performed by interventional radiologists to achieve hemostasis. Successful EUS-guided hemostasis has now been reported for more than 8 years for both variceal and nonvariceal refractory GI bleeding.[2–4] EUS-guided techniques for hemostasis are rapidly evolving and with accumulating evidence may become a useful alternative technique to achieve hemostasis.

ESOPHAGEAL VARICES

Endoscopic band ligation (EBL) is the primary treatment of bleeding esophageal varices and has largely replaced sclerotherapy as the first-line therapy. Sclerotherapy is still used as a rescue technique in cases in which EBL is no longer feasible, but with higher complication and recurrence rates.[5] Refractory bleeding of such varices is probably the result of failure to treat the perforating feeder vessels.[6,7] EUS can target perforating vessels as well as collateral veins to perform sclerotherapy and uses Doppler to assess success. Lahoti and colleagues[8] first reported the use of EUS-guided dynamic sclerotherapy with sodium morrhuate and color Doppler in 5 patients with esophageal varices. Complete obliteration was achieved in 2.2 sessions with no major complication associated with the sclerotherapy. One patient developed an esophageal stricture that responded to balloon dilation. The safety and efficacy of the EUS-guided sclerotherapy were shown in a randomized controlled trial that compared endoscopic sclerotherapy with EUS-guided sclerotherapy.[9] Fifty cirrhotic patients were randomized to undergo either endoscopic sclerotherapy or EUS-guided sclerotherapy, and over a 6-month follow-up posteradication, EUS-guided sclerotherapy was at least as effective as endoscopic sclerotherapy, with a trend toward lower recurrence in the EUS group.

GASTRIC VARICES

The American Association for the Study of Liver Diseases (AASLD) guidelines and expert consensus have endorsed the use of endoscopic cyanoacrylate (CYA) as a preferred treatment modality for bleeding gastric varices.[10,11] Soehendra and colleagues[12] were the first to treat gastric varices using CYA in 1986 in Germany. This approach has shown excellent efficacy in achieving hemostasis of acutely bleeding gastric varices, and lower rebleeding and complication rates compared with other endoscopic hemostatic methods like EBL and sclerotherapy.[13–16] Because gastric fundal varices are located at the submucosa layer, EUS allows visualization and puncture of such varices with great ease. Also, EUS has a higher sensitivity to detect gastric varices compared with esophagogastroduodenoscopy.[17] Even in situations with active bleeding or clots in the stomach, EUS visualization is not impaired, enabling a safer and faster therapeutic hemostatic procedure. In expert hands, EUS may allow observation and treatment of feeder vessels. In addition, the use of Doppler enables confirmation of complete varix obliteration, which may have prognostic significance because incomplete obliteration has been linked with higher risk of rebleeding.[18] CYA injection is associated with an overall mortality of 0.5% when N-butyl-cyanoacrylate is used.[19] The most dreaded complication associated with CYA injection is embolization, which is associated with clinically significant consequences in approximately 0.7% of cases,[19] but has been reported to occur in up to 58% of cases.[20] Romero-Castro and colleagues[20] reported in 2013 on a cohort that retrospectively compared CYA injection with coil deployment. The study revealed fewer adverse events with the coil group (9%) compared with the CYA injection group (58%). Notably, most of the CYA adverse events were confirmed by radiology to be caused by asymptomatic pulmonary embolization. The gastric varices obliteration rate was 94.7% in the CYA group versus 90.9% in coil group (*P* = nonsignificant) (**Table 1**).

ENDOSCOPIC ULTRASONOGRAPHY–GUIDED COIL DELIVERY

As an alternative to CYA or other sclerosant injection, the deployment of coils through standard fine-needle aspiration (FNA) has been reported (**Box 1, Fig. 1**). Levy and colleagues[3] first reported the insertion of a microcoil using a 22-gauge needle in a 50-year-old patient with extensive choledochojejunal anastomotic varices with good results. No sclerosants were used along with the coil. Based on ex-vivo observations, Binmoeller and colleagues[21] proposed the use of intravascular coils just before the EUS-guided CYA injection to decrease the risk of systemic embolization. They positioned the echoendoscope in the distal esophagus to visualize gastric fundus in antegrade fashion, puncture into the fundal varix via transesophageal-transcrural approach, and deliver the coils and CYA into the varix. The coil has attached systemic fibers that may act as a scaffold for CYA, preventing embolization and even decreasing the amount of glue needed to achieve complete varix obliteration. In addition, the coil itself may help to promote thrombosis and obliteration of the targeted varix. Bhat and colleagues[22] published in 2016 a large series of combined CYA and coil for the treatment of gastric fundal varices with more than 150 patients. Seventy-four percent of patients had stigmata of recent bleeding or active bleeding and 26% were treated for primary prophylaxis. Technical success was 99%, mean number of inserted coils was 1.4 (range, 1–4 coils), and mean CYA volume injected was 2 mL (range, 0.5–6 mL). Mild postprocedure abdominal pain occurred in 3% of the patients and signs of pulmonary embolization were seen in 1 patient. During follow-up examination with EUS, 93% of patients had achieved complete obliteration of gastric varices. At present there are no data analyzing the cost of using coils for hemostatic EUS-guided procedures. The cost associated with the use of coils might represent an important issue considering reports of cases that required as many as 13 coils to achieve varix obliteration.[20]

RECTAL BLEEDING

Rectal varices (RVs) are usually a consequence of portal hypertension and are present in 40% of patients with portal hypertension.[23] RVs have no association with the presence or severity of esophageal or gastric varices. In addition, RVs may be a result of

Table 1				
Main published series of endoscopic ultrasonography–guided treatment of gastric varices				
Author	**n**	**Coil/CYA/Coil + CYA (n)**	**Technical Success (%)**	**Complications**
Bhat et al[22]	152	0/0/152	99	9 patients with nonlethal adverse events
Romero-Castro et al[20]	30	11/19/0	100	3 patients with symptomatic embolism
Fujii-Lau et al,[4] 2016	14	4/0/10	100	1 coil migration to liver

Box 1
Technique of endoscopic ultrasonography–guided coil and cyanoacrylate treatment of fundal gastric varices

1. Filling of gastric fundus lumen with water to improve acoustic coupling and visualization of gastric fundal varices.

2. The echoendoscope is retracted to the distal esophagus to sonographically visualize the gastric fundus.

3. The gastric target gastric varix is punctured with an FNA needle using a transesophageal-transcrural approach.

4. A single coil is delivered into the varix through an FNA needle using the stylet as a pusher.

5. After the coil deployment, 1 mL of CYA is immediately injected through the same needle, using normal saline solution to flush the glue through the catheter.

6. Absence of flow in the varix is confirmed with color Doppler.

7. If the varix has a persistent flow, an additional 1 mL of CYA is injected.

Data from Weilert F, Binmoeller KF. EUS-guided vascular access and therapy. Gastrointest Endosc Clin N Am 2012;22(2):303–14.

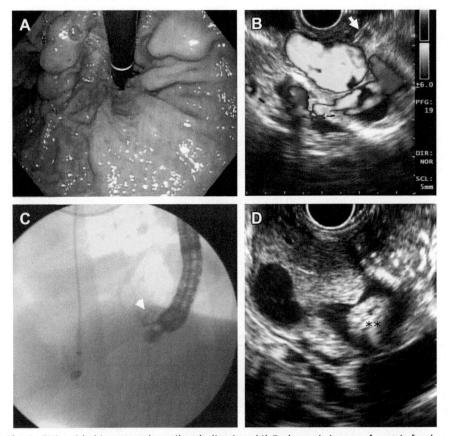

Fig. 1. EUS-guided intravascular coil embolization. (*A*) Endoscopic image of gastric fundus varices. (*B*) EUS color Doppler image showing the fundus varices. The arrow indicates a 19-gauge needle. (*C*) Radiologic image showing the coils (*arrowhead*). (*D*) EUS image showing coil embolization therapy in gastric varices.

vascular anomalies, heart failure, mesenteric venous obstruction, and adhesions.[24,25] RVs are rarely a source of significant lower GI bleeding.[26] Sometimes, RVs are not detected endoscopically, posing a diagnostic challenge to standard endoscopic hemostasis techniques like sclerotherapy and EBL.[24,25,27] Weilert and colleagues[28] reported the first treatment of bleeding rectal varices using EUS-guided coil and CYA injection in a 60-year-old woman awaiting liver transplant with recurrent hematochezia requiring ongoing blood transfusions. Four punctures were performed delivering 1 to 2 coils followed by 1 mL of CYA. Follow-up examination at 4 weeks revealed absence of flow on Doppler. The patient had no recurrent bleeding in a 12-month follow-up.

NONVARICEAL BLEEDING

Currently available endoscopic hemostatic methods successfully treat almost all nonvariceal GI bleeding cases. Reported EUS-guided hemostasis cases for treatment of nonvariceal bleeding are scarce.[29] Levy and colleagues[2] reported 5 cases with EUS-guided injection of absolute alcohol or CYA into the bleeding vessel. Absolute alcohol and/or CYA were injected through standard FNA needles. There were no complications associated with the method and bleeding control was achieved in all cases. Law and colleagues[30] reported an 88% clinical success rate in 17 patients with nonvariceal refractory GI bleeding from 2003 to 2014. Indications for treatment included GIST, colorectal vascular malformations, Dieulafoy lesion, duodenal ulcers, and rectally invasive prostate cancer.

SUMMARY

EUS-guided hemostasis with CYA and/or coils is a highly advanced and promising therapeutic modality that can be used as an adjunct to regular endoscopic management of acutely bleeding and nonbleeding gastric varices for primary prophylaxis. Most published studies are retrospective and the overall quality of the data is suboptimal. More prospective, randomized studies are warranted to better delineate the role of EUS-guided hemostasis in both variceal and nonvariceal bleeding.

REFERENCES

1. DiMagno EP, Buxton JL, Regan PT, et al. Ultrasonic endoscope. Lancet 1980;1: 629–31.
2. Levy MJ, Wong Kee Song LM, Farnell MB, et al. Endoscopic ultrasound (EUS)-guided angiotherapy of refractory gastrointestinal bleeding. Am J Gastroenterol 2008;103:352–9.
3. Levy MJ, Wong Kee Song LM, Kendrick ML, et al. EUS-guided coil embolization for refractory ectopic variceal bleeding (with videos). Gastrointest Endosc 2008; 67:572–4.
4. Fujii-Lau LL, Law R, Wong Kee Song LM, et al. Endoscopic ultrasound (EUS)-guided coil injection therapy of esophagogastric and ectopic varices. Surg Endosc 2016;30:1396–404.
5. Jacques J, Legros R, Chaussade S, et al. Endoscopic haemostasis: an overview of procedures and clinical scenarios. Dig Liver Dis 2014;46:766–76.
6. Irisawa A, Obara K, Bhutani MS, et al. Role of para-esophageal collateral veins in patients with portal hypertension based on the results of endoscopic ultrasonography and liver scintigraphy analysis. J Gastroenterol Hepatol 2003;18:309–14.

7. Irisawa A, Saito A, Obara K, et al. Endoscopic recurrence of esophageal varices is associated with the specific EUS abnormalities: severe periesophageal collateral veins and large perforating veins. Gastrointest Endosc 2001;53:77–84.

8. Lahoti S, Catalano MF, Alcocer E, et al. Obliteration of esophageal varices using EUS-guided sclerotherapy with color Doppler. Gastrointest Endosc 2000; 51:331–3.

9. de Paulo GA, Ardengh JC, Nakao FS, et al. Treatment of esophageal varices: a randomized controlled trial comparing endoscopic sclerotherapy and EUS-guided sclerotherapy of esophageal collateral veins. Gastrointest Endosc 2006; 63:396–402 [quiz: 463].

10. de Franchis R, Baveno V Faculty. Revising consensus in portal hypertension: report of the Baveno V consensus workshop on methodology of diagnosis and therapy in portal hypertension. J Hepatol 2010;53:762–8.

11. Garcia-Tsao G, Sanyal AJ, Grace ND, et al. Prevention and management of gastroesophageal varices and variceal hemorrhage in cirrhosis. Hepatology 2007;46:922–38.

12. Soehendra N, Nam VC, Grimm H, et al. Endoscopic obliteration of large esophagogastric varices with bucrylate. Endoscopy 1986;18:25–6.

13. Binmoeller KF, Soehendra N. "Superglue": the answer to variceal bleeding and fundal varices? Endoscopy 1995;27:392–6.

14. Lo GH, Lai KH, Cheng JS, et al. A prospective, randomized trial of butyl cyanoacrylate injection versus band ligation in the management of bleeding gastric varices. Hepatology 2001;33:1060–4.

15. Sarin SK, Jain AK, Jain M, et al. A randomized controlled trial of cyanoacrylate versus alcohol injection in patients with isolated fundic varices. Am J Gastroenterol 2002;97:1010–5.

16. Khan MA, Kamal F, Ali B, et al. Should cyanoacrylate glue be the treatment of choice for gastric varices? a systematic review and meta-analysis. Am J Gastroenterol 2016;111:S378.

17. Boustiere C, Dumas O, Jouffre C, et al. Endoscopic ultrasonography classification of gastric varices in patients with cirrhosis. Comparison with endoscopic findings. J Hepatol 1993;19:268–72.

18. Lee YT, Chan FK, Ng EK, et al. EUS-guided injection of cyanoacrylate for bleeding gastric varices. Gastrointest Endosc 2000;52:168–74.

19. Cheng LF, Wang ZQ, Li CZ, et al. Low incidence of complications from endoscopic gastric variceal obturation with butyl cyanoacrylate. Clin Gastroenterol Hepatol 2010;8:760–6.

20. Romero-Castro R, Ellrichmann M, Ortiz-Moyano C, et al. EUS-guided coil versus cyanoacrylate therapy for the treatment of gastric varices: a multicenter study (with videos). Gastrointest Endosc 2013;78:711–21.

21. Binmoeller KF, Weilert F, Shah JN, et al. EUS-guided transesophageal treatment of gastric fundal varices with combined coiling and cyanoacrylate glue injection (with videos). Gastrointest Endosc 2011;74:1019–25.

22. Bhat YM, Weilert F, Fredrick RT, et al. EUS-guided treatment of gastric fundal varices with combined injection of coils and cyanoacrylate glue: a large U.S. experience over 6 years (with video). Gastrointest Endosc 2016;83:1164–72.

23. Misra SP, Dwivedi M, Misra V. Prevalence and factors influencing hemorrhoids, anorectal varices, and colopathy in patients with portal hypertension. Endoscopy 1996;28:340–5.

24. Coelho-Prabhu N, Baron TH, Kamath PS. Endoscopic band ligation of rectal varices: a case series. Endoscopy 2010;42:173–6.

25. Sharma M, Somasundaram A. Massive lower GI bleed from an endoscopically inevident rectal varices: diagnosis and management by EUS (with videos). Gastrointest Endosc 2010;72:1106–8.
26. Shudo R, Yazaki Y, Sakurai S, et al. Clinical study comparing bleeding and non-bleeding rectal varices. Endoscopy 2002;34:189–94.
27. Ikeda K, Konishi Y, Nakamura T, et al. Rectal varices successfully treated by endoscopic injection sclerotherapy after careful hemodynamic evaluation: a case report. Gastrointest Endosc 2001;54:788–91.
28. Weilert F, Shah JN, Marson FP, et al. EUS-guided coil and glue for bleeding rectal varix. Gastrointest Endosc 2012;76:915–6.
29. Weilert F, Binmoeller KF. EUS-guided vascular access and therapy. Gastrointest Endosc Clin N Am 2012;22:303–14, x.
30. Law R, Fujii-Lau L, Wong Kee Song LM, et al. Efficacy of endoscopic ultrasonography-guided hemostatic interventions for resistant nonvariceal bleeding. Clin Gastroenterol Hepatol 2015;13:808–12.e1.

Progress in Endoscopic Ultrasonography

Training in Therapeutic or Interventional Endoscopic Ultrasonography

Monica Saumoy, MD, MS, Michel Kahaleh, MD*

KEYWORDS

- Training • Therapeutic endoscopic ultrasound
- Endoscopic retrograde cholangiopancreatography

KEY POINTS

- Only endoscopists with skills in both endoscopic ultrasound (EUS) and endoscopic retrograde cholangiopancreatography should preform EUS-guided biliary and pancreatic drainage.
- Given the risk of complications, the endoscopist must also be comfortable managing potential complications before taking on the responsibility of performing TEUS procedures.
- Trainees should begin with EUS-guided pancreatic fluid collections to become familiar with the technique of needle puncture, tract dilation, and stent placement. This can be performed initially on training models, and eventually under supervision of an expert endoscopist.
- Once trainees are able to show competency with identification and access of larger endoscopic targets, they can proceed to EUS-guided biliary and pancreatic drainage, then EUS-guided gallbladder drainage and creation of gastroenteric anastomosis.

INTRODUCTION

With the rapid expansion of therapeutic endoscopic ultrasound (TEUS), interventional endoscopy is rapidly expanding with additional techniques being continuously added. Initially described in the management of pancreatic fluid collections, the TEUS has expanded to drainage of the biliary and pancreatic duct in the setting of failed endoscopic retrograde cholangiopancreatography (ERCP), drainage of intra-abdominal and mediastinal collections, and, more recently, drainage of the gallbladder and creation of gastrojejunostomy. A key reason that new interventional procedures are

Department of Gastroenterology and Hepatology, Weill Cornell Medicine, New York Presbyterian Hospital, 1305 York Avenue, 4th Floor, New York, NY 10021, USA
* Corresponding author.
E-mail address: mik9071@med.cornell.edu

Gastrointest Endoscopy Clin N Am 27 (2017) 749–758
http://dx.doi.org/10.1016/j.giec.2017.06.012
1052-5157/17/© 2017 Elsevier Inc. All rights reserved.

constantly being developed is the recent explosion in the creation of novel endoscopic devices. Novel stents, delivery systems, improved quality optics and ultrasound visualization, have all led to a tremendous shift in the realm of the therapeutic endoscopist.

However, to accomplish these ever-challenging techniques, TEUS requires additional training beyond the traditional gastroenterology fellowship. The endoscopist must master ERCP and endoscopic ultrasound (EUS) techniques, in addition to conventional endoscopy. Only then can one advance to learning the various therapeutic ultrasound techniques in a step-wise fashion (**Fig. 1**). Despite the skill acquired from performing therapeutic techniques, such procedures are still challenging. Even in expert hands, advanced therapeutic procedures can fail in up to 15% to 30% of cases.[1] Due to the increased complexity of advanced therapeutic procedures, additional endoscopic skills require a further 12 to 24 months of training to develop.[2,3] Despite this requirement, advanced endoscopic training has become one of the most sought-after pathways in gastroenterology, so much so that the American Society of Gastrointestinal Endoscopy created a formal match system for those interested in an advanced endoscopy fellowship (AEF) position.[4] Many tertiary care centers that possess sufficient case volume now have an established advanced endoscopy training program.[5] Participating in a formal AEF allows trainees to receive necessary hands-on exposure to perform these procedures.

Requirements for Training in Therapeutic Endoscopic Ultrasound

Like any other evolving technology, there are no defined guidelines for credentialing a trainee to independently perform TEUS. However, some consensus exists on how to ensure trainees are prepared to become the next generation of advanced endoscopists. First, before starting AEF training, one must achieve proficiency in luminal endoscopy with both upper endoscopy and colonoscopy. This is typically achieved with a minimum of 18 months of a clinical gastroenterology fellowship. Luminal endoscopic training obtained in a gastroenterology fellowship must also include comfort in management of potential complications, such as perforation and hemostasis. Both of these complications occur at a higher iatrogenic rate with therapeutic endoscopy and the endoscopist must be comfortable in managing them. Second, experience in conventional endoscopy from a dedicated fellowship also ensures the trainee becomes versed in other issues, such as patient selection, procedure indication, management of anticoagulation or antiplatelet agents, and so forth.[5] These skills are

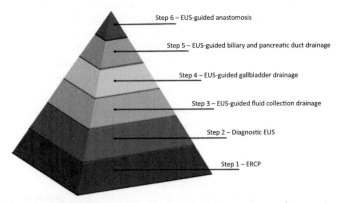

Step 6 – EUS-guided anastomosis

Step 5 – EUS-guided biliary and pancreatic duct drainage

Step 4 – EUS-guided gallbladder drainage

Step 3 – EUS-guided fluid collection drainage

Step 2 – Diagnostic EUS

Step 1 – ERCP

Fig. 1. Step-wise training for therapeutic ultrasound procedures of increasing complexity.

also traditionally learned as part of a standardized gastroenterology fellowship. Finally, it is important for trainees to understand that EUS-guided drainage should not be used to compensate for a lack of ERCP skills. Though TEUS is obviously exciting, there is a great responsibility to ensure that there is a disciplined clinical pathway to use these techniques.

The EUS-guided ERCP consortium meeting of 2011 brought together leading experts to generate recommendations for training in these procedures. Their recommendations on who should perform TEUS techniques included[6]

1. Endoscopists routinely preforming pancreaticobiliary EUS and fine needle aspiration (FNA)
2. Endoscopists with extensive ERCP and EUS experience for nearly 4 to 5 years (at least 200–300 EUS and ERCP each year)
3. Endoscopists with 95% to 98% success rate for standard ERCP with normal anatomy
4. Working in a center with interventional radiology and/or pancreatic-biliary surgery back up.

With sufficient mastery of all the prerequisite skills, a trainee can begin to become adept in new TEUS techniques. In focusing on training in therapeutic and interventional EUS, one must first review training for ERCP and diagnostic EUS.

Training in Endoscopic Retrograde Cholangiopancreatography

Therapeutic EUS-guided procedures require extensive knowledge of ERCP techniques. In particular, using fluoroscopy-guided interpretation and manipulation of a guidewire, dilation, and stent placement. Obtaining competency in ERCP requires experience and technical skill. Initially when ERCP was developed in the 1960s and 1970s, cannulation rates were poor, documented at only 25%.[7] With advances such as videoendoscopy, as well as noninvasive imaging modalities, the use and success of ERCP expanded dramatically.[5] Becoming more of a therapeutic, rather than a solely diagnostic, technique, ERCP credentialing guidelines with a threshold of 100 ERCPs were initially published in 1996 to create guidelines for reaching competency.[8] However, a learning curve analysis by Jowell and colleagues[9] suggested at least 180 procedures with an 80% success rate are required for competency. This led to the revised Gastroenterology Core Curriculum recommendations to increase the competency threshold to 200 ERCPs to achieve competency.[10] Even this updated minimum threshold seems to be insufficient in anticipation of advanced TEUS, and may even be insufficient for independent practice for therapeutic ERCP techniques. Therefore, the British Society of Gastroenterology recommends that trainees complete 300 to 400 ERCPs for competency.[11] Recently, there has been a change in mindset from a raw number procedure threshold to objective measures of competency, particularly in advanced endoscopy training. However, the definition of competency by achieving successful cannulation has been varied in the literature, ranging from contrast injection, deep common bile duct cannulation, to cannulation with a native papilla.[12] Given the varied societal recommendations and the lack of objective cognitive and motor skill competency parameters, it is generally accepted that a range of 200 to 500 procedures with at least a 90% success rate, is necessary.[12–14]

More importantly, because ERCP is no longer being used as a diagnostic procedure, cannulation is not the only component of a successful ERCP. In addition to cannulation, techniques such as wire manipulation and stent placement must also be learned in anticipation of preforming TEUS techniques. The Accreditation

Council for Graduate Medical Education recommends that practice using simulation models be incorporated in training programs.[15] Simulators provide a risk-free environment for trainees to learn device management, as well as gain confidence in using a duodenoscope. ERCP simulator models have been developed to supplement live ERCP training. Different models, such as the ERCP mechanical simulator (EMS) and the ERCP computer simulator (ECS), have been studied for hands-on practice of the basic maneuvers. EMS uses a standard duodenoscope and accessories to practice scope movements, as well as coordinated wire exchanges. ECS uses a mannequin with stored modules that are performed using sensors attached to the adapted duodenoscope (**Fig. 2**). Both modalities have demonstrated enhanced trainee procedural confidence after using simulated models.[16–18] Though head-to-head trials suggest that EMS is rated higher than ECS when used for supplementation of ERCP training, because actual accessories are used for a more realistic simulation, both methods are accepted and have a role in improving basic ERCP skills.[19]

Emphasis is placed on training for ERCP is because it is important to acknowledge the potential serious risk of complications from ERCP, especially as endoscopic capabilities have increased, such as direct cholangioscopy and pancreatoscopy, intraductal lithotripsy, and so forth. The American Society of Gastrointestinal Endoscopists developed a grading scale to describe the inherent difficulty of these diagnostic and therapeutic ERCP procedures (**Table 1**). Because there is significant technical complexity, as well as a wide range of therapeutic procedures that can be accomplished via ERCP, TEUS should not be used to replace ERCP. However, training for ERCP is clearly an important first step to mastering the TEUS.

Training in Endoscopic Ultrasound

Trainees must also achieve a level of competency with diagnostic EUS before tackling TEUS. EUS is a minimally invasive endoscopic modality to evaluate luminal and extraluminal structures, as well as provide real-time, accurate, in-depth tumor staging and tissue acquisition. The learning curve for EUS is known to be difficult, especially for pancreatic and biliary diseases. Previous studies have looked at learning

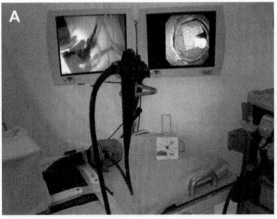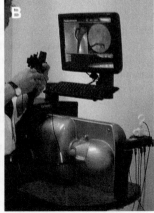

Fig. 2. ECS (*A*) and EMS (*B*) for simulated training of ERCP. (*Data from* Leung JW, Lee JG, Rojany M, et al. Development of a novel ERCP mechanical simulator. Gastrointest Endosc 2007;65(7):1058; with permission.)

Table 1
Grading scale for endoscopic retrograde cholangiopancreatography procedures based on inherent difficulty

	Biliary Procedure	Pancreatic Procedure
Grade 1	• Diagnostic cholangiogram • Biliary brush cytology • Sphincterotomy • Removal of stones <10 mm • Stricture dilation, stent, or nasobiliary drain for extrahepatic stricture or bile leak	• Diagnostic pancreatogram • Pancreatic cytology
Grade 2	• Diagnostic cholangiogram with Billroth II anatomy • Removal of stones >10 mm • Stricture dilation, stent, nasobiliary, or drain for hilar tumors or benign intrahepatic strictures	• Diagnostic pancreatogram with Billroth II anatomy • Minor papilla cannulation
Grade 3	• Sphincter of Oddi manometry • Cholangioscopy • Therapy in patient with Billroth II anatomy • Removal of intrahepatic stones or lithotripsy	• Sphincter of Oddi manometry • Pancreatoscopy • All pancreatic therapy including pseudocyst drainage

Adapted from the ASGE Training Committee ERCP Core Curriculum.[2]

curves for reaching competency for EUS. For example, EUS competency for diagnostic staging of subepithelial masses requires 150 supervised cases.[20,21] Of those procedures, 25 to 75 use sampling techniques with FNA to reach competency.[22–25] Competency of the EUS-FNA technique requires simultaneous endoscopic manipulation, interpretation, and needle manipulation for sampling. Mastery of the EUS-FNA with needle puncture is the foundation for TEUS. To improve experience with this key technique, simulated models have been developed to enhance trainee education.

Multiple types of simulated models have been developed over the years for trainees to master EUS. For example, computer-based simulation models are often implemented to augment training of therapeutic endoscopists. Such computer simulations, including the GI-Mentor (Simbionix, Airport City, Israel), contain an additional model for both radial and linear-array EUS called EUS Mentor.[26] This machine is used for EUS image interpretation and identification of landmarks, though the ECS does not simulate diagnostic or therapeutic techniques (**Fig. 3**).

Another commonly used technique for trainees is ex vivo models using explanted animal organs supplemented with plastic parts to create EUS conditions. EUS equipment is used, with actual echoendoscopes and the associated needles, wires, and so forth.[27] The model can be manipulated to simulate both diagnostic and therapeutic procedures. Finally, in vivo models, typically live pig animal models because the anatomy and ultrasonographic echo texture is similar to humans, have been used for training therapeutic techniques.[28] Animal models have been used for hands-on training of therapeutic techniques, such as pseudocyst drainage and celiac axis neurolysis.[29] However, these models require a large investment with dedicated animal facilities and equipment. In addition to the high cost, there are also ethical issues that limit their use in routine training.

Both advantages and disadvantages are associated with any of the described models. Despite most studies demonstrating improved efficiency when using simulated models, only a few studies demonstrate that these training techniques actually

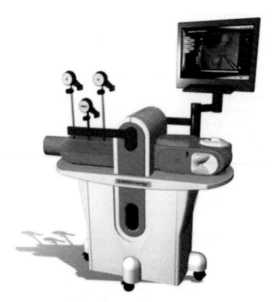

Fig. 3. Photo of EUS GI-Mentor (Simbionix, Airport City, Israel) for simulated training with computer models. (Simbionix GI Mentor from 3D Systems; with permission.)

improve clinical practice.[30] It is clear that the knowledge gained by using any of these models is only to augment the training gained from supervised clinical experience under the guidance of experts.[23]

Training in Therapeutic and Interventional Endoscopic Ultrasound

Once ERCP and EUS-FNA techniques are mastered, trainees can advance to other models developed specifically for TEUS. The initial challenge to becoming proficient in TEUS is the limited number of opportunities for training cases in addition to the challenging learning curve. Because of the ever rapidly advancing tools and techniques, learning on real patients is associated with ethical problems as well.[31] Therefore, endoscopic simulated models are a good alternative to trial new equipment or techniques.

A previously described example of a live animal model developed for EUS-guided biliary drainage, is a porcine model with a clipped papilla to dilate intrahepatic biliary ducts. However, this model is costly and can require 10 days for maturation. Though this model routinely causes common bile duct dilation, it is not always reliable for intrahepatic ductal dilation. Alcaide and colleagues[32] reported that, when using this live animal simulated model for EUS-guided biliary ductal access and cholangiography, there was only a 30.5% rate of successful anastomoses, which is a lower success rate than observed in humans. A newly developed simulated model was described by Dhir and colleagues.[33] Their novel ex vivo model using a 3-dimensional (3D) printed dilated polycarbonate biliary system was developed as a cost-effective alternative to practice EUS-guided biliary drainage. The Mumbai EUS 3D printing bile duct prototype allows for practice with standard equipment for both antegrade procedures and choledochoduodenostomy. The synthetic models have limited imitation in their tissue properties, and cannot be used with electrocautery for fistula creation, but they are still useful for learning the technical aspects of a procedure (**Fig. 4**). Published

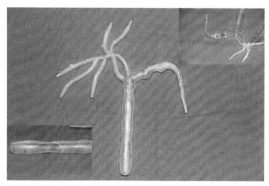

Fig. 4. TEUS machine using a 3D printing system of a polycarbonate bile duct for simulated training of EUS-guided biliary drainage. (*Data from* Dhir V, Itoi T, Fockens P, et al. Novel ex vivo model for hands-on teaching of and training in EUS-guided biliary drainage: creation of "Mumbai EUS" stereolithography/3D printing bile duct prototype (with videos). Gastrointest Endosc 2015;81(2):442; with permission.)

success rates seem to more accurately reflect published technical success rates of 82.4% for wire manipulation and 80% for stent placement.[33]

Of course, training solely on simulated models cannot ensure competence in a procedure. Trainees much also have in vivo experience to show competency under proctored cases by experienced endoscopists. After a trainee has demonstrated success in EUS-FNA sampling, as well as ERCP techniques, interventional cases such as EUS-guided pseudocyst drainage can be attempted under supervision. Fellows should be given the opportunity to participate in some part of the interventional procedure, either puncture, guide wire placement, fistula creation, stent deployment, or other. This piecemeal approach gives confidence to the trainee while preserving success and safety of the procedure. Eventually, a trainee is able to perform the whole procedure under supervision.[34] Ideally, trainees should independently perform 25 EUS-guided pancreatic fluid collection drainage procedures to be proficient.[35] However, a dedicated learning curve for TEUS procedures has not been specifically characterized. Once a trainee is comfortable with the pancreatic fluid collection drainage procedure, they can progress to more technically challenging procedures, such as EUS-guided biliary and, eventually, pancreatic drainage. The smaller target requires improved endoscopic manipulation, as well as understanding of anatomy, to ensure the safest angle for fistula creation.

EUS-guided biliary and pancreatic drainage has developed as an effective salvage technique after failed conventional ERCP. Even in the most expert hands, EUS-guided biliary drainage has been associated with a 10% to 20% adverse event rate.[36,37] This emphasizes the need for adequate training to ensure optimal patient safety and outcomes. Like many innovative endoscopic techniques, universal dissemination into the community is difficult. For example, a Spanish national survey of endoscopists who performed EUS-guided biliary drainage showed only a 62.7% technical success rate, much lower than reported in larger volume centers.[38] These endoscopists were beginners, working at low-volume centers with an average experience of less than 20 procedures. The investigators suggested that intraductal guidewire manipulation was the most challenging part of the procedure, associated with 68.2% of the documented complications. The technical challenges associated with equipment manipulation, incorrect access, or failed stent deployment, can lead to complications, such as leakage of intestinal material into the peritoneum, hemorrhage, or even death.

Because of these potentially devastating complications, it is important that inexperienced endoscopists learn TEUS under a mentor's supervision for at least the first 20 cases.[39]

Disseminated application of TEUS is, therefore, likely not realistic unless trainees are able to perform sufficient cases and are able to manage the complications. Most institutions do not provide sufficient training given high technical success rates of conventional ERCP procedures and failure to offer advanced complex TEUS cases. However, strong advanced endoscopy programs can offer TEUS training for the next generation of endoscopists.

SUMMARY

With the development of TEUS, endoscopists are able to use minimally invasive techniques to manage patients previously treated via percutaneous drainage or open or laparoscopic approach. In the subset of patients in whom conventional access is not possible, or patients who are at too high risk for surgery, endoscopists now have the ability to manage these patients without the need for other morbid procedures. However, EUS-guided therapeutic procedures have higher risks and, if unsuccessful, can lead to devastating complications. Early experience with in vitro models is beneficial to trainees to master the initial concept of EUS and ERCP, and allow them to progress to TEUS techniques. Though there are no set guidelines to determine competency for these procedures, trainees who choose to participate in an AEF at high-volume centers will have sufficient clinical experience to learn and preform TEUS.

REFERENCES

1. Perez-Miranda M, Barclay RL, Kahaleh M. Endoscopic ultrasonography-guided endoscopic retrograde cholangiopancreatography: endosonographic cholangiopancreatography. Gastrointest Endosc Clin N Am 2012;22(3):491–509.
2. Committee AT, Jorgensen J, Kubiliun N, et al. Endoscopic retrograde cholangiopancreatography (ERCP): core curriculum. Gastrointest Endosc 2016;83(2): 279–89.
3. Rosenthal LS. Is a fourth year of training necessary to become competent in EUS and ERCP? Notes from the 2008 class of advanced endoscopy fellows. Gastrointest Endosc 2008;68(6):1150–2.
4. Coyle WJ, Kedia PS, Kahaleh M. The advanced endoscopy fellowship match: an update and perspectives. Gastrointest Endosc 2012;76(6):1211–3.
5. Feurer ME, Draganov PV. Training for advanced endoscopic procedures. Best Pract Res Clin Gastroenterol 2016;30(3):397–408.
6. Kahaleh M, Artifon EL, Perez-Miranda M, et al. Endoscopic ultrasonography guided biliary drainage: summary of consortium meeting, May 7th, 2011, Chicago. World J Gastroenterol 2013;19(9):1372–9.
7. McCune WS, Shorb PE, Moscovitz H. Endoscopic cannulation of the ampulla of vater: a preliminary report. Ann Surg 1968;167(5):752–6.
8. Training the gastroenterologist of the future: the gastroenterology core curriculum. The Gastroenterology Leadership Council. Gastroenterology 1996;110(4): 1266–300.
9. Jowell PS, Baillie J, Branch MS, et al. Quantitative assessment of procedural competence. A prospective study of training in endoscopic retrograde cholangiopancreatography. Ann Intern Med 1996;125(12):983–9.

10. A journey toward excellence: training future gastroenterologists - the gastroenterology core curriculum, third edition. Gastrointest Endosc 2007;65(6):875–81.

11. Wilkinson M. ERCP - the way forward, a standards framework. British Society of Gastroenterology, UK: 2014.

12. Shahidi N, Ou G, Telford J, et al. When trainees reach competency in performing ERCP: a systematic review. Gastrointest Endosc 2015;81(6):1337–42.

13. Cote GA, Keswani RN, Jackson T, et al. Individual and practice differences among physicians who perform ERCP at varying frequency: a national survey. Gastrointest Endosc 2011;74(1):65–73.e12.

14. Cote GA, Singh S, Bucksot LG, et al. Association between volume of endoscopic retrograde cholangiopancreatography at an academic medical center and use of pancreatobiliary therapy. Clin Gastroenterol Hepatol 2012;10(8):920–4.

15. ACGME. Program director guide to the common program requirement. Cersion 2.2. 2009. Available at: http://www.acgme.org/Portals/0/PDFs/commonguide/Complete Guide_v2%20.pdf. Accessed July 14, 2017.

16. Lim BS, Leung JW, Lee J, et al. Effect of ERCP mechanical simulator (EMS) practice on trainees' ERCP performance in the early learning period: US multicenter randomized controlled trial. Am J Gastroenterol 2011;106(2):300–6.

17. Leung JW, Lee JG, Rojany M, et al. Development of a novel ERCP mechanical simulator. Gastrointest Endosc 2007;65(7):1056–62.

18. Fayez R, Feldman LS, Kaneva P, et al. Testing the construct validity of the Simbionix GI Mentor II virtual reality colonoscopy simulator metrics: module matters. Surg Endosc 2010;24(5):1060–5.

19. Leung JW, Wang D, Hu B, et al. A head-to-head hands-on comparison of ERCP mechanical simulator (EMS) and ex-vivo porcine stomach model (PSM). J Interv Gastroenterol 2011;1(3):108–13.

20. Eisen GM, Dominitz JA, Faigel DO, et al. Guidelines for credentialing and granting privileges for endoscopic ultrasound. Gastrointest Endosc 2001;54(6):811–4.

21. Park CH, Park JC, Kim EH, et al. Learning curve for EUS in gastric cancer T staging by using cumulative sum analysis. Gastrointest Endosc 2015;81(4):898–905.e1.

22. Polkowski M, Larghi A, Weynand B, et al. Learning, techniques, and complications of endoscopic ultrasound (EUS)-guided sampling in gastroenterology: European society of gastrointestinal endoscopy (ESGE) technical guideline. Endoscopy 2012;44(2):190–206.

23. Barthet M. Endoscopic ultrasound teaching and learning. Minerva Med 2007; 98(4):247–51.

24. Gonzalez JM, Cohen J, Gromski MA, et al. Learning curve for endoscopic ultrasound-guided fine-needle aspiration (EUS-FNA) of pancreatic lesions in a novel ex-vivo simulation model. Endosc Int Open 2016;4(12):E1286–91.

25. Committee AT, DiMaio CJ, Mishra G, et al. EUS core curriculum. Gastrointest Endosc 2012;76(3):476–81.

26. Bar-Meir S. A new endoscopic simulator. Endoscopy 2000;32(11):898–900.

27. Kim GH, Bang SJ, Hwang JH. Learning models for endoscopic ultrasonography in gastrointestinal endoscopy. World J Gastroenterol 2015;21(17):5176–82.

28. Bhutani MS, Wong RF, Hoffman BJ. Training facilities in gastrointestinal endoscopy: an animal model as an aid to learning endoscopic ultrasound. Endoscopy 2006;38(9):932–4.

29. Barthet M, Gasmi M, Boustiere C, et al. EUS training in a live pig model: does it improve echo endoscope hands-on and trainee competence? Endoscopy 2007; 39(6):535–9.

30. Parra-Blanco A, Gonzalez N, Gonzalez R, et al. Animal models for endoscopic training: do we really need them? Endoscopy 2013;45(6):478–84.
31. Van Dam J, Brady PG, Freeman M, et al. Guidelines for training in electronic ultrasound: guidelines for clinical application. From the ASGE. American Society for Gastrointestinal Endoscopy. Gastrointest Endosc 1999;49(6):829–33.
32. Alcaide N, Lorenzo-Pelayo S, Ruiz-Zorrilla R, et al. Su1353 endoscopic porcine model of biliary obstruction using over-the-scope clips: feasibility and applicability to training in EUS-guided drainage procedures. Gastrointestinal Endoscopy 2013;77(5):AB294–5.
33. Dhir V, Itoi T, Fockens P, et al. Novel ex vivo model for hands-on teaching of and training in EUS-guided biliary drainage: creation of "Mumbai EUS" stereolithography/3D printing bile duct prototype (with videos). Gastrointest Endosc 2015; 81(2):440–6.
34. Kahaleh M. Training the next generation of advanced endoscopists in EUS-guided biliary and pancreatic drainage: learning from master endoscopists. Gastrointest Endosc 2013;78(4):638–41.
35. Varadarajulu S, Tamhane A, Blakely J. Graded dilation technique for EUS-guided drainage of peripancreatic fluid collections: an assessment of outcomes and complications and technical proficiency (with video). Gastrointest Endosc 2008;68(4):656–66.
36. Dhir V, Bhandari S, Bapat M, et al. Comparison of EUS-guided rendezvous and precut papillotomy techniques for biliary access (with videos). Gastrointest Endosc 2012;75(2):354–9.
37. Khashab MA, Dewitt J. EUS-guided biliary drainage: is it ready for prime time? Yes! Gastrointest Endosc 2013;78(1):102–5.
38. Vila JJ, Perez-Miranda M, Vazquez-Sequeiros E, et al. Initial experience with EUS-guided cholangiopancreatography for biliary and pancreatic duct drainage: a Spanish national survey. Gastrointest Endosc 2012;76(6):1133–41.
39. Hara K, Yamao K, Mizuno N, et al. Endoscopic ultrasonography-guided biliary drainage: who, when, which, and how? World J Gastroenterol 2016;22(3): 1297–303.

Future Directions for Endoscopic Ultrasound
Where Are We Heading?

Sahin Coban, MD[a], Omer Basar, MD[b],*, William R. Brugge, MD[b]

KEYWORDS

- Endoscopic ultrasonography • Elastography • Confocal endomicroscopy
- Contrast-enhanced • Device • Drainage • Future directions

KEY POINTS

- Technological advances have provided an expansion of the therapeutic potential of endoscopic ultrasound.
- New imaging modalities, including tissue harmonic echo, elastography, and contrast-enhanced harmonic endoscopic ultrasound, have enhanced the diagnostic capabilities of endoscopic ultrasound.
- Innovations in stent technology and new accessories, as well as echoendoscopes, such as the forward-viewing linear echoendoscopes, offer a broad range of indications for therapeutic endosonography.

DIAGNOSTIC ENDOSCOPIC ULTRASOUND

Endoscopic ultrasound (EUS) is a useful technique for the diagnosis and treatment of gastrointestinal (GI) tract diseases, particularly for the detection of small lesions, tissue acquisition, tumor staging, tumor ablation, and various drainage techniques.[1,2] The recent improvements in EUS technology have enhanced the diagnostic capabilities of EUS. Most recently, a new EUS processor, EU-ME2 Premier Plus (Olympus Medical Systems Corp, Tokyo, Japan) has been introduced to the market. This processor is capable of 3 new functions, including tissue harmonic echo (THE), elastography, and contrast-enhanced harmonic EUS (CH-EUS). The efficacy of THE has been has recently been reported, particularly in providing high-quality images of pancreatic cystic and solid lesion.[3,4] On the other hand, elastography is an important feature of EUS that may enable imaging to differentiate between benign and malignant lesions.[5]

Disclosure Statement: The authors declare they have no conflicts of interest.
[a] Department of Medicine, University of Massachusetts Medical School, 55 N Lake Avenue, Worcester, MA 01655, USA; [b] Pancreas Biliary Center, Gastrointestinal Unit, Massachusetts General Hospital, 55 Fruit Street, Boston, MA 02114, USA
* Corresponding author.
E-mail address: obasar@mgh.harvard.edu

Gastrointest Endoscopy Clin N Am 27 (2017) 759–772
http://dx.doi.org/10.1016/j.giec.2017.06.013
1052-5157/17/Published by Elsevier Inc.
giendo.theclinics.com

CH-EUS is another useful technology for the differential diagnosis of pancreatic tumors. However, the usefulness of these 3 new functions for the diagnosis and management of GI tract lesions is still not clear.

Tissue Harmonic Echo

THE imaging is a newly developed sonographic technique that can potentially provide higher quality images compared with conventional B-mode images.[3] THE seems to be an important examination modality because it is superior for imaging of pancreatic cystic lesions and ductal structures. In a consensus meeting, THE function of EU-ME2 Premier Plus was found to be useful in the diagnosis of both cystic lesions and solid lesions of the pancreas. Most participants stated that THE was useful for all pancreas-biliary lesions, including for the bile duct and gallbladder indications.[6] THE might provide more clear images delineating the borders of benign and malignant lesions. It is most likely to gain widespread acceptance in the near future due to its ease of use. Although THE provides an effective enhancement of EUS imaging, its utility in differential diagnosis and tumor staging, or to what extent it would provide information to distinguish between benign and malignant changes is still unclear. These issues should be clarified with further studies. THE provides the maximum intensity at an optimum depth below the surface. It is not useful for the visualization of the superficial tissues because the harmonic waves that are generated within the tissue increase with depth to a point of maximum intensity and then decrease with further depth as a result of attenuation. Therefore, the maximum intensity is achieved at an optimum depth below the surface.[7] However, by the development of new harmonics and technological modifications in the future, THE might be used for identification of the superficial submucosal tumors such as GI stromal tumors and gastric cancer.

Endoscopic Ultrasound–Elastography

Elastography is a new imaging technique that was developed to improve diagnostic EUS examinations.[5] Tissue stiffness is assessed and the differences between various lesions were used for differential diagnosis. In this modality, the elastic features of tissues are evaluated by doing slight compression of the tissue and the differences were compared before and after compression images. It can be useful in the differential diagnosis of a pancreatic solid mass from the normal parenchyma by identifying the margin of a solid mass.[8] However, the elastographic features of some tissues still remain unclear.

There are still some limitations of elastography. Commercially available EUS-elastography is not able to assess tissues quantitatively. It may assess relative stiffness compared with the surrounding tissue, which is a subjective evaluation with operator dependency. The new generation EUS-elastography devices are able to measure the mean strain ratio within a selected area between the targeted lesion and the surrounding tissue, providing a numeric value, but multiple measurements are needed to be performed in each patient for obtaining an optimal evaluation.[9] Furthermore, EUS-elastography has a high sensitivity but a low specificity (**Table 1**). It is usually able to diagnose solid masses, but it is not able to differentiate a mass from fibrotic tissue. That is why many endosonographers think that it is still very difficult to differentiate a pancreatic cancer from chronic pancreatitis based on elastography.[6] Shear wave elastography, including acoustic radiation force impulse imaging and supersonic shear wave imaging, may offer new imaging modalities to assess the stiffness of lymph nodes and the pancreas.[10]

Table 1
Selected prospective studies reporting endoscopic ultrasound–elastography evaluation of the solid pancreatic lesions and lymph nodes

Author	Lesion Type	Final Diagnosis	Number of Subjects	EUS-Elastography Evaluation	Diagnostic Rate Sensitivity or Specificity
Giovannini et al,[5] 2006	PSLs	Surgery or EUS-FNA	24	Color pattern	Sn: 100%, Sp: 67%
	Lymph node	EUS-FNA	31	Color pattern	Sn: 100%, Sp: 50%
Iglesias-Garcia et al,[13] 2009	PSLs	Surgery or EUS-FNA	130	Color pattern	Sn: 100%, Sp: 85%, Acc: 94%
Giovannini et al,[16] 2009	PSLs	Surgery or EUS-FNA	121	Color pattern	Sn: 92%, Sp: 80%
	Lymph node	Surgery or EUS-FNA	101	Color pattern	Sn: 91.8%, Sp: 82.5%
Iglesias-Garcia et al,[17] 2010	PSLs	Surgery or EUS-FNA	86	SR: 4.62	Sn: 100%, Sp: 92%
Saftoiu et al,[8] 2011	PSLs	Surgery or EUS-FNA	258	Hue histogram cut off value of 175	Sn: 93%, Sp: 66%, Acc: 85%
Larsen et al,[18] 2012	Lymph node	Surgery	56	Color pattern	Sn: 55%–59%, Sp: 82%–85%
Paterson et al,[19] 2012	Lymph node	EUS-FNA	53	SR for malignancy	Sn: 83%, Sp: 96%, Acc: 90%
Knabe et al,[20] 2013	Lymph node	EUS-FNA	40	Color pattern Computed analysis	Sn: 100%, Sp: 64% Sn: 88.9, Sp: 86.7%
Rustemovic et al,[21] 2014	PSLs	Surgery or EUS-FNA	149	SR: 7.59	Sn: 100%, Sp: 45%
Mayerle et al,[12] 2016	PSLs	Surgery or EUS-FNA	85	SR: 24.82 SR: 10	Sn: 77%, Sp: 65% Sn: 96%, Sp: 43%

Abbreviations: Acc, accuracy; FNA, fine-needle aspiration; PSLs, pancreatic solid lesions; Sn, sensitivity; Sp, specificity; SR, Cut-off value of the strain ratio.

In a recent study, quantitative EUS-elastography was shown to differentiate between benign and malignant pancreatic lesions with a high sensitivity.[11] Furthermore, pancreatic neuroendocrine tumors could also be differentiated by EUS-elastography.

EUS-elastography can also assess the degree and extent of pancreatic steatosis, especially in patients with obesity, diabetes, or alcoholism. It can also be used for the evaluation of the degree of steatosis before and after a treatment.

One of the major limitations of elastography is the use of tissue compression and the subjective nature of the compression during EUS. Motion artifacts can be seen because of respiratory and heart movements.[12,13] Interposition of adjacent structures, such as heart and major vessels, and cysts or dilated ducts, should be avoided because these structures interfere with obtaining optimal images.[14] Moreover, the negative predictive value is still low, which is around 60% to 70%. The procedure is somewhat operator-dependent and poorly reproducible.[15] To overcome these problems in EUS-elastography, it will be necessary to develop a method to measure tissue stiffness quantitatively.

Contrast-Enhanced Harmonic Endoscopic Ultrasound

CH-EUS is an imaging modality used for assessment of blood flow inside tissue. The aim of CH-EUS is to improve detectability and understand the nature of a tumor based

Table 2
Selected prospective studies reported contrast-enhanced harmonic endoscopic ultrasonography assessment for solid pancreatic masses

Author	Contrast Agent	Number of Subjects	Mechanical Index	Diagnostic Rate for Hypoenhancement (a Sign of Adenocarcinoma)
Napoleon et al,[40] 2010	Sonovue	35 (PC: 18, NET: 9, CP: 7, stromal tumor: 1)	0.4	89% sensitivity, 88% specificity, 88.5% accuracy
Fusaroli et al,[23] 2010	Sonovue	90 (PC: 51, CP: 13, NET: 13)	0.36 radial, 0.28 linear	96% sensitivity, 64% specificity, 82% accuracy
Hocke et al,[41] 2012	Sonovue	58	NA	84% sensitivity, 76% specificity
Kitano et al,[22] 2012	Sonazoid	277 (PC: 204, CP: 46, NET: 19, Other: 8)	0.3	95% sensitivity, 89% specificity
Lee et al,[42] 2013	Sonovue	37 (PC: 28, NET: 5, CP: 2)	NA	93% sensitivity, 86% specificity
Gincul et al,[43] 2014	Sonovue	100 (PC: 69, CP: 13, NET: 10, Other: 8)	0.4	96% sensitivity, 94% specificity

Abbreviations: CP, chronic pancreatitis; NA, not available; NET, neuroendocrine tumor; PC, pancreatic cancer.

on its vascularity. Whereas a Doppler image detects only large vessels, CH-EUS is able to identify small vessels using microbubbles by the high-resolution image capacity of EUS.[6] Thus, CH-EUS may provide additional information compared with a Doppler or a computed tomography (CT) image. Kitano and colleagues[22] have proposed a diagnostic classification of pancreatic tumors as follows: no-enhancement, necrotic tissue; hypoenhancement, ductal carcinoma; isoenhancement, focal pancreatitis; and hyperenhancement, neuroendocrine tumor. However, it can be difficult to diagnose mass-forming autoimmune pancreatitis because CH-EUS cannot distinguish between focal inflammatory lesions and the normal pancreatic parenchyma. The diagnosis of intraductal papillary neoplasm is another challenge for endosonographers. The differentiation between a mural nodule and a mucus clot can be difficult in conventional EUS examination. Contrast-enhanced CT can reveal the vascularity of a large mural nodule, but the assessment of a small nodule is very difficult. One of the advantages of CH-EUS is the ability to identify and characterize small nodular lesions and to provide a more accurate diagnosis. When it is compared with pancreatic indications, the indications for the use of CH-EUS are lower for biliary diseases.[6] However, the differentiation of gallbladder polyps and cancer is a major strength of CH-EUS. These types of lesions are not amenable to EUS–fine-needle aspiration (FNA) or CT imaging. Conventional EUS sometimes fails to identify margins of the target for EUS-FNA. CH-EUS provides full identification of these difficult lesions, including solid lesions of the pancreas and lymph nodes[23,24] (**Table 2**). CH-EUS is found useful for distinguishing malignant from benign lymph nodes in patients with pancreatobiliary carcinomas.[24] Moreover, fewer needle passes are needed to obtain diagnostic samples from solid pancreatic lesions using CH-EUS guidance compared with conventional sampling during EUS-FNA.[25] Therefore, CH-EUS seems to be a useful imaging modality for EUS-FNA guidance by defining the lesion, selecting the target, and avoiding vascular structures and/or necrotic tissue.[26]

Besides the tissue acquisition, some interventional applications can be performed using CH-EUS. CH-EUS may be applied to the treatment of cancer in the near future.

CH-EUS is useful to assess the grade of tumor before chemotherapy and to evaluate the state of tumor perfusion. Chemotherapy-induced changes in vascularity may be predictive of successful tumor ablation. It was shown that in cases in which the intratumoral blood flow is abundant, it may predict a better response to chemotherapy and improved survival.[27] Matsui and colleagues[28] showed the change in size and vascularity of a tumor during chemotherapy in subjects with gastric cancer using CH-EUS. Tumors with abundant intratumoral vessels were chemosensitive because the drugs were able to penetrate tumors via vessels.[29] These important principles of tumor vascularity in gastric cancer can be applied to other types of gastrointestinal cancers. Also, GI stromal tumor and leiomyoma can be differentiated accurately using by CH-EUS,[30] and it can be useful for making a diagnosis of sarcoidosis.[31] Furthermore, in the near future, it may be used for the evaluation of the therapy for other digestive tract tumors, such as esophagus, gastric, colon, and rectal cancers.

Microbubbles, which have a high affinity to specific molecules, can image sites of inflammation, angiogenesis, and cancer to provide more precise information related to disease. In many experimental models, it has been shown that vascular endothelial growth factor receptor (VEGFR) type 2, which is overexpressed on angiogenic vascular endothelial cells of cancer, was visualized by USG using VEGFR2-targeted ultrasound (US) microbubbles for pancreatic adenocarcinoma, colon carcinoma, and breast cancer. These molecules have been used for monitoring the response to anticancer therapy.[32–35] Moreover, recently, Bachawal and colleagues[36] showed that expression of B7-H3 (CD276) is intensely and selectively accumulated in tumor vessels of breast cancer, compared with VEGFR. They suggested that the use of B7-H3–targeted US molecular imaging might be applied for more selective tumor detection.

Using US-targeted microbubbles improves not only tumor characterization but also efficacy and selectivity of the treatment to reduce the side effects of chemotherapy. A novel doxorubicin-loaded or plasmid DNA-loaded microbubble formulation has the potential to markedly improve the local therapies by driving the delivery of these cytotoxic agents to malignant tissues.[37,38] These promising results show that molecular-targeted US microbubbles may be used in clinical practice in near future, along with EUS, making characterization of lesions easier and improving efficacy of local therapies.

CH-EUS can also be applied for local ablation of tumors. Recently, phase-changed nanodroplets (PCNDs) were reported as a sensitizer for the mechanical effects of pulsed high-intensity focused US.[39] PCND enhanced mechanical tissue separation by pulsed high-intensity focused US combination may be a new approach to the treatment of locally advanced cancer. A specific echoendoscope producing high-powered US waves may be able to allow local ablation using US contrast agents.[26]

However, limited availability of US contrast media in many countries and its cost are important challenges for the use of CH-EUS. Indications for CH-EUS remain controversial and prospective comparative studies are needed.

Confocal Endomicroscopy

Confocal laser endomicroscopy (CLE) is an endoscopic modality that has the capability of obtaining high-resolution magnified images.[44] CLE works based on tissue illumination with a low-power laser, with subsequent capturing of the fluorescence of light reflected from the tissue via a pinhole. Because the illumination and detection systems are in the same focal plane, it is called confocal. At first, light is focused at a selected depth in the tissue, then the reflected light is refocused onto the detection system by the same lens. Therefore, CLE offers to obtain real-time cellular imaging and evaluation of tissue architecture during endoscopy. There have been 2 types of CLE catheter developed and studied to date. The first is the probe-based CLE system, Cellvizio confocal probes (Mauna Kea Technologies, Paris, France), which makes it possible to obtain cross-sectional imaging at different depths. The second is needle-based CLE (nCLE), which uses the AQ-Flex 19 probe through a 19-gauge EUS needle. EUS guides the placement of the needle and the confocal probe into the pancreas, lymph nodes, or other lesions. Konda and colleagues[45] demonstrated the effectiveness of nCLE in subjects with pancreatic lesions, with a technical success in 17 out of 18 of subjects. Subsequently, these outcomes were validated in a prospective, multicenter study comprising 65 subjects (**Table 3**). The study showed that detection of papillary (finger-like) projections had 100% specificity for intraductal papillary mucinous neoplasms, but a low sensitivity of 59% because of variations in the location of the probe within a cyst.[46] Napoleon and colleagues[47] defined the superficial vascular network as a new imaging criterion to diagnose serous cystadenomas. The superficial vascular network was found to be 100% specific for serous cystadenomas; however, nCLE was only 69% sensitive to detect serous cystadenomas.

Recently, Samarasena and colleagues[48] proposed that nCLE may be used for visualization of the Meissner and Auerbach plexus after the submucosal injection of NeuroTrace (Molecular Probes, Invitrogen, Carlsbad, CA, USA). This type of imaging may allow a new modality for the evaluation of functional and motility disorders of GI tract.

Currently, EUS-guided nCLE is mostly used in research trials despite its high accuracy and the presence of different clinical applications (see **Table 3**). Because it still has some shortcomings, including a lack of standardization of imaging results, its availability and reimbursement is limited in some countries.

THERAPEUTIC ENDOSCOPIC ULTRASOUND

Several new applications for EUS have been developed to provide drainage of fluid collections, the biliary tree, and tissue ablation therapy.

Table 3
Diagnostic rates of endoscopic ultrasound–guided needle confocal laser endomicroscopy of the different cystic pancreatic lesions in selected prospective studies

Selected Studies or Author	Number of Samples	Modality	Lesion Type	Diagnostic Rate Accuracy or Sensitivity or Specificity
Napoleon et al,[47] 2015	31	EUS-FNA + nCLE	SCA	87% accuracy, 69% sensitivity, 100% specificity
Napoleon et al,[49] 2016	33	EUS FNA + nCLE	SCA MCN	100% specificity >90% specificity
Karia et al,[50] 2016	15	nCLE	PCLs	Mean 46% accuracy
Konda et al,[46] 2013	66	nCLE	PCLs	59% sensitivity, 100% specificity
Giovannini et al,[51] 2016	32 (23 PC, 6 CP, 3 NET)	EUS FNA + nCLE	PSLs	96% accuracy
Kadayifci et al,[52] 2017	20	EUS FNA + nCLE	PCLs	66% sensitivity, 100% specificity, 80% accuracy

Abbreviations: CP, chronic pancreatitis; FNA, fine-needle aspiration; MCN, mucinous cystic neoplasm; nCLE, needle-based confocal laser endomicroscopy; NET, neuroendocrine tumor; PC, pancreatic cancer; PSLs, pancreatic solid lesions; SCA, serous cystadenoma.

Forward-Viewing Linear Echoendoscope

The standard curvilinear array (CLA)-EUS scope has an oblique view of 100° and an endoscopic view that is rotated 55° from the axis of the endoscope and the US probe. A forward-viewing linear (FV)-EUS (Olympus America, Center Valley, PA, USA) was developed to eliminate the disadvantages of the standard EUS scope. FV-EUS shifts the orientation of both the endoscopic and US views from oblique to forward and may make the passage of accessories easier by allowing for better visualization and increasing application of mechanical force. It has the capability of reaching areas of the GI lumen that are not easily accessible with the CLA-EUS. Nevertheless, it has some shortcomings: the US scanning area is limited to only 90° (it is 180° in standard CLA-EUS scopes) and the 3.7 mm working channel lacks an elevator. In this context, the reported studies have not demonstrated a significant clinical benefit of FV-EUS compared with the CLA-EUS.[53,54] However, it can be useful for evaluating difficult to reach lesions, such as duodenum third portion and upper genu, and gastric fundus greater curvature. Also, it could be used in patients who have undergone surgery and have anatomic changes. In such cases, FNA can be performed more easily by using an FV-EUS rather than a CLA-EUS. In addition, FV-EUS can be used for evaluating subepithelial lesions placed at the gastric, small intestine, or colonic wall. It is hoped that there will be new FV echoendoscopes with elevators for therapeutic procedures, as well as additional tools that expand the use of EUS beyond its current limits.

Lumen Apposing Metal Stents

The lumen apposing metal stent (LAMS) was designed specifically for transluminal drainage and to reduce the side effects of traditional plastic and metal stents, including leakage, perforation, tissue damage, and migration.[55] One of the important advantages of the stents is allowing for debridement of pseudocysts and pancreatic necrosis.

Axios stent

The Axios stent (Boston Scientific, Natick, MA, USA) is composed of double-walled flanges with diameters that are double the stent lumen and keep the tissue walls in apposition.[56] The stent is available in 10 and 15 mm diameter. The flexibility of the stent is a result of a braided nitinol wire and is responsible for ease of deployment and removal. The covering of the stent ensures a leak-proof seal and drainage. The large flanges and a short stent length are designed to distribute pressure on the luminal wall and to provide tissue apposition.

Spaxus stent

The Niti-S Spaxus stent (Taewoong Medical Co Ltd, Goyang, Korea) is similar to Axios stent. It also composed of nitinol wire, is fully covered, and has large diameter flanges providing pressure on the lumen wall to prevent migration. The diameter of the flanges at the both ends is 25 mm. A different feature of this stent is the use of folding flaps that add additional security. Stents of 8, 10, and 16 mm, with a length of 20 mm are available.

Endoscopic Ultrasound–Guided Drainage and Indications for Lumen Apposing Metal Stents

Pancreatic fluid collections

Historically, double-pigtail plastic stents have been the cornerstone of therapy for pancreatic fluid collections (PFCs). However, plastic stents may be occluded by necrotic material or secondary infection due to their small caliber. Therefore, fully covered self-expanding metal stents and, recently, LAMSs were used to overcome these limitations. Endoscopic necrosectomy can be performed directly using these devices due to their wider diameter; thus a quicker resolution of the symptoms can be provided. There are multiple studies evaluating the safety and efficacy of LAMS (mostly with Axios stents), in which they were applied to drain PFCs.[57–59] In these studies, treatment success rate of LAMSs have been reported to be high, ranging from 93% to 100%, but in relatively small subject groups.[57–59] In a prospective study that compared Axios stents with plastic pigtail stents, technical and clinical success of Axios stent were similar. However, the subjects with double-pigtail stents had higher rates of complications, recurrences, and stent migration rates.[59] There is no agreement regarding which type of stent should be used for the drainage of PFCs. In the future, some specialized LAMSs could be produced for specific purposes. For example, a longer LAMS (at least 3 cm in diameter) could be used for the pseudocysts that are localized a distance from the GI track, or a larger and thicker LAMS can be used for endoscopic necrosectomy of larger necrotic and viscous materials from the necrotic pancreas. Further randomized studies, including larger subject groups, are needed to justify the use of these stents for PFC drainage.

Endoscopic ultrasound–guided gallbladder drainage

EUS-guided gallbladder drainage (GBD) is a relatively new modality with scarce published data. This approach could be indicated in patients who are not suitable for surgery and have not responded to antibiotics.[60] In a retrospective study evaluating 15 nonsurgical candidates who underwent EUS-GBD with a LAMS to decompress the gallbladder, the technical success rate was reported as 93%.[61] A larger, multicenter, prospective study assessed the safety of LAMSs for EUS-GBD in 30 subjects. It revealed the technical success rate as 90% and clinical success as 96% in the subjects.[62] In another study, the modified lumen apposing stent (Hot AXIOS, Xlumena Inc, Mountainview, Calif) with cautery-tipped stent delivery system was used without the need for tract dilation before stent deployment.[63] In the future, a specialized LAMS with larger diameter could be used for large gallbladder stones in cases that are not suitable for surgery. Also, an anchor-type LAMS could be produced for transgastric biliary drainage that might provide prevention against migration of the stent.

Endoscopic ultrasound–guided gastrojejunostomy

This technique uses a specially created double-balloon enteric tube, Tokyo Medical University Type (Create Medic, Yokohama, Japan) for stabilizing the small bowel adjacent to the stomach and LAMS placement. Itoi and colleagues[64] conducted a prospective study evaluating the efficacy of this technique using LAMSs in 20 subjects. They reported that the technical success rate was 90%. In the future, a specialized anchor-type LAMS could be produced to provide better apposition of the lumens.

Endoscopic ultrasound–directed transgastric endoscopic retrograde cholangiopancreatography

After a Roux-en-Y gastric bypass, the ampulla cannot be accessed through a standard endoscopic retrograde cholangiopancreatography (ERCP) procedure because of the altered anatomy. Recently, Kedia and colleagues[65] reported EUS-guided construction of a gastrogastric or jejunogastric fistula through the placement of LAMSs. Their aim was to provide access to the ampulla after creating a passage using LAMS for a duodenoscope. The initial results are promising but large trials are awaited.

Formation of multiple drainage routes

Providing a single enteral drainage route may not provide sufficient drainage in the management of walled-off necrosis. Therefore, opening multiple access sites into the cavity can provide better drainage and irrigation of the cavity. Dual-modality drainage, including percutaneous and endoscopic drainage simultaneously, has been proposed for achieving better clinical results[66,67]; however, prospective randomized trials are needed to validate the success of this modality.

Access into the cavity can be difficult because of a thick wall and the tract can be difficult for dilatation. A wire-guided bent needle knife to provide a wider access has been used to overcome this issue.[68] A double-guidewire technique for using a double-lumen catheter has been proposed to eliminate the need for cannulation of pseudocysts.[69] To allow placement of multiple stents, a modification of the dual-lumen biliary brush catheter has been used to place multiple guidewires.[70] An exchange-free access device with an inner trocar for puncture and an outer dual balloon for dilatation of the tract has also been proposed for EUS-guided drainage of PFCs.[71] Wider and longer stents connecting one side to the other side of huge cysts could be produced in the future. Better drainage could be provided for cysts with a thick wall using this approach. Additionally, many innovative approaches, such as using hydrogen peroxide and streptokinase have been reported; however, prospective randomized studies are needed to validate the use of these approaches in daily practice.

Endoscopic ultrasound–guided intra-abdominal abscess drainage

A modality of EUS-guided internal drainage of abdominal and pelvic abscess has emerged in recent years as an alternative option to the traditional percutaneous approach. Abscesses in areas adjacent to GI lumen, such as mediastinum, perihepatic and subphrenic space, and pelvis, might be drained using EUS. Recently, mediastinal abscesses have been drained by EUS guidance using LAMSs.[72,73] Similarly, splenic or liver abscesses can also be drained under EUS guidance with LAMS.[74,75] In the future, specialized LAMSs could be designed to access distant abscesses. Or wider LAMSs that might discharge the abscesses faster, or spiral-shaped stents that could be placed into the abscess, could be produced.

Preloaded fiducial needle

Recently, multiple studies have been reported evaluating the utility of fiducial marker placement under EUS guidance to facilitate radiation therapy in pancreatic cancer.[76,77] Usually 3 to 4 markers are needed to outline a pancreatic malignancy. These landmarks are used for guiding radiation therapy in intra-abdominal malignancy. Currently, preloaded needles have been developed that do not require the reloading of fiducial markers. Echotip fiducial needle is a 22-gauge needle that contains 4 gold fiducial markers (Cook Medical, Bloomington, IN, USA). Another preloaded needle is newly developed by Medtronic (Sunnyvale, CA, USA) in both 19-gauge and 22-gauge needles containing 2 fiducial markers. However, further studies with large subject groups are warranted to assess its feasibility and safety.

SUMMARY

In conclusion, EUS is an indispensable tool for the diagnosis and therapy for a wide spectrum of lesions in and adjacent to the GI tract. Many EUS-guided therapies have become widely accepted interventions, such as pseudocyst drainage. It is hoped that, as its role expands, its availability will increase and it will play a crucial role in both diagnosis and treatment of many other GI diseases.

REFERENCES

1. Kaufman AR, Sivak MV Jr. Endoscopic ultrasonography in the differential diagnosis of pancreatic disease. Gastrointest Endosc 1989;35(3):214–9.
2. Brugge WR. EUS. Gastrointest Endosc 2013;78(3):414–20.
3. Ishikawa H, Hirooka Y, Itoh A, et al. A comparison of image quality between tissue harmonic imaging and fundamental imaging with an electronic radial scanning echoendoscope in the diagnosis of pancreatic diseases. Gastrointest Endosc 2003;57(7):931–6.
4. Matsumoto K, Katanuma A. Novel tissue harmonic imaging clearly visualizes a case of intraductal papillary mucinous neoplasm with mural nodules. JOP 2014;15(3):274–5.
5. Giovannini M, Hookey LC, Bories E, et al. Endoscopic ultrasound elastography: the first step towards virtual biopsy? Preliminary results in 49 patients. Endoscopy 2006;38(4):344–8.
6. Katanuma A, Isayama H, Bapaye A. Endoscopic ultrasonography using new functions for pancreatobiliary diseases: current status and future perspectives. Dig Endosc 2015;27(Suppl 1):47–54.
7. Ohno E, Kawashima H, Hashimoto S, et al. Current status of tissue harmonic imaging in endoscopic ultrasonography (EUS) and EUS-elastography in pancreatobiliary diseases. Dig Endosc 2015;27(Suppl 1):68–73.
8. Saftoiu A, Vilmann P, Gorunescu F, et al. Accuracy of endoscopic ultrasound elastography used for differential diagnosis of focal pancreatic masses: a multicenter study. Endoscopy 2011;43(7):596–603.
9. Dietrich CF, Saftoiu A, Jenssen C. Real time elastography endoscopic ultrasound (RTE-EUS), a comprehensive review. Eur J Radiol 2014;83(3):405–14.
10. Cui XW, Chang JM, Kan QC, et al. Endoscopic ultrasound elastography: current status and future perspectives. World J Gastroenterol 2015;21(47):13212–24.
11. Iglesias-Garcia J, Lindkvist B, Larino-Noia J, et al. Differential diagnosis of solid pancreatic masses: contrast-enhanced harmonic (CEH-EUS), quantitative-elastography (QE-EUS), or both? United Eur Gastroenterol J 2017;5(2):236–46.
12. Mayerle J, Beyer G, Simon P, et al. Prospective cohort study comparing transient EUS guided elastography to EUS-FNA for the diagnosis of solid pancreatic mass lesions. Pancreatology 2016;16(1):110–4.
13. Iglesias-Garcia J, Larino-Noia J, Abdulkader I, et al. EUS elastography for the characterization of solid pancreatic masses. Gastrointest Endosc 2009;70(6):1101–8.
14. Itokawa F, Itoi T, Sofuni A, et al. EUS elastography combined with the strain ratio of tissue elasticity for diagnosis of solid pancreatic masses. J Gastroenterol 2011;46(6):843–53.
15. Seicean A, Mosteanu O, Seicean R. Maximizing the endosonography: The role of contrast harmonics, elastography and confocal endomicroscopy. World J Gastroenterol 2017;23(1):25–41.
16. Giovannini M, Thomas B, Erwan B, et al. Endoscopic ultrasound elastography for evaluation of lymph nodes and pancreatic masses: a multicenter study. World J Gastroenterol 2009;15(13):1587–93.
17. Iglesias-Garcia J, Larino-Noia J, Abdulkader I, et al. Quantitative endoscopic ultrasound elastography: an accurate method for the differentiation of solid pancreatic masses. Gastroenterology 2010;139(4):1172–80.

18. Larsen MH, Fristrup C, Hansen TP, et al. Endoscopic ultrasound, endoscopic so-noelastography, and strain ratio evaluation of lymph nodes with histology as gold standard. Endoscopy 2012;44(8):759–66.
19. Paterson S, Duthie F, Stanley AJ. Endoscopic ultrasound-guided elastography in the nodal staging of oesophageal cancer. World J Gastroenterol 2012;18(9): 889–95.
20. Knabe M, Gunter E, Ell C, et al. Can EUS elastography improve lymph node staging in esophageal cancer? Surg Endosc 2013;27(4):1196–202.
21. Rustemovic N, Opacic D, Ostojic Z, et al. Comparison of elastography methods in patients with pancreatic masses. Endosc Ultrasound 2014;3(Suppl 1):S4.
22. Kitano M, Kudo M, Yamao K, et al. Characterization of small solid tumors in the pancreas: the value of contrast-enhanced harmonic endoscopic ultrasonography. Am J Gastroenterol 2012;107(2):303–10.
23. Fusaroli P, Spada A, Mancino MG, et al. Contrast harmonic echo-endoscopic ultrasound improves accuracy in diagnosis of solid pancreatic masses. Clin Gastroenterol Hepatol 2010;8(7):629–34.e1-2.
24. Miyata T, Kitano M, Omoto S, et al. Contrast-enhanced harmonic endoscopic ultrasonography for assessment of lymph node metastases in pancreatobiliary carcinoma. World J Gastroenterol 2016;22(12):3381–91.
25. Sugimoto M, Takagi T, Hikichi T, et al. Conventional versus contrast-enhanced harmonic endoscopic ultrasonography-guided fine-needle aspiration for diagnosis of solid pancreatic lesions: a prospective randomized trial. Pancreatology 2015;15(5):538–41.
26. Kitano M, Kamata K. Contrast-enhanced harmonic endoscopic ultrasound: future perspectives. Endosc Ultrasound 2016;5(6):351–4.
27. Sofuni A, Itoi T, Itokawa F, et al. Usefulness of contrast-enhanced ultrasonography in determining treatment efficacy and outcome after pancreatic cancer chemotherapy. World J Gastroenterol 2008;14(47):7183–91.
28. Matsui S, Kudo M, Kitano M, et al. Evaluation of the response to chemotherapy in advanced gastric cancer by contrast-enhanced harmonic EUS. Hepatogastroenterology 2015;62(139):595–8.
29. Yamashita Y, Ueda K, Itonaga M, et al. Tumor vessel depiction with contrast-enhanced endoscopic ultrasonography predicts efficacy of chemotherapy in pancreatic cancer. Pancreas 2013;42(6):990–5.
30. Ignee A, Jenssen C, Hocke M, et al. Contrast-enhanced (endoscopic) ultrasound and endoscopic ultrasound elastography in gastrointestinal stromal tumors. Endosc Ultrasound 2017;6(1):55–60.
31. Rahimi E, Younes M, Zhang S, et al. Endoscopic ultrasound elastography to diagnose sarcoidosis. Endosc Ultrasound 2016;5(3):212–4.
32. Pochon S, Tardy I, Bussat P, et al. BR55: a lipopeptide-based VEGFR2-targeted ultrasound contrast agent for molecular imaging of angiogenesis. Invest Radiol 2010;45(2):89–95.
33. Korpanty G, Carbon JG, Grayburn PA, et al. Monitoring response to anticancer therapy by targeting microbubbles to tumor vasculature. Clin Cancer Res 2007;13(1):323–30.
34. Anderson CR, Rychak JJ, Backer M, et al. scVEGF microbubble ultrasound contrast agents: a novel probe for ultrasound molecular imaging of tumor angiogenesis. Invest Radiol 2010;45(10):579–85.
35. Pysz MA, Foygel K, Rosenberg J, et al. Antiangiogenic cancer therapy: monitoring with molecular US and a clinically translatable contrast agent (BR55). Radiology 2010;256(2):519–27.

36. Bachawal SV, Jensen KC, Wilson KE, et al. Breast Cancer Detection by B7-H3-Targeted Ultrasound Molecular Imaging. Cancer Res 2015;75(12):2501–9.
37. Hernot S, Klibanov AL. Microbubbles in ultrasound-triggered drug and gene delivery. Adv Drug Deliv Rev 2008;60(10):1153–66.
38. Tinkov S, Coester C, Serba S, et al. New doxorubicin-loaded phospholipid microbubbles for targeted tumor therapy: in-vivo characterization. J Control Release 2010;148(3):368–72.
39. Ashida R, Kawabata K, Maruoka T, et al. New approach for local cancer treatment using pulsed high-intensity focused ultrasound and phase-change nanodroplets. J Med Ultrason (2001) 2015;42(4):457–66.
40. Napoleon B, Alvarez-Sanchez MV, Gincoul R, et al. Contrast-enhanced harmonic endoscopic ultrasound in solid lesions of the pancreas: results of a pilot study. Endoscopy 2010;42(7):564–70.
41. Hocke M, Ignee A, Dietrich CF. Advanced endosonographic diagnostic tools for discrimination of focal chronic pancreatitis and pancreatic carcinoma–elastography, contrast enhanced high mechanical index (CEHMI) and low mechanical index (CELMI) endosonography in direct comparison. Z Gastroenterol 2012;50(2):199–203.
42. Lee TY, Cheon YK, Shim CS. Clinical role of contrast-enhanced harmonic endoscopic ultrasound in differentiating solid lesions of the pancreas: a single-center experience in Korea. Gut Liver 2013;7(5):599–604.
43. Gincul R, Palazzo M, Pujol B, et al. Contrast-harmonic endoscopic ultrasound for the diagnosis of pancreatic adenocarcinoma: a prospective multicenter trial. Endoscopy 2014;46(5):373–9.
44. ASGE Technology Committee, Thosani N, Abu Dayyeh BK, Sharma P, et al. Confocal laser endomicroscopy. Gastrointest Endosc 2014;80(6):928–38.
45. Konda VJ, Aslanian HR, Wallace MB, et al. First assessment of needle-based confocal laser endomicroscopy during EUS-FNA procedures of the pancreas (with videos). Gastrointest Endosc 2011;74(5):1049–60.
46. Konda VJ, Meining A, Jamil LH, et al. A pilot study of in vivo identification of pancreatic cystic neoplasms with needle-based confocal laser endomicroscopy under endosonographic guidance. Endoscopy 2013;45(12):1006–13.
47. Napoleon B, Lemaistre AI, Pujol B, et al. A novel approach to the diagnosis of pancreatic serous cystadenoma: needle-based confocal laser endomicroscopy. Endoscopy 2015;47(1):26–32.
48. Samarasena JB, Ahluwalia A, Shinoura S, et al. In vivo imaging of porcine gastric enteric nervous system using confocal laser endomicroscopy &molecular neuronal probe. J Gastroenterol Hepatol 2016;31(4):802–7.
49. Napoleon B, Lemaistre AI, Pujol B, et al. In vivo characterization of pancreatic cystic lesions by needle-based confocal laser endomicroscopy (nCLE): proposition of a comprehensive nCLE classification confirmed by an external retrospective evaluation. Surg Endosc 2016;30(6):2603–12.
50. Karia K, Waxman I, Konda VJ, et al. Needle-based confocal endomicroscopy for pancreatic cysts: the current agreement in interpretation. Gastrointest Endosc 2016;83(5):924–7.
51. Giovannini M, Caillol F, Monges G, et al. Endoscopic ultrasound-guided needle-based confocal laser endomicroscopy in solid pancreatic masses. Endoscopy 2016;48(10):892–8.
52. Kadayifci A, Atar M, Basar O, et al. Needle-Based Confocal Laser Endomicroscopy for Evaluation of Cystic Neoplasms of the Pancreas. Dig Dis Sci 2017; 62:1346–53.

53. Voermans RP, Ponchon T, Schumacher B, et al. Forward-viewing versus oblique-viewing echoendoscopes in transluminal drainage of pancreatic fluid collections: a multicenter, randomized, controlled trial. Gastrointest Endosc 2011;74(6): 1285–93.

54. Chapman CG, Matthews JB, Siddiqui UD. EUS-guided internal drainage of a deep abdominal postoperative abscess after Whipple procedure. Gastrointest Endosc 2015;82(6):1132–3 [discussion: 1133].

55. Yamamoto N, Isayama H, Kawakami H, et al. Preliminary report on a new, fully covered, metal stent designed for the treatment of pancreatic fluid collections. Gastrointest Endosc 2013;77(5):809–14.

56. Binmoeller KF, Shah J. A novel lumen-apposing stent for transluminal drainage of nonadherent extraintestinal fluid collections. Endoscopy 2011;43(4):337–42.

57. Itoi T, Binmoeller KF, Shah J, et al. Clinical evaluation of a novel lumen-apposing metal stent for endosonography-guided pancreatic pseudocyst and gallbladder drainage (with videos). Gastrointest Endosc 2012;75(4):870–6.

58. Gornals JB, De la Serna-Higuera C, Sanchez-Yague A, et al. Endosonography-guided drainage of pancreatic fluid collections with a novel lumen-apposing stent. Surg Endosc 2013;27(4):1428–34.

59. Shah RJ, Shah JN, Waxman I, et al. Safety and efficacy of endoscopic ultrasound-guided drainage of pancreatic fluid collections with lumen-apposing covered self-expanding metal stents. Clin Gastroenterol Hepatol 2015;13(4): 747–52.

60. Subtil JC, Betes M, Munoz-Navas M. Gallbladder drainage guided by endoscopic ultrasound. World J Gastrointest Endosc 2010;2(6):203–9.

61. Irani S, Baron TH, Grimm IS, et al. EUS-guided gallbladder drainage with a lumen-apposing metal stent (with video). Gastrointest Endosc 2015;82(6): 1110–5.

62. Walter D, Teoh AY, Itoi T, et al. EUS-guided gall bladder drainage with a lumen-apposing metal stent: a prospective long-term evaluation. Gut 2016;65(1):6–8.

63. Teoh AY, Binmoeller KF, Lau JY. Single-step EUS-guided puncture and delivery of a lumen-apposing stent for gallbladder drainage using a novel cautery-tipped stent delivery system. Gastrointest Endosc 2014;80(6):1171.

64. Itoi T, Ishii K, Ikeuchi N, et al. Prospective evaluation of endoscopic ultrasonography-guided double-balloon-occluded gastrojejunostomy bypass (EPASS) for malignant gastric outlet obstruction. Gut 2016;65(2):193–5.

65. Kedia P, Tyberg A, Kumta NA, et al. EUS-directed transgastric ERCP for Roux-en-Y gastric bypass anatomy: a minimally invasive approach. Gastrointest Endosc 2015;82(3):560–5.

66. Varadarajulu S, Phadnis MA, Christein JD, et al. Multiple transluminal gateway technique for EUS-guided drainage of symptomatic walled-off pancreatic necrosis. Gastrointest Endosc 2011;74(1):74–80.

67. Ross AS, Irani S, Gan SI, et al. Dual-modality drainage of infected and symptomatic walled-off pancreatic necrosis: long-term clinical outcomes. Gastrointest Endosc 2014;79(6):929–35.

68. Azar RR, Oh YS, Janec EM, et al. Wire-guided pancreatic pseudocyst drainage by using a modified needle knife and therapeutic echoendoscope. Gastrointest Endosc 2006;63(4):688–92.

69. Itoi T, Itokawa F, Tsuchiya T, et al. EUS-guided pancreatic pseudocyst drainage: simultaneous placement of stents and nasocystic catheter using double-guidewire technique. Dig Endosc 2009;21(Suppl 1):S53–6.

70. Khashab MA, Lennon AM, Singh VK, et al. Endoscopic ultrasound (EUS)-guided pseudocyst drainage as a one-step procedure using a novel multiple-wire insertion technique (with video). Surg Endosc 2012;26(11):3320–3.

71. Binmoeller KF, Smith I, Gaidhane M, et al. A kit for EUS-guided access and drainage of pancreatic pseudocysts: efficacy in a porcine model. Endosc Ultrasound 2012;1(3):137–42.

72. Consiglieri CF, Escobar I, Gornals JB. EUS-guided transesophageal drainage of a mediastinal abscess using a diabolo-shaped lumen-apposing metal stent. Gastrointest Endosc 2015;81(1):221–2.

73. Saxena P, Kumbhari V, Khashab MA. EUS-guided drainage of a mediastinal abscess. Gastrointest Endosc 2014;79(6):998–9.

74. Rana SS, Chaudhary V, Sharma V, et al. Infected pancreatic pseudocyst of spleen successfully treated by combined endoscopic transpapillary stent placement and transmural aspiration. Gastrointest Endosc 2014;79(2):360–1.

75. Alcaide N, Vargas-Garcia AL, de la Serna-Higuera C, et al. EUS-guided drainage of liver abscess by using a lumen-apposing metal stent (with video). Gastrointest Endosc 2013;78(6):941–2 [discussion: 942].

76. Choi JH, Seo DW, Park DH, et al. Fiducial placement for stereotactic body radiation therapy under only endoscopic ultrasonography guidance in pancreatic and hepatic malignancy: practical feasibility and safety. Gut Liver 2014;8(1):88–93.

77. Fuccio L, Lami G, Guido A, et al. EUS-guided gold fiducial placement and migration rate. Gastrointest Endosc 2014;80(3):533–4.

UNITED STATES POSTAL SERVICE ®

Statement of Ownership, Management, and Circulation
(All Periodicals Publications Except Requester Publications)

1. Publication Title	2. Publication Number	3. Filing Date
GASTROINTESTINAL CLINICS OF NORTH AMERICA	012 – 603	9/18/2017

4. Issue Frequency	5. Number of Issues Published Annually	6. Annual Subscription Price
JAN, APR, JUL, OCT	4	$342

7. Complete Mailing Address of Known Office of Publication (Not printer) (Street, city, county, state, and ZIP+4®)

ELSEVIER INC.
230 Park Avenue, Suite 800
New York, NY 10169

Contact Person
STEPHEN R. BUSHING

Telephone (Include area code)
215-239-3688

8. Complete Mailing Address of Headquarters or General Business Office of Publisher (Not printer)

ELSEVIER INC.
230 Park Avenue, Suite 800
New York, NY 10169

9. Full Names and Complete Mailing Addresses of Publisher, Editor, and Managing Editor (Do not leave blank)

Publisher (Name and complete mailing address)

ADRIANNE BRIGIDO, ELSEVIER INC.
1600 JOHN F KENNEDY BLVD. SUITE 1800
PHILADELPHIA, PA 19103-2899

Editor (Name and complete mailing address)

KERRY HOLLAND, ELSEVIER INC.
1600 JOHN F KENNEDY BLVD. SUITE 1800
PHILADELPHIA, PA 19103-2899

Managing Editor (Name and complete mailing address)

PATRICK MANLEY, ELSEVIER INC.
1600 JOHN F KENNEDY BLVD. SUITE 1800
PHILADELPHIA, PA 19103-2899

10. Owner (Do not leave blank. If the publication is owned by a corporation, give the name and address of the corporation immediately followed by the names and addresses of all stockholders owning or holding 1 percent or more of the total amount of stock. If not owned by a corporation, give the names and addresses of the individual owners. If owned by a partnership or other unincorporated firm, give its name and address as well as those of each individual owner. If the publication is published by a nonprofit organization, give its name and address.)

Full Name	Complete Mailing Address
WHOLLY OWNED SUBSIDIARY OF REED/ELSEVIER US HOLDINGS	1600 JOHN F KENNEDY BLVD. SUITE 1800 PHILADELPHIA, PA 19103-2899

11. Known Bondholders, Mortgagees, and Other Security Holders Owning or Holding 1 Percent or More of Total Amount of Bonds, Mortgages, or Other Securities. If none, check box ▶ ☐ None

Full Name	Complete Mailing Address
N/A	

12. Tax Status (For completion by nonprofit organizations authorized to mail at nonprofit rates) (Check one)
The purpose, function, and nonprofit status of this organization and the exempt status for federal income tax purposes:
☒ Has Not Changed During Preceding 12 Months
☐ Has Changed During Preceding 12 Months (Publisher must submit explanation of change with this statement)

13. Publication Title	14. Issue Date for Circulation Data Below
GASTROINTESTINAL ENDOSCOPY CLINICS OF NORTH AMERICA	JULY 2017

PS Form **3526**, July 2014 [Page 1 of 4 (see instructions page 4)] PSN: 7530-01-000-9931   PRIVACY NOTICE: See our privacy policy on www.usps.com.

---

15. Extent and Nature of Circulation			Average No. Copies Each Issue During Preceding 12 Months	No. Copies of Single Issue Published Nearest to Filing Date
a. Total Number of Copies (Net press run)			231	186
b. Paid Circulation (By Mail and Outside the Mail)	(1)	Mailed Outside-County Paid Subscriptions Stated on PS Form 3541 (Include paid distribution above nominal rate, advertiser's proof copies, and exchange copies)	88	94
	(2)	Mailed In-County Paid Subscriptions Stated on PS Form 3541 (Include paid distribution above nominal rate, advertiser's proof copies, and exchange copies)	0	0
	(3)	Paid Distribution Outside the Mails Including Sales Through Dealers and Carriers, Street Vendors, Counter Sales, and Other Paid Distribution Outside USPS®	38	50
	(4)	Paid Distribution by Other Classes of Mail Through the USPS (e.g., First-Class Mail®)	0	0
c. Total Paid Distribution (Sum of 15b (1), (2), (3), and (4))		▶	126	144
d. Free or Nominal Rate Distribution (By Mail and Outside the Mail)	(1)	Free or Nominal Rate Outside-County Copies included on PS Form 3541	42	42
	(2)	Free or Nominal Rate In-County Copies Included on PS Form 3541	0	0
	(3)	Free or Nominal Rate Copies Mailed at Other Classes Through the USPS (e.g., First-Class Mail)	0	0
	(4)	Free or Nominal Rate Distribution Outside the Mail (Carriers or other means)	0	0
e. Total Free or Nominal Rate Distribution (Sum of 15d (1), (2), (3) and (4))		▶	42	42
f. Total Distribution (Sum of 15c and 15e)		▶	168	186
g. Copies not Distributed (See Instructions to Publishers #4 (page 4))		▶	63	0
h. Total (Sum of 15f and g)		▶	231	186
i. Percent Paid (15c divided by 15f times 100)		▶	75%	77.42%

* If you are claiming electronic copies, go to line 16 on page 3. If you are not claiming electronic copies, skip to line 17 on page 3.

16. Electronic Copy Circulation	Average No. Copies Each Issue During Preceding 12 Months	No. Copies of Single Issue Published Nearest to Filing Date
a. Paid Electronic Copies ▶	0	0
b. Total Paid Print Copies (Line 15c) + Paid Electronic Copies (Line 16a) ▶	126	144
c. Total Print Distribution (Line 15f) + Paid Electronic Copies (Line 16a) ▶	168	186
d. Percent Paid (Both Print & Electronic Copies) (16b divided by 16c × 100) ▶	75%	77.42%

☒ I certify that 50% of all my distributed copies (electronic and print) are paid above a nominal price.

17. Publication of Statement of Ownership

☒ If the publication is a general publication, publication of this statement is required. Will be printed

in the OCTOBER 2017 issue of this publication.   ☐ Publication not required.

18. Signature and Title of Editor, Publisher, Business Manager or Owner

[signature]   Date 9/18/2017

STEPHEN R. BUSHING - INVENTORY DISTRIBUTION CONTROL MANAGER

I certify that all information furnished on this form is true and complete. I understand that anyone who furnishes false or misleading information on this form or who omits material or information requested on the form may be subject to criminal sanctions (including fines and imprisonment) and/or civil sanctions (including civil penalties).

PS Form **3526**, July 2014 (Page 3 of 4)   PRIVACY NOTICE: See our privacy policy on www.usps.com.

Moving?

Make sure your subscription moves with you!

To notify us of your new address, find your **Clinics Account Number** (located on your mailing label above your name), and contact customer service at:

Email: journalscustomerservice-usa@elsevier.com

800-654-2452 (subscribers in the U.S. & Canada)
314-447-8871 (subscribers outside of the U.S. & Canada)

Fax number: 314-447-8029

Elsevier Health Sciences Division
Subscription Customer Service
3251 Riverport Lane
Maryland Heights, MO 63043

*To ensure uninterrupted delivery of your subscription, please notify us at least 4 weeks in advance of move.

Printed and bound by CPI Group (UK) Ltd, Croydon, CR0 4YY

08/05/2025

01864703-0003